MAKING MEANING OF DATA IN PHARMACEUTICAL AND CLINICAL RESEARCH

MAKING MEANING OF DATA IN PHARMACEUTICAL AND CLINICAL RESEARCH

Susan J. Blalock, MPH, PhD
Chapel Hill, NC

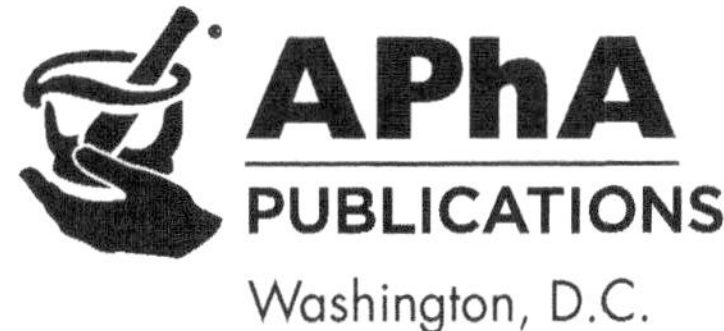

Washington, D.C.

Acquiring Editor: Janan Sarwar
Managing Editors: John Fedor and Janan Sarwar
Composition Services: Circle Graphics, Inc.
Cover Design: Richard Muringer, APhA Integrated Design and Production Center
Editorial Services: J&J Editorial LLC and Publications Professionals LLC

APhA was founded in 1852 as the American Pharmaceutical Association

Published by the American Pharmacists Association
2215 Constitution Avenue, NW
Washington, DC 29937-2985
www.pharmacist.com www.pharmacylibrary.com

To comment on this book via e-mail, send your message to the publisher at aphabooks@aphanet.org.

Library of Congress Cataloging-in-Publication Data

Names: Blalock, Susan J., author. | American Pharmacists Association, issuing body.
Title: Making meaning of data in pharmaceutical and clinical research / Susan J. Blalock.
Description: Washington, D.C. : American Pharmacists Association, [2019] | Includes bibliographical references.
Identifiers: LCCN 2019006370 | ISBN 9781582123103
Subjects: | MESH: Pharmaceutical Research | Statistics as Topic | Problems and Exercises
Classification: LCC RM301.27 | NLM QV 18.2 | DDC 615.1072/4-dc23 LC record available at https://lccn.loc.gov/2019006370

Dedicated to the memory of my brother Harold Bernard (Bernie) Blalock and my grandmother Minnie Hattie Baringer who taught me to dream big, work hard, and never give up.

Table of Contents

FINISHING TOUCHES

Preface

This book is the product of having taught the statistics portion of an evidence-based medicine class for PharmD students for about 15 years. I think it is fair to say that relatively few students enter pharmacy school with a burning desire to learn more about statistics. Nonetheless, knowledge of statistical principles is needed to be able to read the pharmaceutical literature and make meaning of the data reported. Without the skills and confidence needed to read the literature, pharmacists cannot stay abreast of the most recent findings concerning experimental therapies that may be on the horizon or emerging safety concerns regarding medications that are currently on the market.

The primary target audience for this book is pharmacists and pharmacy students who want to be able to better understand the methods and results sections of published papers so that they are able to judge for themselves whether the conclusions reached by the author(s) are supported by the data presented. Therefore, most of the examples used throughout the book pertain to pharmacotherapy. However, students and health professionals in other areas are also likely to find the book helpful.

The book covers a broad range of topics, from descriptive statistics in Chapter 1 to survival analysis in Chapter 9 and meta-analysis in Chapter 12. Appendix A provides a summary of the statistical tests reviewed. By design, the book provides a 40,000-foot view of these topic. It does not include the type of detail needed by those responsible for developing the analytic strategy for a study or crunching the numbers themselves. There are hundreds, if not thousands, of books that provide this type of detail—usually accompanied by mind-numbing formulas. However, this book might provide a good starting point for novices to gain a better understanding of basic statistical concepts before tackling the more complex math that underlies many statistical procedures.

My teaching experience has helped me understand the concepts that students are most likely to struggle with when learning the procedures that underlie statistical inference. I hope that this experience has helped me learn to explain these concepts in simple terms, avoiding as much jargon as possible. That was my primary goal in writing this book.

Over the years, my biggest struggle in teaching has been how much detail students need. Often, when I have tried to gloss over topics (e.g., degrees of freedom), students have wanted more detail. Therefore, in this book, I provide more detail in some places than I think is absolutely necessary to understand the basic concepts involved. However, where possible, I have put that detail in "boxed" examples. This makes the information readily available to those who want it, yet readers may skip over the boxed examples if they do not feel a need for that level of detail. In most chapters, I have also included examples from the literature to allow readers to see how the statistical procedures discussed are used in practice.

A final caveat. Although I sometimes discuss methodological issues that should be considered when interpreting the findings from a study (e.g., the distinction between control and comparison groups, correlation versus causality, control for potential confounders), this book does not include a detailed description of the strengths and weaknesses associated with different study designs (e.g., randomized controlled trials, cohort studies). Therefore, students will want to consult other sources to learn more about the methodological issues that affect the inferences that can be drawn from the results of a study.

I hope that readers enjoy this book. Most important, I hope that it enhances readers' ability to understand the findings reported in published papers in the pharmaceutical literature and think critically about the inferences that can be drawn from those findings.

List of Abbreviations

1-way ANOVA, one-way analysis of variance
ADL, activities of daily living
AHRF, Area Health Resources Files
ANCOVA, analysis of covariance
ANOVA, analysis of variance
AOR, adjusted odds ratio
ARI, absolute risk increase
ARR, absolute risk reduction
BMD, bone mineral density
BMI, body mass index
BRFSS, Behavioral Risk Factor Surveillance System
CDC, Centers for Disease Control and Prevention
CER, control event rate
CHC, community health clinic
CI, confidence interval
CS+GH, chondroitin sulfate plus glucosamine hydrochloride
CV, critical value
DBP, diastolic blood pressure
df, degrees of freedom
EER, experiment event rate
FDA, Food and Drug Administration
GEE, generalized estimating equations
GP, glycoprotein
HR, hazard ratio
ICC, intraclass correlation coefficient
ID, identification
IDU, injection drug user
IQR, interquartile range
IRF, independent review facility
LDL, low-density lipoprotein
LMWH, low molecular weight heparin
LR, likelihood ratio
MMAS-8, Morisky Medication Adherence Scale
MTM, medication therapy management
NHATS, National Health and Aging Trends Study

NNH, number needed to harm
NNT, number needed to treat
NPV, negative predictive value
NSOC, National Study of Caregiving
OR, odds ratio
PDC, proportion of days covered
PFS, progression-free survival
PICOS, Patient population, Intervention, Comparator, Outcome, Study design
PPV, positive predictive value
PRISMA, Preferred Reporting Items for Systematic Reviews and Meta-Analyses
PSA, prostate-specific antigen
QR, quick response
RCT, randomized controlled trial
ROC, receiver operating characteristic
RR, relative risk
RRI, relative risk increase
RRR, relative risk reduction
SBP, systolic blood pressure
SD, standard deviation
SE, standard error
SEAMS, Self-Efficacy for Appropriate Medication Use Scale
SMD, standardized mean difference
SS, sums of squares
WOMAC, Western Ontario and McMaster Universities (osteoarthritis index)

THE BASICS

Descriptive Statistics

1

After reading this chapter, you should be able to do the following:

1. Identify, describe, and differentiate between the two broad areas of statistics.
2. Explain what a variable is, and differentiate between independent and dependent variables.
3. Describe three measures of central tendency and two measures of dispersion, explain the situations in which different measures are used, and interpret data presented using these measures.
4. Given a set of data, compute a mean, mode, median, and standard deviation.
5. Use the z-transformation to convert a raw value into a z-score and interpret the results.
6. Given a clinical variable, determine if it was assessed at the nominal, ordinal, interval, or ratio level of measurement.
7. Given a histogram or the mean and standard deviation of a variable, assess whether the variable is normally distributed.
8. Interpret data presented in the form of histograms and box plots.

Biostatistics is a branch of mathematics that focuses on issues involving the collection, presentation, analysis, and interpretation of health-related data. Biostatistics can be divided into two broad areas: descriptive statistics and inferential statistics.

Descriptive statistics are used to describe the characteristics of people and things. The **purpose** of descriptive statistics is simply to describe something. Often descriptive statistics are used to describe the characteristics of a sample in a study (e.g., mean age of study participants). Once a statistic is used to make an inference (e.g., whether the participants in one group are older than participants in another group), it is no longer a descriptive statistic.

Inferential statistics are used to make inferences about the characteristics of a large group of people (i.e., a population) based on data collected from some of the people (i.e., a sample) who belong to the large group. Inferential statistics involve drawing conclusions based on the results of hypothesis tests or estimation of confidence intervals. These issues will be discussed in later chapters. This chapter focuses exclusively on issues involving the presentation, analysis, and interpretation of descriptive statistics.

Understanding Variables

In research studies, the characteristics of interest are called **variables**. A variable is anything that is measured or manipulated in a study. For example, the age of study participants might be **measured** by asking them how old they are or what year they were born. Similarly, the weight of study participants might be measured by weighing them on an accurate scale. Variables are **manipulated** in experimental studies, where people in different groups receive different treatments. For example, people in one group might receive an experimental medication, whereas people in another group receive a medication that is currently on the market. In this experimental study, "medication" is a manipulated variable with two levels: (1) experimental medication and (2) currently available medication.

Types of Variables. There are two main types of variables in research studies: independent variables and dependent variables. Independent variables are used to **predict** things or explain the variation in a dependent variable. For example, an investigator might believe that study participants who receive the experimental medication in a study will be more likely to get better than the people who receive the currently available medication. Thus, the type of medication participants receive would be used to predict treatment outcomes. In another study, independent variables such as age and weight might be used to explain variation in health status among people with a particular health problem such as osteoarthritis. Independent variables are often called **predictor variables**. They may also be called **risk factors** (when they are thought to predict bad outcomes) or **treatments** (when they are thought to predict good outcomes).

Dependent variables are the **outcomes** of interest in a research study (i.e., the variables you are trying to affect or whose variation you are trying to explain). For example, an investigator may want to know if participants who receive an experimental medication live longer than people who receive a currently available medication. Thus, survival time following the initiation of therapy might be the dependent variable or outcome of interest. As you may have guessed by now, in medical research, dependent variables are often called **outcomes**.

One of the first things you should do when reading a research paper is to figure out what the investigators considered the primary independent and dependent variables in the study. You can often determine this from the abstract that appears on the first page of most scientific papers. Table 1-1 presents abridged abstracts from two different hypothetical studies. See if you can determine what the independent and dependent variables were in each study. Answers are provided in Appendix B.

Scales of Measurement. Variables may also be classified according to their **scale of measurement**. The way in which a variable is measured has major implications for how investigators present information concerning the variable in tables and charts and the types of statistical procedures they use to analyze the data. So, when you are reading a research paper, be sure you know the type of scale used to measure each variable of interest.

There are four major types of measurement scales:

1. **Nominal** scales can be characterized as **named categories**. Each category may be given a number, but the numbers are chosen arbitrarily and serve only to identify the category. For example, in one study, "0" might be used to identify men and "1" might be used to identify women. However, these numbers are arbitrary. The investigators might just as easily have used "0" to identify women and "1" to identify men. In this example, the variable "sex" has only two possible levels (i.e., male or female). However, nominal scales can involve many categories (i.e., levels). For example, if an investigator wanted to compare the effectiveness of four different antihypertensive medications (i.e., Medication A, Medication B, Medication C, Medication D), the variable "Medication" would have four levels.

TABLE 1-1. Hypothetical Abridged Abstract

Some studies have found that bisphosphonates increase the risk of atypical femur fracture. In this study, we attempted to better quantify the magnitude of this risk. From a large claims database, we identified 100,000 patients who began using an oral bisphosphonate between 2005 and 2010. Bisphosphonate users were matched to 100,000 individuals of similar age and sex but with no history of bisphosphonate use. We compared the risk of atypical femur fracture between these two groups. A total of 214 atypical femur fractures were experienced by study participants between January 1, 2011, and December 31, 2017.

What are the primary independent and dependent variables in this study?

Obesity is a major public health problem. Individuals who are obese are more likely than the nonobese to experience a variety of health problems (e.g., stroke, heart attack, chronic obstructive pulmonary disease) and die prematurely. This study compared the amount of weight loss experienced by obese individuals who were prescribed either (1) a very low carbohydrate diet, (2) a prescription weight-loss medication, or (3) a placebo. Three hundred obese individuals participated, with 100 of these participants assigned to each arm of the study. The weight of each participant was recorded at the start of the study and at the end of a 6-month treatment period.

What are the primary independent and dependent variables in this study?

Each drug could be assigned a number. However, again, the numbers assigned would be chosen arbitrarily and their only purpose would be to facilitate reference.

If a nominal variable only has two levels, it is often referred to as a **dichotomous** or **binary** variable. These types of variables are common in the medical literature. Often investigators want to know if a specific treatment increases or decreases the risk of different health outcomes (e.g., fractures, heart attacks, strokes). At the simplest level, participants might be classified according to whether or not they experienced the outcome (0 = did not experience the outcome, 1 = experienced the outcome). Thus, you will encounter many dichotomous (i.e., binary) measures as you read the medical literature.

2. **Ordinal scales** can be characterized as **ordered categories**. Thus, the characteristic being measured increases or decreases in magnitude from one end of the scale to the other (e.g., no pain, mild pain, moderate pain, severe pain). For example, the stages of breast cancer are commonly measured on a 4-point scale (i.e., I, II, III, IV), where higher numbers reflect more advanced disease. However, there is no assumption that the increase in disease progression when one moves from Stage I to Stage II is equal to the increase in disease progression when one moves from Stage II to Stage III, or from Stage III to Stage IV. The absence of this assumption differentiates ordinal scales from interval and ratio scales.
3. **Interval scales** are characterized by a series of numbers where the **intervals between adjacent numbers are equal** across the full range of the scale. For example, temperature measured on a Fahrenheit or Celsius scale has interval properties. An increase in temperature from 20 to 30°F is an increase of 10 degrees. Likewise, an increase from 70 to 80°F is an increase of 10 degrees. This characteristic allows investigators to perform mathematical procedures (e.g., addition and subtraction) on variables measured on an interval scale.
4. **Ratio scales** have the same characteristics as interval scales. In addition, for a measure to have ratio properties, "0" must reflect the absence of the attribute being assessed. Thus, "0" on a ratio scale is often called a "**true zero**." Many physiological characteristics have a true zero. For example, a heart rate of 0 would indicate the absence of a heart rate. A diastolic blood pressure (DBP) of 0 would indicate the absence of blood pressure. A weight of 0 would indicate the absence of weight. In contrast, temperature when measured on a Fahrenheit or Celsius scale does not have a true zero, because "0" on these scales does not reflect the absence of temperature.

Typically, the same types of statistical procedures are used to analyze variables assessed on either interval or ratio scales. Therefore, they are sometimes discussed together under the general term "**numerical scales**." Following this convention, I will use the term "numerical variables" to describe variables measured on either an interval scale or a ratio scale.

It is very important to remember that the scale of measurement of a variable is not an inherent characteristic of the attribute of interest (e.g., blood pressure). **Scale of measurement reflects how the attribute was measured.** For example, blood pressure may be measured on a numerical scale (i.e., mmHg), an ordinal scale (e.g., normal, borderline high, high), or a nominal scale (e.g., normal, high). Thus, investigators have a lot of control over how variables are measured. Moreover, how a particular attribute is measured will differ across studies. Therefore, when reading a scientific paper, you must pay careful attention to how each variable was measured in the study being reported.

One final point. Numerical variables (i.e., variables measured on an interval or a ratio scale) may also be described as either continuous or discrete. **Continuous variables** can have fractional values at the individual level and, theoretically, can assume any value across the range of the variable. For example, we could express the age of a person as 29.37 years old or, if we had a very sensitive scale, measure the person's weight as 135.8642 pounds. In contrast, **discrete variables** can only have integer values at the individual level; fractions are not possible. For example, a person cannot have 2.5 children, break 1.2 bones, or have 3.7 heart attacks. As these examples suggest, discrete variables are often assessed by counting things (e.g., number of children, fractures, myocardial infarctions). Table 1-2 shows a list of variables measured in a hypothetical study. See if you can determine the type of scale used to measure each variable and whether the variable is continuous or discrete. Answers are provided in Appendix B.

TABLE 1-2. Identify the Scale of Measurement (i.e., Nominal, Ordinal, Numerical) for Each of the Following Variables

Age, measured in years
Age (categorized as: under 18, 18–65, over 65)
Age (categorized as: under 65, 65 or older)
Number of broken bones experienced
Bone mineral density, measured in g/cm^2
Bone mineral density (categorized as: normal, osteopenia, osteoporosis)
Sex (male, female)
Race (white, African American, Asian, Native American, other)
Diagnosed with osteoporosis (yes, no)
Taking a bisphosphonate (yes, no)

Summarizing the Data Collected in a Study

The first task that investigators must do when analyzing data from a study involves describing the characteristics of the sample from which data were collected. This information is often presented in "Table 1" of scientific papers. When you are reading a scientific paper, it is important to look at this information carefully. It often contains valuable clues about the generalizability of study findings. For example, if a study investigating a new antihypertensive medication were limited to patients under the age of 60, a reader might question whether study findings would generalize (i.e., be applicable) to older adults.

Nominal Variables. In most cases, data from nominal variables are summarized using percentages. For example, if a study had 200 participants and 90 were men, an investigator might describe the sex distribution in the study by saying that 45% of study participants were male and that 55% were female. The investigator might also put this information in a frequency table like the one shown in Table 1-3. In this table, "n" refers to the number of participants in the study with the characteristic described. From this table, one can also see that most study participants were white, 25% had been diagnosed with osteoporosis, and 5% were taking a bisphosphonate. This information can help readers assess the amount of variability in the sample with respect to each characteristic measured. For example, there was a high level of variability in sex, with men and women being fairly equally represented. However, there was little variability in race or bisphosphonate use.

Ordinal and Numerical Variables. Describing the distribution of ordinal and numerical variables is more complex. Typically, the distributions of these types of variables have three characteristics that are of

TABLE 1-3. Summary of Nominal Variables

Characteristic	% (n)
Male	45 (90)
White	90 (180)
Diagnosed with osteoporosis	25 (50)
Taking a bisphosphonate	5 (10)

interest: (1) the center, (2) the amount of dispersion of observations around the center, and (3) the shape of the distribution of observations around the center. Measures used to assess these characteristics are described below.

1. **The Center.** Measures of **central tendency** are used to describe where the center of the distribution of a variable lies. The three most frequently used measures of central tendency are as follows:
   a. **Arithmetic Mean.** The arithmetic mean of a variable is determined by summing the values for each observation in the sample and dividing by the number of observations. For example, if a study had only 4 subjects and their ages were 13, 14, 15, and 16, the mean age in the sample would be $\frac{13+14+15+16}{4}=14.5$. (Note: Although there are different types of means [e.g., geometric mean, harmonic mean], in clinical papers, it is fairly safe to assume that the term "mean" refers to the arithmetic mean, unless stated otherwise.)
   b. **Median.** The median is the point in the distribution of a variable at which half of the observations are smaller and half are larger. For example, if a study had only three subjects and their ages were 13, 14, and 15, the median age in the sample would be 14. If a sample has an even number of observations, the median is calculated by averaging the middle two values. For example, if a study had four subjects and their ages were 13, 14, 15, and 16, the median age in the sample would be $\frac{14+15}{2}=14.5$.
   c. **Mode.** The mode is the value within a distribution that appears most often. This measure of central tendency is used much less frequently than the mean and median. It is mostly used to describe the distribution of an ordinal variable. For example, imagine a study in which bone density was categorized as normal, osteopenia, or osteoporosis. When presenting the data, the investigators would calculate the percentage of participants in each of these three categories. If 60% of the participants were classified as having osteopenia, the investigators might state that the mode (or modal category) was osteopenia.
2. **Dispersion.** Measures of dispersion are used to describe how observations are distributed around the center of the distribution. The two most frequently used measures of dispersion are the standard deviation (SD) and the interquartile range (IQR). The SD is used as a measure of dispersion around the mean. The IQR is used as a measure of dispersion around the median. Thus, the mean and SD go hand in hand, as do the median and IQR.
   a. **SD.** The formula for calculating the SD of a variable is shown in Figure 1-1, where (X_i) is the value for each observation, $\bar{X}$ is the sample mean, n is the number of observations in the sample, and Σ indicates that you sum the squares of the differences between each observation in the sample and the sample mean. At an intuitive level, the SD of a variable can be thought of as the average distance of a person in a sample from the sample mean. For example, if a study has three subjects with the ages 13, 14, and 15, the SD is 1.0. If the ages of subjects are 12, 14, and 16, the SD is 2.0. What do you think the SD is if the ages of the subjects are 9, 14, and 19? If you are thinking it would be 5.0, you are correct! Note that the bigger the SD, the greater the variability of observations around the mean.
   b. **IQR.** The IQR is calculated by ordering observations from those with the smallest values on the variable of interest to those with the largest values. Then, the 25th percentile of the distribution is

FIGURE 1-1. Standard Deviation Formula

$$SD=\sqrt{\frac{\sum\left(X_i-\bar{X}\right)^2}{n-1}}$$

found by multiplying the number of observations in the sample by 0.25, and the 75th percentile is found by multiplying the number of observations in the sample by 0.75. Finally, the IQR is calculated by subtracting the value of the observation at the 25th percentile from the value of the observation at the 75th percentile.

For example, consider the following sample of ages:

10 11 12 13 (14) 15 16 17 18 19 20 21 22 (23) 24 25 26 27 years

This sample has a total of 18 observations. Thus, the 25th percentile is at the fifth observation (i.e., 18*0.25 = 4.5), and the 75th percentile is at the 14th observation (i.e., 18*0.75 = 13.5). (Note: Always round up to the nearest integer.) The IQR is 23 – 14 = 9 years. By definition, the IQR captures 50% of the observations in the sample. As the variability of a characteristic in a sample increases, the IQR will increase as well.

3. **Shape.** Many statistical tests make the assumption that the distribution of the variable being analyzed is symmetrical. A variable has a symmetrical distribution if the observations on one side of the mean is the mirror image of the distribution on the other side. Note that if a variable has a symmetrical distribution, the mean and median will be equal.

   The histogram in Figure 1-2 shows a hypothetical symmetrical distribution of age in a sample of 1,100 people. Note that the mean and median are both 55. If you imagine folding the histogram at the mean, you can see that the distribution of observations on the left side of the mean is the mirror image of the distribution on the right side, confirming that the distribution is symmetrical. If the data distribution is not symmetrical, it is called "skewed." The direction of the skew is described as the direction in which the "tail" of the distribution points. The left panel in Figure 1-3 shows a histogram in which the data are skewed to the left. This is sometimes called a negative skew. The right panel in Figure 1-3 shows a histogram in which the data are skewed to the right. This type of distribution is sometimes called a positive skew. Notice that the median remains at 55 regardless of the distribution of the data; however, the mean changes. In general, the mean is more sensitive than the median to changes in the distribution of a variable.
4. **When to Use the Mean (SD) Versus the Median (IQR).** As stated previously, the mean and SD are used in combination to describe the distribution of a variable. Similarly, the median and IQR are used in combination. This raises the following question: "When describing the distribution of

FIGURE 1-2. Symmetrical Distribution of Age

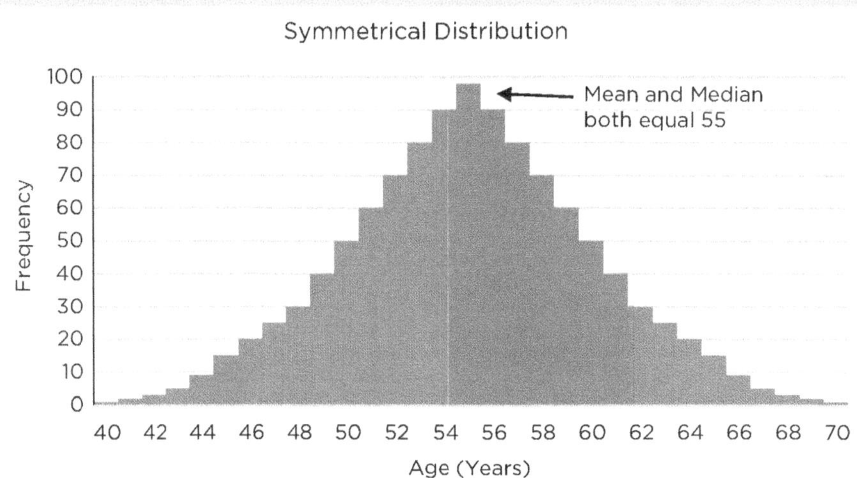

FIGURE 1-3. **Asymmetrical Distribution**

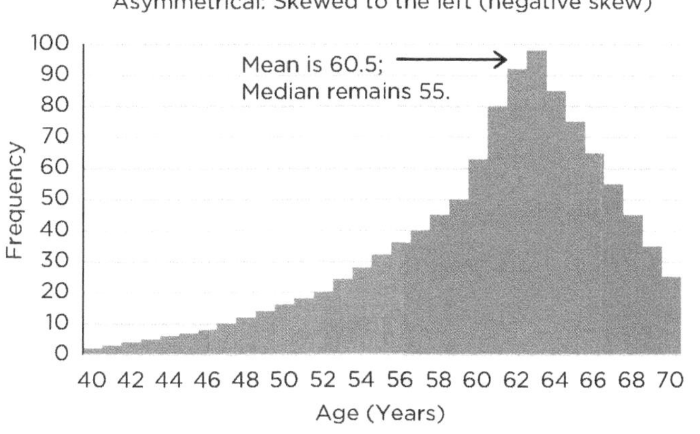

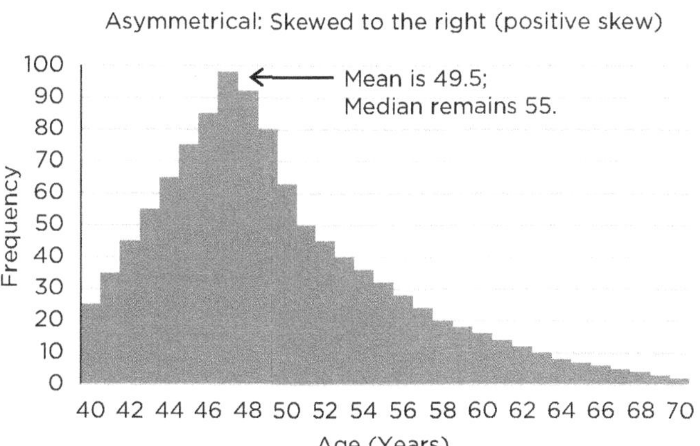

a specific variable, which combination should be used?" The following guidelines provide the answer to this question.

a. **Mean (SD) Should Be Used.** The mean (SD) should only be used if the investigator is describing (1) a variable measured on a numerical scale (i.e., has interval or ratio properties) *and* (2) the distribution of the variable is symmetrical. If a variable has an asymmetrical distribution, the mean (SD) may not accurately describe where the center of the distribution lies and the amount of dispersion that exists around the center.
b. **Median (IQR) Should Be Used.** The median (IQR) should be used if the investigator is describing (1) a variable measured on an ordinal scale *or* (2) the distribution of the variable is not symmetrical. This is because the median (IQR) is less sensitive than the mean (SD) to changes in the distribution of a variable, including the presence of extreme values (i.e., outliers).
c. **Example.** Below are 2 hypothetical distributions depicting the ages of study participants (sample size, n = 18). The distributions are identical except that one distribution contains an individual who is 27 years old. In the other distribution, this person is replaced by an individual who is 87 years old. The mean age (SD) in the first sample is 18.5 (5.34). The mean age (SD) in the second sample is 21.8 (16.99). In contrast, the median (IQR) is 18.5 (9.0) for both distributions. This example shows the sensitivity of the mean to violations in the distribution of a variable, especially when extreme values (i.e., outliers) are present, such as the person aged 87 in the second distribution. The smaller the sample size, the more the mean (SD) will be affected by these types of issues.

Distribution 1

10 11 12 13 (14) 15 16 17 18 19 20 21 22 (23) 24 25 26 **27** years

Distribution 2

10 11 12 13 (14) 15 16 17 18 19 20 21 22 (23) 24 25 26 **87** years

Interpreting Normal and Standard Normal Distributions

The normal distribution is a probability distribution that is defined by its mean and SD. As shown in Figure 1-4, the normal distribution is symmetrical (i.e., the shape of the distribution on one side of the mean is identical to the shape of the distribution on the other side of the mean) and "bell shaped."

FIGURE 1-4. Normal Distribution

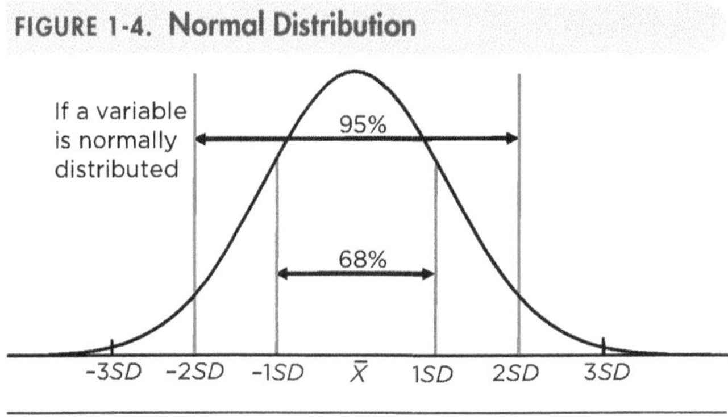

SD, standard deviation

Variables are often described in terms of whether they are normally distributed. If a variable is normally distributed and the mean and SD of the variable are known, one can calculate the probability of observing any particular value in the distribution. For example, if a variable is normally distributed, (1) approximately 68% of all observations will be within 1 SD of the mean, (2) approximately 95% of all observations will be within 2 SDs of the mean, and (3) approximately 99.7% of all observations will be within 3 SDs of the mean. If the distribution of observations in a sample departs from these percentages, the variable is not normally distributed.

Few variables are perfectly normally distributed. However, when reading scientific papers, you should be alert to major departures from normality. Fortunately, there are a few things you can look at to determine whether a variable is likely to be normally distributed. If a variable is normally distributed, the following qualities are present:

1. The mean of the variable will be halfway between the highest and lowest observed values. For example, if a variable ranges from 40 to 80, the mean should be around 60 (i.e., $\frac{40+80}{2}$).
2. The mean and median should be equal.
3. The mean ± 2 SDs should be a valid number. This is because 5% of the observations in the sample should have values greater than 2 SDs away from the mean (2.5% in the tail on the right-hand side of the distribution and 2.5% in the tail on the left-hand side of the distribution). What is an invalid number you ask? The easiest example involves variables that are assessed by counting (e.g., number of myocardial infarctions). These types of variables cannot have values less than zero. Other examples are more subjective. One might argue that values of attributes such as weight (in adults) must be above a certain point (e.g., 60 pounds) to be valid. For example, imagine that 5 people are in a sample and they have the following weights in pounds: 120, 130, 140, 150, and 200. The mean weight is 168 (SD = 74.6). Therefore, mean ± 2 SDs = 168–2(74.6) to 168+2(74.6) = 18.8 to 317.2. One could conclude that this variable is not normally distributed because 18.8 is not a valid weight for an adult.
4. In a relatively small sample (e.g., 100 or less), no observations should be greater than 3 SDs away from the mean. Based on the probabilities provided previously, 99.7% of all observations should be within 3 SDs of the mean. Only 0.3% of observations should be 3 SDs or more away from the mean. Thus, in a sample of 100 or fewer, one would not expect to see any observations 3 SDs or more away from the mean. In larger samples, one would expect to see a few observations in this range. For example, in a sample of 1,000, a normally distributed variable will contain about three observations 3 SDs or more away from the mean.

Often, it is useful to know where an individual observation in a sample lies within the overall distribution (e.g., whether a person 45 years old is one of the youngest in the sample or one of the oldest). This may be difficult to determine, however, because it requires knowledge of the mean and SD of the variable of interest. This problem can be overcome by converting the original values of the variable (i.e., the raw scores) into z-scores. Z-scores indicate how many SD units the observation is from the sample mean. When the z-score is greater than 0, it indicates that the observation is above the mean. When the z-score is less than 0, it indicates the observation is below the mean. The formula for converting a raw score into a z-score is $z = \frac{Raw\ Score - \bar{X}}{SD}$.

Z-scores follow a z-distribution, also called a standard normal distribution. By definition, a standard normal distribution has a mean of 0 and an SD of 1.

Example 1: Imagine that the mean age in a sample is 45 years (SD = 5 years). The z-score for someone aged 45 is $z = \frac{45-45}{5} = 0$. This tells you that the person's age is identical to the sample mean. Because the standard normal distribution is symmetrical around the mean, this also tells you that about 50% of the other people in the sample are younger than this person and that about 50% are older.

Example 2: Imagine that the mean age in a sample is 45 years (SD = 5 years). The z-score for someone aged 60 is $z = \frac{60-45}{5} = 3$. Thus, this person's age is 3 SD units above the sample mean. Because about 99.7% of the people in the sample are within 3 SDs of the mean, this tells you that this person is one of the oldest people in the sample.

Example 3: Imagine that the mean age in a sample is 45 years (SD = 5 years). The z-score for someone aged 30 is $z = \frac{30-45}{5} = -3$. Thus, this person's age is 3 SD units below the sample mean. This tells you that this person is one of the youngest people in the sample.

The formula provided previously can be used to convert any value on the original variable into a z-score. The exact location of each observation within the distribution can then be determined by consulting a z-table. An abbreviated z-table is provided in Table 1-4. More detailed z-tables can be found in introductory statistics books and from a wide variety of sources online.

TABLE 1-4. Z-Table

z-Score	% of Distribution Greater Than z	z-Score	% of Distribution Less Than z
0.0	0.50	0.0	0.50
0.5	0.31	−0.5	0.31
1.0	0.16	−1.0	0.16
1.5	0.07	−1.5	0.07
1.6	0.05	−1.6	0.05
1.9	0.03	−1.9	0.03
2.0	0.02	−2.0	0.02
2.5	0.01	−2.5	0.01
2.6	0.005	−2.6	0.005
3.0	0.001	−3.0	0.001
3.5	0.0002	−3.5	0.0002
4.0	0.00003	−4.0	0.00003

Reading Tables and Figures

Often, the most important findings reported in a paper are highlighted in tables and figures. We introduce three types of tables and figures often used to present the results of descriptive statistical analyses. In later chapters, we will introduce many other types of tables and figures used to summarize the results of inferential analyses.

1. **Frequency Tables.** Ordinal and numerical variables can be summarized in frequency tables, just like nominal variables. When dealing with numerical variables, investigators make the tables digestible by aggregating individual values into a limited number of categories, with each category corresponding to a different range of values. Investigators then compute (1) the number of observations within each category and (2) the percentage of all observations that are within each category. For example, the frequency table in Table 1-5 presents information concerning bone mineral density (BMD) at the hip and spine in a sample of 427 women. Specific BMD scores were aggregated into categories, with each category spanning an interval of 0.1 g/cm^2. The table shows the number of people in each category, the percentage of the total sample within each category, and the cumulative percentage of the sample, with BMD values either within the category or within a lower category.
2. **Histograms.** Histograms, like the one shown in Figure 1-5, look like bar charts, but with no spaces between the bars. The values of the observed variable are presented on the x-axis. The frequency or percentage of observations within each interval is presented on the y-axis. Histograms provide a great deal of information about the distribution of a variable because the area under each bar corresponds to the percentage of the sample within that interval. As discussed previously, histograms can be used to determine if the distribution of a variable is symmetrical.
3. **Box and Whisker Plots.** Figure 1-6 shows three box and whisker plots. These plots correspond to the 3 histograms presented in the subsection titled "Shape." From left to right, the plots show the distribution that was (1) skewed to the left (i.e., negatively skewed), (2) skewed to the right (i.e., positively skewed), and (3) symmetrical. The bottom of each box corresponds to the 25th percentile of the distribution. The top of each box corresponds to the 75th percentile. Thus, the area within each

TABLE 1-5. Frequency Table

BMD (g/cm^2)	Hip			Spine		
	#	%	Cum. %	#	%	Cum. %
.5–.59	1	0.2	0.2	0	0.0	0.0
.6–.69	19	4.4	4.7	1	0.2	0.2
.7–.79	45	10.5	15.2	3	0.7	0.9
.8–.89	124	29.0	44.3	9	2.1	3.0
.9–.99	105	24.6	68.9	30	7.0	10.1
1.0–1.09	79	18.5	87.4	71	16.6	26.7
1.1–1.19	37	8.7	96.0	113	26.5	53.2
1.2–1.29	11	2.6	98.6	98	23.0	76.1
1.3–1.39	3	0.7	99.3	64	15.0	91.1
1.4–1.49	3	0.7	100.0	24	5.6	96.7
1.5–1.59	0	0.0	100.0	13	3.0	99.8
1.6–1.69	0	0.0	100.0	1	0.2	100.0

FIGURE 1-5. **Histogram**

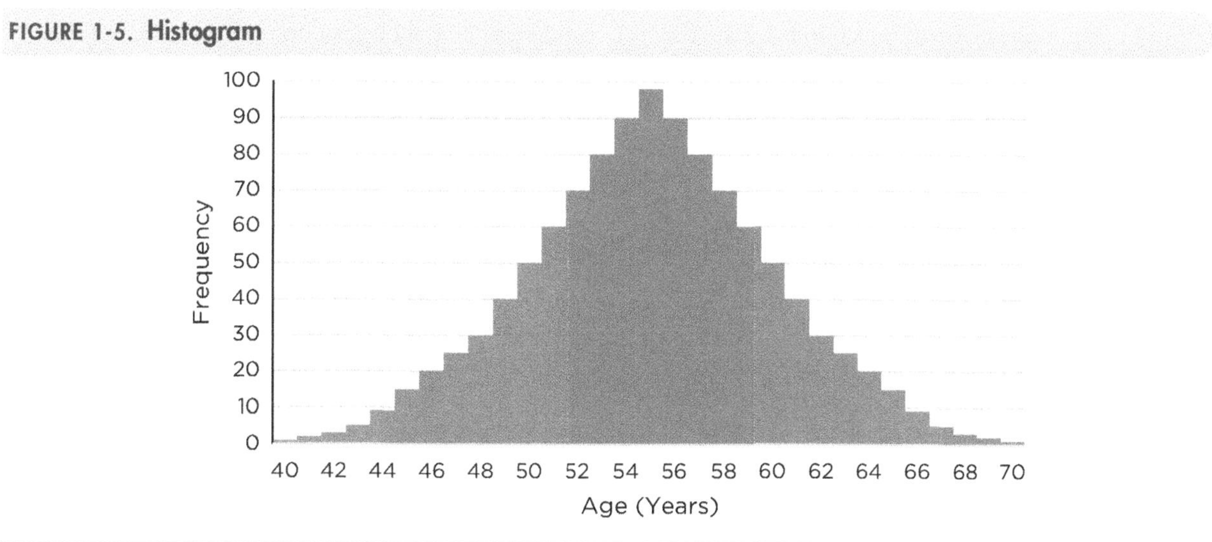

FIGURE 1-6. **Box and Whisker Plots**

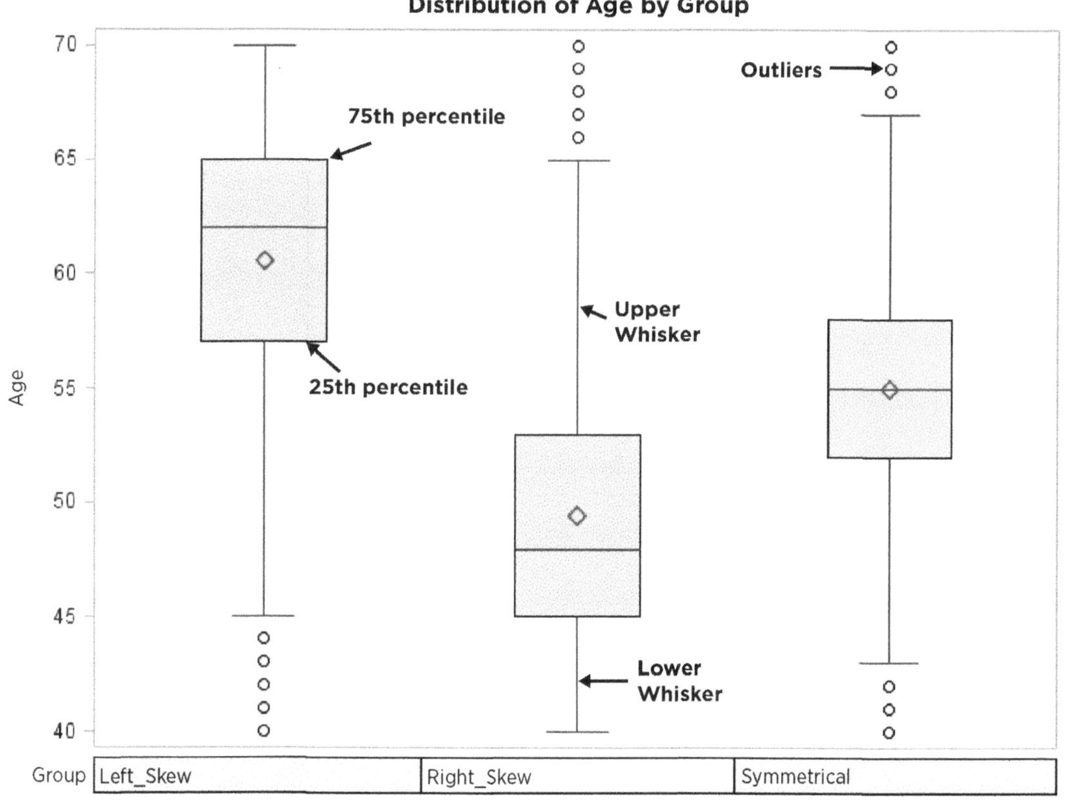

box identifies the IQR. Remember that, by definition, 50% of the observations in the sample fall within the IQR. The line in the middle of each box shows the median. The small triangle within each box indicates the mean. Note that the mean and median are identical in the symmetrical distribution. Each whisker extends 1.5 times the IQR in each direction away from the box unless the highest/lowest value in the distribution is reached first. In that case, the whisker ends at the highest/lowest value in the distribution, creating whiskers that differ in length. One would expect the whiskers to capture almost all of the observations in the distribution. Values that lie beyond the whiskers are considered outliers (i.e., extreme values). They are depicted by the small circles in the box and whisker plots. Outliers can distort the results of inferential statistics. Therefore, when reading the literature, you should look to see if outliers are present and whether the investigators assessed the impact of any outliers on the results of their primary analyses. Box and whisker plots can also be used to examine whether the distribution of a particular variable is similar across the different groups in a study.

Self-Study Questions

1. Which of the following sets of numbers has the largest SD?

   A. 5, 10, 15, 20, 25
   B. 5, 15, 25, 35, 45
   C. 5, 20, 35, 50, 65
   D. 5, 20, 35, 50, 85

2. Which of the following statistics is most commonly used to describe the central tendency of a normally distributed numerical variable?

   A. Mean
   B. Median
   C. Mode
   D. SD

3. Imagine that you know a person's systolic blood pressure (SBP) and DBP. You also know the mean and SD of SBP and DBP in the general population. You use this information to convert the person's blood pressure readings into z-scores. The z-scores obtained are –0.45 for DBP and –0.85 for SBP. Based on this information, what would you conclude?

   A. The person appears to have abnormally low blood pressure.
   B. The person appears to have abnormally high blood pressure.
   C. The person's blood pressure appears to be about normal.
   D. These data cannot be correct because z-scores cannot take negative values.

4. The SD of a measure is:

   A. Where the center of the distribution of observations lies
   B. The difference between the median and the mean
   C. The average distance of an observation in a sample from the sample mean
   D. The probability that the measure is normally distributed

5. If data from a sample are normally distributed, approximately 95% of the observations will lie within how many SDs of the mean?

   A. Plus or minus 1
   B. Plus or minus 2
   C. Plus or minus 3
   D. Plus or minus 4

6. If the distribution of a variable is symmetrical, the most appropriate statistics to use to describe the sample are:

   A. Mean and SD
   B. Mean and standard error of the mean
   C. Median and IQR
   D. Median and range
   E. Mode

Assessing Rates and Risks

2

After reading this chapter, you should be able to do the following:

1. Differentiate between raw (crude) and adjusted rates and explain why adjusted rates are often needed.
2. Describe the type of information conveyed by the following statistics: (a) relative risk ratio, (b) relative risk reduction, (c) absolute risk reduction, (d) number needed to treat, and (e) odds ratio.
3. Interpret raw and adjusted incidence and prevalence rates.
4. Given a set of data, compute the following statistics: (a) relative risk ratio, (b) relative risk reduction/increase, (c) absolute risk reduction/increase, (d) number needed to treat/harm, and (e) odds ratio.
5. Given the results of a study, interpret the various measures used to assess risk.

Many of the questions addressed in medical research involve assessing the risk of experiencing a specific health outcome (e.g., dying from a certain illness) or the rate at which specific health outcomes occur (e.g., rate of falls among older adults taking a particular medication). Often, investigators are interested in learning if treatment or preventive actions can reduce the rate or risk of deleterious health outcomes. Therefore, before turning to inferential statistics, it is helpful to better understand the different types of measures used to assess rates and risks in the medical literature.

Assessing Rates

Rates are used to summarize data from nominal variables. To determine the rate at which a particular health outcome occurs, one must first know the proportion of people who experience the outcome. Remember that proportions simply indicate the number of people with a particular characteristic relative to the total number of people in the group of interest (i.e., $\frac{\text{\# of People with Characteristic}}{n}$). Proportions can range from 0 to 1.0. For example, imagine that you have a sample of 200 people aged 40 to 50. If 24 of these people had diabetes, the proportion of people with diabetes would be 0.12 (i.e., 24 of 200). Proportions can be converted to percentages by multiplying by 100%. This conversion allows one to talk about the percentage of people in a group who have a particular characteristic. In the sample described previously, 12% of study participants have diabetes. Percentages can range from 0% to 100%.

Rates provide information about how often an outcome occurs over a specified period of time. Rates can range from 0 to infinity. They are computed by multiplying the proportion of people in a group who experience the outcome by a base (i.e., $\left(\frac{\text{\# of People Who Experience Outcome}}{n}\right) * \textit{Base}$). Multiplication by the base makes it easier to interpret how frequently the event occurs. Potentially, any base can be used. However, bases are usually selected to maximize interpretability. The base must always be included in any expression of a rate. Without the base, the rate is uninterpretable. Box 2-1 provides an example of how a rate might be computed and communicated.

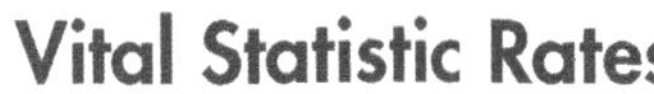

Vital Statistic Rates

Information concerning vital statistics is often presented as rates. This includes information concerning both mortality and morbidity. **Mortality** rates convey information about the frequency of death. Often, mortality rates are reported within specific population subgroups (e.g., neonates, people aged 85–94). Rates of death from specific causes (e.g., myocardial infarction, stroke, breast cancer, motor vehicle crashes) may also be reported. **Morbidity** rates convey information about illness frequency. Morbidity rates are usually expressed in terms of the prevalence or incidence of disease.

Prevalence statistics provide information about the number of people in a population who have a particular health problem **at a given point in time.** Although people talk about prevalence **rates**, prevalence statistics are really just **proportions**. Prevalence is calculated by dividing the number of people in the population who have the health problem of interest by the total number of people in the population who are at risk for the health problem (e.g., the number of men in the population with prostate cancer divided by the total number of men in the population). Prevalence statistics are often used within the context of chronic conditions that are not rapidly fatal (e.g., diabetes mellitus). Prevalence statistics reflect the burden of the condition on society. If treatments improve, prevalence of a chronic illness can increase even as incidence decreases, because people with the condition live longer.

Incidence statistics provide information about the number of people **who develop a health problem over a specified period of time** relative to the number of people who were at risk for the health problem at

BOX 2-1. Expression of Rate Example

Imagine that 23,250 patients take a particular medication, each for exactly 1 year. Twelve of these people develop aplastic anemia.

The proportion of people who develop aplastic anemia during the 1-year follow-up period is:

$$\frac{12}{23{,}250} = 0.00052$$

To express the rate with which patients developed aplastic anemia, this proportion must be multiplied by a base. Below, the proportion is multiplied by bases ranging from 100 to 1,000,000. Which base do you think leads to the most interpretable rate?

Proportion	Base	Expression of Rate
0.00052	100	0.052 cases per 100 patient-years of treatment
0.00052	1,000	0.52 cases per 1,000 patient-years of treatment
0.00052	10,000	5.2 cases per 10,000 patient-years of treatment
0.00052	100,000	52 cases per 100,000 patient-years of treatment
0.00052	1,000,000	520 cases per 1,000,000 patient-years of treatment

Any of the bases are acceptable, but I think that, in this particular case, the base of 10,000 yields the most interpretable expression of the rate. It is fairly easy to visualize both 5.2 patients with aplastic anemia and a population of 10,000 patients.

the start of the time period. Incidence can be measured in two different ways: cumulative incidence (i.e., incidence proportion) or incidence rate. To calculate either of these two measures, investigators first must identify the relevant time period. **Cumulative incidence** is calculated by dividing the number of people who develop the health problem during that period of time by the number of people at risk for the health problem at the beginning of the time period (i.e., $\frac{\text{\# of New Cases During a Specified Period}}{\text{\# of People at Risk at the Start of the Period Specified}}$). Note that the denominator in this formula includes all people at risk at the start of the period specified and does not consider the exact point in time when each new case was identified. **Incidence rates** are calculated by dividing the number of people who develop the health problem during the period of time specified by the total time of observation (i.e., $\frac{\text{\# of New Cases During a Specified Period}}{\text{Total Observation Time for At-Risk Individuals}}$). Here, the denominator is expressed in person-time (e.g., person-years). Note that once a person develops the health problem of interest, that person is no longer at risk. Therefore, the person stops contributing observation time to the denominator in the calculation of incidence rate. (Box 2-2 provides an example of the calculation of prevalence, cumulative incidence, and incidence rates.) Cumulative incidence and incidence rates are often used to express the frequency at which acute conditions are occurring (e.g., medication side effects, injuries, new cases of influenza during the winter months). They are particularly appropriate to use for conditions that either are short-term (e.g., respiratory infections) or have a high mortality rate (e.g., cancer). They can be useful in identifying areas where prevention efforts are needed.

Raw (Crude) Versus Adjusted Rates

Often, investigators want to compare rates in two different groups. For example, an investigator might want to know if the mortality rate among people with a certain type of cancer varies as a function of the medications they use. The investigator might form groups of people treated with different medications (e.g., Medication A or Medication B) and determine the incidence of death during the first year following the initiation of therapy. To calculate the raw (crude) incidence rates in the different groups, the investigator would just need to determine the number of people within each group who died during the specified period divided by the number of people treated. For example, in Table 2-1, the mortality rate among people taking Medication A is $\frac{9{,}545}{230} = 41.5$ per 1,000 person-years; whereas, the mortality rate among people taking Medication B is $\frac{5{,}688}{175} = 32.5$ per 1,000 person-years. These are raw (crude) mortality rates. They suggest that Medication A may be less effective than Medication B because patients taking Medication A experience a higher mortality rate. (The term person-years reflects both the number of people under investigation and the length of time they are followed. In this example, I made the math easy by assuming each person was followed for 1 year. If one person was followed for exactly 2 years, he or she would contribute a total of 2 person-years of data. If one person was followed for exactly 6 months, he or she would contribute a total of 0.5 person-years of data.)

However, if you look at the data presented in Table 2-1 more closely, you will see that **within each age group**, the mortality rates are the same (e.g., 50 per 1,000 person-years among people aged 60–79). The difference in the crude rates is caused by the fact that the mortality rate is highest in the older age group **and** people taking Medication A tend to be older (i.e., 75% versus 50% are aged 60–79 among people taking Medication A versus Medication B, respectively). This difference in the age distribution between the two groups makes it difficult to determine if the effectiveness of the medications differ. In this example, age is a **confounder**. Confounders alter the relationship between the primary variables of interest.

To overcome this type of problem, investigators often calculate **adjusted rates**. There are different ways of calculating adjusted rates. At an intuitive level, all methods involve calculating rates that impose the same distribution of the confounding factor on all groups. In Tables 2-2A through 2-2C, I calculated

BOX 2-2. Example of Calculation of Prevalence and Incidence

Imagine that an investigator is interested in the prevalence and incidence of Health Problem A, a chronic condition that can be treated but not cured. The following data are available for 2017.

Population on January 1, 2017	100,000
Existing cases of Health Problem A on January 1, 2017	1,000
New cases of Health Problem A reported during 2017	500
Births during 2017	20,000
Deaths among people with Health Problem A during 2017	200
Deaths from all other causes during 2017	10,000

To calculate the **prevalence** of Health Problem A on January 1, 2018:

$$\frac{\textit{(Existing Cases + New Cases − Death Among Cases)}}{\textit{Total \# of People in Population on January 1, 2018}}$$

$$\frac{1{,}000 + 500 - 200}{100{,}000 + 20{,}000 - 200 - 10{,}000} = 0.0118 \text{ or } 1.18\%$$

Note that prevalence only includes information about people who are in the population at a specific point in time (in this case on January 1, 2018). Further, "cases" are people who have the health problem at that time. Thus, people who die before that point in time are not included.

To calculate the **cumulative incidence** of Health Problem A during 2017:

$$\frac{\textit{\# of New Cases During a Specified Period}}{\textit{\# of People at Risk at the Start of the Period Specified}} = \frac{500}{100{,}000 - 1{,}000} = 0.005$$

Multiplying this value by a base of 1,000 yields a cumulative incidence of five new cases of Health Problem A per year for every 1,000 people in the at-risk population.

To calculate the **incidence rate** of Health Problem A during 2017:

$$\frac{\textit{\# of New Cases During a Specified Period}}{\textit{Total Observation Time for At-Risk Individuals}}$$

$$= \frac{500}{100{,}000 - 1{,}000 + \left(\frac{20{,}000}{2}\right) - \left(\frac{10{,}000}{2}\right) - \left(\frac{200}{2}\right) - \left(\frac{500}{2}\right)}$$

$$= \frac{\textit{500 Cases}}{\textit{103,650 Person-Years}} = 0.0048$$

Multiplying this value by a base of 1,000 yields an incidence rate of 4.8 new cases of Health Problem A per every 1,000 person-years of observation.

Note that incidence rate only includes information about people who develop the condition during the study period, regardless of whether people die or recover before the end of the study period. In addition, people who already have the condition at the start of the study period must be excluded from the denominator, because they are **not at risk** for developing the condition. Finally, in the calculations, I made the simplifying assumption that all births, deaths, and new cases of Health Problem A occurred midway through the year, putting everyone who was born, died, or developed Health Problem A during the year at risk for 6 months. Therefore, I divided the number of births, deaths, and new cases of Health Problem A that occurred during 2017 by 2.

TABLE 2-1. 1-Year Crude Mortality Rates Among Patients Treated with Medications A and B

	Medication A				Medication B			
	Patients Treated		Deaths		Patients Treated		Deaths	
Age	N (in 1000s)	%	#	Rate Per 1,000	N (in 1000s)	%	#	Rate Per 1,000
20–39	23.0	10	230	10.0	43.75	25	438	10.0
40–59	34.5	15	690	20.0	43.75	25	875	20.0
60–79	172.5	75	8,625	50.0	87.5	50	4,375	50.0
Total	230	100	9,545	41.5	175	100	5,688	32.5

the adjusted mortality rate among people taking Medication A by imposing the same age distribution observed among people taking Medication B. I did this by doing the following:

1. Substituting the percentage of patients within each age group taking Medication A with the percentages observed for Medication B (Table 2-2A).
2. Calculating the number of people (N) within each age group, keeping the total number of people treated with Medication A fixed at 230,000 (Table 2-2B).
3. Calculating the number of deaths that would have occurred among patients treated with Medication A if the age distribution had been identical to Medication B by multiplying the number of patients treated within each age group by the age-specific mortality rate (Table 2-2C).
4. Summing the number of deaths across age groups, which yielded a total of 7,475 deaths, and dividing this total by 230 to yield the adjusted mortality rate of 32.5 per 1,000 person-years—identical to that observed among patients taking Medication B. Thus, Medications A and B appear to be equally effective. The difference in the raw (crude) rates was an artifact of Medication A being more likely than Medication B to be used among older patients.

We will discuss problems caused by confounding more in later chapters, as well as analytic strategies used to address these problems. For now, the take-home message is simply that crude rates can be misleading. In presenting rates, investigators should **adjust** for any factors that may differ between the groups being compared. As a reader of the literature, pay attention to the factors that are included when investigators calculate **adjusted rates**. Be sure to think about whether they adjusted for all potentially important factors.

TABLE 2-2A. Calculating 1-Year-Adjusted Mortality Rates Among Patients Treated with Medications A and B (Step 1)

	Medication A				Medication B			
	Patients Treated		Deaths		Patients Treated		Deaths	
Age	N (in 1000s)	%	#	Rate Per 1,000	N (in 1000s)	%	#	Rate Per 1,000
20–39		25		10.0	43.75	25	438	10.0
40–59		25		20.0	43.75	25	875	20.0
60–79		50		50.0	87.5	50	4,375	50.0
Total	230	100			175	100	5,688	32.5

TABLE 2-2B. Calculating 1-Year-Adjusted Mortality Rates Among Patients Treated With Medications A and B (Step 2)

	Medication A				Medication B			
	Patients Treated		Deaths		Patients Treated		Deaths	
Age	N (in 1000s)	%	#	Rate Per 1,000	N (in 1000s)	%	#	Rate Per 1,000
20–39	57.5	25		10.0	43.75	25	438	10.0
40–59	57.5	25		20.0	43.75	25	875	20.0
60–79	115.0	50		50.0	87.5	50	4,375	50.0
Total	230	100			175	100	5,688	32.5

TABLE 2-2C. Calculating 1-Year-Adjusted Mortality Rates Among Patients Treated With Medications A and B (Step 3)

	Medication A				Medication B			
	Patients Treated		Deaths		Patients Treated		Deaths	
Age	N (in 1000s)	%	#	Rate Per 1,000	N (in 1000s)	%	#	Rate Per 1,000
20–39	57.5	25	575	10.0	43.75	25	438	10.0
40–59	57.5	25	1,150	20.0	43.75	25	875	20.0
60–79	115.0	50	5,750	50.0	87.5	50	4,375	50.0
Total	230	100	7,475	32.5	175	100	5,688	32.5

Assessing Risks

In medicine, we are often interested in determining if the risk of a particular health outcome varies between two groups. For example, we might want to know if people who smoke are more likely than nonsmokers to experience a particular health problem (e.g., myocardial infarction, stroke). In this case, smoking would be considered a possible risk factor for certain adverse health outcomes. In contrast, we might want to know if people who take a particular medication are more likely than others to survive at least 5 years following the initiation of treatment. In this case, pharmacotherapy would be considered a treatment that is hoped to improve health outcomes.

There are several different statistics that can be used to express estimates of risk. All of these estimates are based on values contained in the 2 × 2 contingency table shown in Table 2-3. This table shows the relationship between exposure to a particular treatment (risk factor) and development of a specific health outcome. The table can be used to calculate statistics that assess whether exposure to the treatment (risk factor) is associated with a decreased (or increased) risk of the outcome. In the table, "A" indicates the number of people who were exposed to the treatment (risk factor) **and** who developed the disease of interest. "B" indicates the number of people who were exposed to the treatment (risk factor) but who did not develop the disease. Thus, the total number of people who were exposed to the treatment (or risk factor) equals "A" + "B." Similarly, "C" indicates the number of people who were **not** exposed but who developed the disease; "D" indicates the number of people who were neither exposed nor developed the

TABLE 2-3. Structure of Contingency Table to Calculate Risk Measures

	Outcome		
Treatment (Risk Factor)	**Disease**	**No Disease**	**TOTAL**
Exposed	A	B	A+B
Not Exposed	C	D	C+D
Total	A+C	B+D	A+B+C+D

disease. Thus, the total number of people who were **not** exposed to the treatment (or risk factor) equals "C" + "D." You can also see from the table that the total number of people who developed the disease equals "A" + "C" and that the total number of people did not develop the disease equal "B" + "D." Finally, the total number of people observed equals "A" + "B" + "C" + "D."

The contingency table can be used to compute the following two event rates:

1. The **experiment event rate (EER)** is the probability of developing the disease among those exposed to the treatment (risk factor).
   The EER is calculated as: A / (A + B).
2. The **control event rate (CER)** is the probability of developing the disease among those who were **not** exposed to the treatment (risk factor). People who are not exposed to the treatment (risk factor) are often referred to as the "reference group."
   The CER is calculated as: C / (C + D).

The EER and CER form the building blocks for four of the five basic measures used to estimate risk. These five measures are described below, and their computational formulae are summarized in Box 2-3. Boxes 2-7 and 2-8 later in this chapter illustrate calculation of all five risk measures within the context of two fictitious studies.

1. **Absolute Risk Reduction (ARR); Absolute Risk Increase (ARI).** This statistic is computed by subtracting the CER from the EER and is expressed as an absolute value (i.e., $|EER - CER|$). The term ARR is used if exposure is associated with a lower risk (i.e., the EER is less than the CER). The term ARI is used if exposure is associated with an increased risk (i.e., the EER is higher than the CER). To enhance interpretability, the ARR (or ARI) can be multiplied by a base. Thus, if the ARR is computed to be 0.009, one might say that exposure is associated with nine fewer cases of the disease per every 1,000 people exposed.
2. **Relative Risk Reduction (RRR); Relative Risk Increase (RRI).** This statistic indicates the percent reduction (increase) in risk in the exposed group relative to the reference group. It is computed as $\left(\frac{|EER - CER|}{CER}\right) * 100\%$. From this formula, you should be able to see that if the EER is 0, risk would be completely eliminated and the RRR would be 100%.
3. **Number Needed to Treat (NNT); Number Needed to Harm (NNH).** This is the number of people who would need to be exposed in order for (a) one person to benefit (NNT) assuming that exposure decreases risk or (b) one person to be harmed (NNH) assuming that exposure increases risk. It is computed as $\frac{1}{|EER - CER|}$. As a clinician, you would like the NNT to be small and the NNH to be large. That is, you would like almost everyone to benefit from treatment. If everyone benefited from a treatment, the NNT would be "1." You would also like almost no one to be harmed by treatment. If almost no one were harmed by a treatment, it would mean that you could treat an infinite number of patients without harming one.

BOX 2-3. Computational Formulae for Risk Measures

Absolute Risk Reduction (ARR) Absolute Risk Increase (ARI)	$\lvert EER - CER\rvert$
Relative Risk Reduction (RRR) Relative Risk Increase (RRI)	$\left(\frac{\lvert EER - CER\rvert}{CER}\right) * 100\%$ *OR* $\lvert 1 - RR\rvert * 100\%$
Number Needed to Treat Number Needed to Harm	$\frac{1}{\lvert EER - CER\rvert}$
Relative Risk (RR)	$\frac{A/(A+B)}{C/(C+D)} = \frac{EER}{CER}$
Odds Ratio	$\frac{A/B}{C/D}$

4. **Relative Risk (RR).** This statistic is the ratio of the risk in the exposed group relative to the risk in the unexposed group. RR is computed as: $\frac{A/(A+B)}{C/(C+D)} = \frac{EER}{CER}$ and has a possible range from 0 to ∞. If RR is "1," the risk in the two groups is equal. The closer RR is to "1," the weaker the association between the exposure and outcome variables; the further away RR is from "1," the stronger the association. If the EER is larger than the CER, exposure increases risk and the RR will be greater than 1. In contrast, if the CER is larger than the EER, exposure decreases risk and the RR will be less than 1. Note that RR is only meaningful in cohort and experimental studies (e.g., randomized controlled trials). In both of these designs, all members of the different study groups are followed over time, allowing the risk of experiencing the outcome of interest to be calculated in each study group.

   The RRI (or RRR) can be computed easily from the RR using the formula: $\lvert 1 - RR \rvert$. Thus, an RR of 0.90 corresponds to a 10% reduction in relative risk; whereas, an RR of 0.10 corresponds to a 90% reduction in relative risk. Notice that **if RR is less than 1**, the RRR increases as the RR moves toward 0. **If RR is between 1.0 and 2.0**, the fractional value of the RR conveys information about the RRI. Thus, an RR of 1.3 indicates a 30% increase in relative risk. An RR of 1.99 indicates a 99% increase in relative risk. An RR of 2.0 indicates a 100% increase in relative risk. **If RR is greater than 2**, remember to subtract the RR from 1 (e.g., RR = 3 corresponds to a 200% increase in risk, RR = 4 corresponds to a 300% increase in risk) when calculating RRI.

   People sometimes have difficulty understanding why RRs near 0 can indicate a strong association. It may be helpful to remember that although RR is usually expressed as a single value (e.g., 0.25) it would be more accurate to express it as RR:1 (e.g., 0.25 to 1). Here, 1 reflects the risk in the reference group, which is the denominator in the RR computational formula. If you have difficulty interpreting RRs less than 1.0, you can imagine "flipping" the groups using the formula: $\frac{RR}{1} = \frac{1}{x}$. I have done this in Table 2-4. From these calculations, you should be able to see that an RR = 0.90 corresponds to a fairly small increase in risk and that the magnitude of the association between the exposure and outcome variables increases as one approaches 0.

TABLE 2-4. Interpreting Relative Risks (RRs) between 0 and 1

RR	"Flipping" Groups	Interpretation
0.90	$\frac{0.9}{1}=\frac{1}{x}; 0.9x=1; x=\frac{1}{0.9}; x=1.1$	1.11-fold decrease in risk
0.50	$\frac{0.5}{1}=\frac{1}{x}; 0.5x=1; x=\frac{1}{0.5}; x=2.0$	2-fold decrease in risk
0.25	$\frac{0.25}{1}=\frac{1}{x}; 0.25x=1; x=\frac{1}{0.25}; x=4.0$	4-fold decrease in risk
0.10	$\frac{0.1}{1}=\frac{1}{x}; 0.1x=1; x=\frac{1}{0.1}; x=10.0$	10-fold decrease in risk
0.01	$\frac{0.01}{1}=\frac{1}{x}; 0.01x=1; x=\frac{1}{0.01}; x=100.0$	100-fold decrease in risk

A final note of caution regarding interpretation of the RR. It is important for readers of the medical literature to understand the distinction between risk estimates conveyed in absolute terms (ARR/ARI) versus relative terms (RR). RR estimates tend to lead to exaggerated perceptions of risk. For example, imagine that a medication increases the risk of a certain form of cancer from 0.010% to 0.013%. This could be expressed in relative terms, as a 30% increase in risk (i.e., $RR=\frac{0.013}{0.010}=1.3$), which seems like a fairly large increase in risk. However, this risk could also be expressed in absolute terms as an increase of 3 cases per every 100,000 patients treated (i.e., $0.013\% - 0.010\% = 0.003\%$; $0.003\% * 100{,}000 = 3$ cases per 100,000), which seems like a fairly small increase in risk. In addition, absolute risk measures such as the ARR/ARI provide a direct estimate of the likelihood that a patient will experience a particular health outcome. Therefore, when making patient care decisions, absolute risk measures are more informative than RR measures.

5. **Odds Ratio (OR).** This statistic is the ratio of the odds that a person exposed to the treatment (risk factor) developed the disease relative to the odds that a person not exposed to the treatment (risk factor) developed the disease. It is computed as $\frac{A/B}{C/D}$. Note that odds relate the probability that a particular outcome occurs to the probability that it does not occur (see Box 2-4). Thus, the odds that a person exposed to the treatment (risk factor) would develop the outcome is $\frac{A}{B}$, and the odds that a person not exposed to the treatment (risk factor) would develop the outcome is $\frac{C}{D}$. ORs are created by calculating the ratio of these two odds.

   ORs are often used to approximate RR, especially in case-control studies where the RR cannot be calculated directly (see Box 2-5). If the proportion of people who develop the outcome of interest is small (e.g., less than 10%), ORs and RRs yield fairly comparable values. This can be seen by comparing the computational formulae for these statistics: $RR=\frac{A/(A+B)}{C/(C+D)}$ *versus* $OR=\frac{A/B}{C/D}$. If few people develop the outcome of interest, A and C are small and the terms (A+B) and (C+D) in the RR formula differ little from the terms B and D, respectively, in the OR formula. However, as the number of people who develop the outcome of interest increases, RR and OR values diverge, and the OR becomes a poor estimate of RR (see Box 2-6).

BOX 2-4. Risk Ratios (Proportions) Versus Odds Ratios (Odds)

In a fictitious study involving 150 people diagnosed with metastatic cancer, imagine that 100 people received an experimental drug and 50 received a placebo. All study participants are followed for 1 year. At the end of the year, the investigators determine whether participants have died or are still alive. Data from the study are presented below.

	Outcome		
Treatment	**Died**	**Survived**	**Total**
Experimental Drug	20	80	100
Placebo	5	45	50
Total	25	125	150

To estimate the relative risk of dying during the 1-year follow-up period among people who received the experimental drug compared to those who received the placebo, one starts by calculating the proportion of people who died in each group.

The proportion of people who died among those who received the experimental drug: $EER = \frac{A}{A+B} = \frac{20}{100} = 0.20$

The proportion of people who died among those who received the placebo: $CER = \frac{C}{C+D} = \frac{5}{50} = 0.10$

RR is then calculated as the ratio of these two proportions.

The RR of death among those who took the experimental medication versus placebo: $RR = \frac{EER}{CER} = \frac{0.20}{0.10} = 2.0$

To estimate the odds of dying during the 1-year follow-up period among people who received the experimental drug compared to those who received the placebo, one starts by calculating the odds of dying in each group.

The odds of that a person who received the experimental drug would die: $\frac{A}{B} = \frac{20}{80} = 0.25$

The odds of that a person who received the placebo would die: $\frac{C}{D} = \frac{5}{45} = 0.11$

Odds ratio is then calculated as the ratio of these two odds.

The odds of death among those who took the experimental medication versus placebo: $OR = \frac{A/B}{C/D} = \frac{0.25}{0.11} = 2.27$

BOX 2-5. Case-Control Studies and Odds Ratios (ORs)

In a prospective study, individuals are enrolled in a study and then followed forward in time to determine if they experience a particular health outcome of interest. Prospective studies include randomized controlled trials (RCTs) and prospective cohort studies. In RCTs, participants are randomly assigned to a specific treatment. In cohort studies, investigators simply assess participants' status on the exposure variable (i.e., type of treatment, presence of suspected risk factor) at the outset of the study.

The table below depicts the structure of a fictitious prospective cohort study designed to assess whether a suspected risk factor increases the risk of a particular health outcome. Note that in this design, the investigators know the number of participants who have the risk factor (A+B) and the number of participants who do not have the risk factor (C+D) at the outset of the study. This allows them to calculate the experiment event rate (EER) and control event rate (CER), which form the basis for the RR.

	Outcome		
Group	**Occurs**	**Does Not Occur**	**Total**
Risk factor present	A	B	100
Risk factor absent	C	D	400
Total	A+C	B+D	500

Another study design used in medical research is called a case-control study. Case-control studies are often used to study rare health outcomes. In this study design, the investigators enroll a group of people who already have the outcome of interest. These are the "cases." They also enroll a group of people who do not have the outcome. These are the "controls." They then look backward in time to determine if the cases and controls were exposed to a suspected risk factor in the past.

The table below depicts the structure of a fictitious case-control study designed to assess whether people with a particular health outcome (i.e., cases) are more likely than those without the health outcome (i.e., controls) to have been exposed to a suspected risk factor. In this study, one control was enrolled for each case. Note that in a case-control study, the investigator knows the number of cases (A+C) and controls (B+D) at the outset of the study.

	Outcome		
Group	**Cases**	**Controls**	**Total**
Risk factor present	A	B	A+B
Risk factor absent	C	D	C+D
Total	500	500	1,000

(continued)

BOX 2-5. Case-Control Studies and Odds Ratios (ORs) *(Continued)*

Case-control studies may enroll multiple controls for each case. The table below depicts the structure of a fictitious case-control study in which four controls were enrolled for each case.

	Outcome		
Group	**Cases**	**Controls**	**Total**
Risk factor present	A	B	A+B
Risk factor absent	C	D	C+D
Total	500	2,000	2,500

In an RCT, the number of people enrolled in the study does not affect the EER or CER. The table shows the results of a study in which 100 people with a particular risk factor and 400 people without the risk factor were enrolled. The CER was 0.01 and the EER was 0.02.

	Outcome		
Group	**Occurs**	**Does Not Occur**	**Total**
Risk factor present	2	98	100
Risk factor absent	4	396	400
Total	6	494	500

As you can see from the calculations below, both the RR and the OR are 2.0.

$$RR = \frac{EER}{CER} = \frac{0.02}{0.01} = 2.0; OR = \frac{A/B}{C/D} = \frac{2/98}{4/396} = 2.0$$

If the number of people in the study were doubled, as shown below, one would simply expect all of the values in Cells A–D to double because changing the number of people enrolled in the study has no effect on the EER and CER.

	Outcome		
Group	**Occurs**	**Does Not Occur**	**Total**
Risk factor present	4	196	200
Risk factor absent	8	792	800
Total	12	988	1,000

BOX 2-5. Case-Control Studies and Odds Ratios (ORs) *(Continued)*

Consequently, the RR and OR would still be 2.0.

$$RR = \frac{EER}{CER} = \frac{0.02}{0.01} = 2.0; OR = \frac{A/B}{C/D} = \frac{4/196}{8/792} = 2.0$$

In a case-control study, the EER and CER are affected by the ratio of cases to controls. The table below shows the results of a study in which 500 cases and 500 controls were enrolled.

	Outcome		
Group	**Cases**	**Controls**	**Total**
Risk factor present	57	30	87
Risk factor absent	443	470	913
Total	500	500	1,000

Here, the RR and OR yield different values.

$$RR = \frac{EER}{CER} = \frac{0.655}{0.485} = 1.35; OR = \frac{A/B}{C/D} = \frac{1.9}{0.94} = 2.0$$

Finally, below are the results from a case-control study in which 500 cases and 2,000 controls were enrolled. I calculated the values for the controls by multiplying the values in the previous table by four.

	Outcome		
Group	**Cases**	**Controls**	**Total**
Risk factor present	57	120	177
Risk factor absent	443	1,880	2,323
Total	500	2,000	2,500

In the calculations below, notice that both the EER and the CER have changed from the study in which only one control was enrolled in the study for each case. This is totally an artifact of the study design. The bottom line message is that because the row totals in a case-control study vary with the number of cases and controls enrolled, these values cannot be used to compute EER, CER, or RR. Thus, the RRs that I calculated for the case-control studies described in this example are meaningless.

However, in the calculations below, you can also see that the OR does not vary as a function of the number of cases and controls enrolled. That is, it was 2.0 in the study where there was 1 control for every case, and it remains at 2.0 when four controls are enrolled for each case. This is because calculation of ORs does not depend on the row totals.

Therefore, in case-control studies, ORs must be used to estimate RR.

$$RR = \frac{EER}{CER} = \frac{0.322}{0.191} = 1.69; OR = \frac{A/B}{C/D} = \frac{0.475}{0.236} = 2.0$$

BOX 2-6. Divergence of Relative Risk (RR) and Odds Ratio (OR) When Outcome Is Common

In Box 2-9, I presented the results of the randomized controlled trial shown below. In this example, note that the outcome is fairly uncommon, affecting only 1% of people without the risk factor and 2% of people with the risk factor.

Group	Outcome		Total
	Occurs	Does Not Occur	
Risk factor present	2	98	100
Risk factor absent	4	396	400
Total	6	494	500

As we calculated in Box 2-9, both the RR and the OR are 2.0.

$$RR = \frac{EER}{CER} = \frac{0.02}{0.01} = 2.0; OR = \frac{A/B}{C/D} = \frac{2/98}{4/396} = 2.0$$

Now, we will imagine that the outcome is a bit more common, affecting 5% of people without the risk factor and 10% of people with the risk factor. These data are shown below.

Group	Outcome		Total
	Occurs	Does Not Occur	
Risk factor present	10	90	100
Risk factor absent	20	380	400
Total	30	470	500

Here, we find that the RR remains 2.0, but the OR, which is an estimate of the RR, has increased a bit.

$$RR = \frac{EER}{CER} = \frac{0.1}{0.05} = 2.0; OR = \frac{A/B}{C/D} = \frac{10/90}{20/380} = 2.11$$

Finally, we will imagine that the outcome is considerably more common, affecting 20% of people without the risk factor and 40% of people with the risk factor. These data are shown below.

Group	Outcome		Total
	Occurs	Does Not Occur	
Risk factor present	40	60	100
Risk factor absent	80	320	400
Total	120	380	500

Here, we find that the RR remains 2.0, but that the OR has increased from 2.0 in the original study to 2.67, even though the EER and CER have not changed.

$$RR = \frac{EER}{CER} = \frac{0.4}{0.2} = 2.0; OR = \frac{A/B}{C/D} = \frac{40/60}{80/320} = 2.67$$

This example illustrates that ORs provide reasonably good estimates of RR **if the prevalence of the outcome is fairly uncommon.** However, when the outcome is more common, ORs provide biased estimates of RR.

BOX 2-7. Calculation of the Five Risk Measures in a Study Where Treatment Reduces Risk

Imagine that a new medication is available to treat a rare and aggressive form of cancer. A study is conducted to evaluate the effectiveness of the drug. A total of 1,000 people receive the new medication, and 1,000 people receive standard care. All patients are followed for 1 year. During the follow-up period, 12% of patients treated with the new medication died, and 22% of those who received standard care died. I used this information to create the following contingency table.

	Outcome		
Group	**Died**	**Did Not Die**	**Totals**
New medication	120	880	1,000
Standard care	220	780	1,000
Totals	340	1,660	2,000

Calculate experiment event rate (EER) and control event rate (CER) as:

$$EER = \frac{A}{A+B} = \frac{120}{1{,}000} = 0.12;\ CER = \frac{C}{C+D} = \frac{220}{1{,}000} = 0.22$$

Calculate absolute risk reduction (ARR) as: $ARR = |EER - CER| = |0.12 - 0.22| = 0.10$

To help interpret this statistic, I multiplied it by 100% (i.e., 0.10 $*$ 100% = 10%). Thus, treatment with the new medication rather than standard care results in a 10% reduction in absolute risk.

Calculate relative risk reduction (RRR) as:

$$RRR = \left(\frac{|EER - CER|}{CER}\right) * 100\% = \left(\frac{|0.12 - 0.22|}{0.22}\right) * 100\% = 45.45\%$$

Thus, the new medication results in a 45.45% reduction in relative risk.

Calculate number needed to treat (NNT) as: $NNT = \frac{1}{|EER - CER|} = \frac{1}{0.10} = 10$

Thus, 1 death would be prevented by treating 10 patients with the new drug rather than standard care.

Calculate relative risk (RR) as: $RR = \frac{EER}{CER} = 0.12/0.22 = 0.5455$

Thus, RR is reduced by $|1 - 0.5455| * 100\% = 45.45\%$ by treating with the new medication rather than standard care, just as we calculated for RRR above.

Calculate odds ratio (OR) as: $OR = \frac{A/B}{C/D} = \frac{120/880}{220/780} = 0.4835$

Note that this is a little lower than the RR. Because odds ratio is used to estimate RR, using the RR is preferable when it can be calculated, remembering that RR cannot be calculated in case-control studies.

BOX 2-8. Calculation of the Five Risk Measures in a Study Where Treatment Increases Risk

Data from a large health plan indicate that among a group of 5,000 patients who took Drug X during 2017, 25 people had a stroke within 6 months of therapy initiation. Among a comparison group of 5,000 patients who did not take Drug X, four people had a stroke during the same time period. This information was used to create the following contingency table.

	Outcome		
Group	**Had Stroke**	**Did Not Have Stroke**	**Totals**
Drug X	25	4,975	5,000
No Drug X	4	4,996	5,000
Totals	29	9,931	10,000

Calculate experiment event rate (EER) and control event rate (CER) as:

$$EER = \frac{A}{A+B} = \frac{25}{5{,}000} = 0.005;\ CER = \frac{C}{C+D} = \frac{4}{5{,}000} = 0.0008$$

Calculate absolute risk increase (ARI) as: $ARI = |EER - CER| = |0.005 - 0.0008| = 0.0042$

To help interpret this statistic, I multiplied it by 100% (i.e., 0.0042 ∗ 100% = 0.42%). Thus, treatment with Drug X rather than other therapies results in a 0.42% increase in absolute risk.

Calculate relative risk increase (RRI) as:

$$RRI = \left(\frac{|EER - CER|}{CER}\right) * 100\% = \left(\frac{|0.005 - 0.0008|}{0.0008}\right) * 100\% = 525\%$$

Thus, Drug X results in a 525% increase in relative risk.

Calculate number needed to harm (NNH) as: $NNH = \frac{1}{|EER - CER|} = \frac{1}{0.0042} = 238$

Thus, one stroke would be caused for every 238 patients treated with Drug X rather than other therapies.

Calculate relative risk (RR) as: $RR = \frac{EER}{CER} = \frac{0.005}{0.0008} = 6.25$

Thus, relative risk is increased more than 6-fold by treating with Drug X rather than other therapies. This corresponds to an increase in risk of $|1 - 6.25| * 100\% = 525\%$, just as we calculated for RRI above.

Calculate odds ratio (OR) as: $OR = \frac{A/B}{C/D} = \frac{25/4{,}975}{4/4{,}996} = 6.28$

Note that here the odds ratio is a pretty good estimate of RR. This is because strokes are uncommon. As a result, the terms A and C have little impact on the denominators in the EER and CER formulae.

Self-Study Questions

1. Imagine that a case-control study is conducted to determine if use of Drug A is associated with an increased risk of sudden cardiac death among people under the age of 40. It is found that "young" adults (i.e., aged 18–39) who died of sudden cardiac death (i.e., the cases) were more likely to have taken Drug A during the 24 hours preceding death compared to control subjects in the same age group who died of noncardiac causes. In this case-control study, which of the following statistics would be most appropriate to use to quantify the increased risk observed?

   A. Relative risk ratio
   B. Odds ratio
   C. Experimental event rate
   D. Control event rate

2. Imagine that a study is conducted examining the risk of falls among older adults taking psychotropic medications compared to older adults not taking such medications. It is found that, among those taking psychotropic medications, the annual incidence of falls is 25.6%, whereas among those not taking psychotropic medications, the annual incidence of falls is 23.2%. Based on these findings, what is the ARI associated with the use of psychotropic medications?

   A. 0.256
   B. 0.232
   C. 0.024
   D. 0.103
   E. 1.103

3. Based on the findings described in Question 2, what is the relative risk (RR) of falls among older adults taking psychotropic medications compared to those not taking psychotropic medications?

   A. 0.256
   B. 0.232
   C. 0.024
   D. 0.103
   E. 1.103

4. Based on the findings described in Question 2, what is the relative risk increase associated with use of psychotropic medications among older adults?

   A. 0.256
   B. 0.232
   C. 0.024
   D. 0.103
   E. 1.103

5. Based on the findings described in Question 2, the number needed to harm is:

   A. 14
   B. 42
   C. 82
   D. 232
   E. 256

6. Is the following statement true or false? If a disease is rapidly fatal, prevalence rates will tend to underestimate the true burden of the disease. (True/False)

7. Is the following statement true or false? If a disease is self-limited and usually resolves itself, with or without treatment, within 2 weeks of onset, prevalence rates will tend to underestimate the true burden of the disease. (True/False)

8. Odds ratios provide good estimates of relative risk when:

   A. The disease in question is quite common
   B. The disease in question is quite rare
   C. Odds ratios always provide good estimates of relative risk
   D. Odds ratios never provide good estimates of relative risk

9. A study of a new medication used to prevent myocardial infarctions among those at very high risk reports that the number needed to treat (NNT) is 25. How is this value interpreted?

   A. For every person treated with the new medication, 25 myocardial infarctions will be prevented.
   B. For every 25 people treated with the new medication, 1 myocardial infarction will be prevented.
   C. 25% of people who take the new medication will experience a myocardial infarction.
   D. 25% of people who do not take the new medication will experience a myocardial infarction.
   E. Use of the new medication reduces the risk of myocardial infarction by 25%.

10. Imagine that a Centers for Disease Control and Prevention (CDC) report provided data from two states, Florida and Minnesota, regarding mortality from influenza during the 2017 flu season. Some of the data are presented in Question Table 2-1. For each state, the first column shows the number of patients treated for influenza in each age category, the third column shows the number of deaths among those treated, and the last column shows the age-specific mortality rates among those treated. The crude mortality rates are 8.6 and 5.7 per 1,000 patients treated in Florida and Minnesota, respectively. If the crude rates were adjusted for age, which state would have the highest mortality rate?

    A. Florida
    B. Minnesota
    C. Neither, the adjusted rates would be the same.
    D. The rate cannot be determined from the information provided.

Use Question Table 2-1 to answer Question 10.

QUESTION TABLE 2-1. Fictitious Influenza Mortality for Two States (Original Data)

	Florida				Minnesota			
	Patients Treated		Deaths		Patients Treated		Deaths	
Age	N (in 1000s)	%	#	Rate Per 1,000	N (in 1000s)	%	#	Rate Per 1,000
0–18	6	10	24	4.0	5	25	20	4.0
19–59	6	10	12	2.0	7	35	14	2.0
60–79	48	80	480	10.0	8	40	80	10.0
Total	60	100	516	8.6	20	100	114	5.7

11. Now, imagine that CDC scientists realized that they made a mistake in the original report. The revised data are shown in Question Table 2-2. The crude mortality rates are 8.6 and 8.1 per 1,000 patients treated in Florida and Minnesota, respectively. If the crude rates were adjusted for age, which state would have the highest mortality rate?

A. Florida
B. Minnesota
C. Neither, the adjusted rates would be the same.
D. The rate cannot be determined from the information provided.

13. Based on the findings described in Question 12, what are the odds of developing Stevens-Johnson Syndrome among patients exposed to Drug A compared to those not exposed?

A. 1.0
B. 1.2
C. 1.5
D. 0.103
E. 1.103

14. Is the following statement true or false? NNT/NNH can be computed from data obtained from a case-control study. (True/False)

Use Question Table 2-2 to answer Question 11.

QUESTION TABLE 2-2. Fictitious Influenza Mortality for Two States (Revised Data)

	Florida				Minnesota			
	Patients Treated		Deaths		Patients Treated		Deaths	
Age	N (in 1000s)	%	#	Rate Per 1,000	N (in 1000s)	%	#	Rate Per 1,000
0–18	6	10	24	4.0	5	25	20	4.0
19–59	6	10	12	2.0	7	35	21	3.0
60–79	48	80	480	10.0	8	40	120	15.0
Total	60	100	516	8.6	20	100	161	8.1

12. Imagine that Drug A is suspected to cause Stevens-Johnson Syndrome. A case-control study is conducted. A total of 1,000 patients diagnosed with Stevens-Johnson Syndrome are enrolled in the study. A total of 1,000 control patients without Stevens-Johnson Syndrome are also enrolled. Among the patients with Stevens-Johnson Syndrome, 500 had taken Drug A within the past month. Among the control patients, 400 had taken Drug A within the past month. Based on these findings, what is the relative risk of developing Stevens-Johnson Syndrome among those taking Drug A compared to those not taking Drug A?

A. 1.0
B. 1.2
C. 1.5
D. Cannot determine. Case-control studies do not provide the information needed to calculate the EER and CER, which are needed to calculate RR.

STATISTICAL INFERENCE AND BETWEEN GROUP COMPARISONS

Probability and Statistical Inference

3

Probability Concepts and Basic Rules

After reading this chapter, you should be able to do the following:

1. Explain what is meant by the term "probability" and how a *P* value is interpreted.
2. Distinguish between sample statistics and population parameters.
3. Identify three probability distributions and the factors that determine which distribution to use within a particular analytic context.
4. Explain the difference between the standard deviation of a variable and the standard error of the mean.
5. Explain how the t- and z-distributions differ.
6. Describe the null hypothesis and the relationships between the null hypothesis, Type I (alpha) errors, Type II (beta) errors, and power.
7. Identify acceptable levels for Type I errors, Type II errors, and power.
8. Explain how sample size influences Type I and Type II errors.
9. Distinguish between statistical and clinical significance.

At a conceptual level, probability can be defined as the likelihood that a certain event (i.e., outcome) will occur relative to some other event. In medicine, probabilities are often determined empirically. For example, one might observe a group of patients diagnosed with a certain type of cancer and record the number of people who (1) died within 5 years of diagnosis and (2) survived at least 5 years following diagnosis. Here, there are only two possible events, surviving the time span indicated or not surviving. The probability of survival could then be calculated as:

$$P(Survival) = \frac{\#\ of\ Patients\ Who\ Survived}{Total\ Number\ of\ Patients\ Observed}$$

Probabilities have a possible range from 0 to 1. The lower the probability of a particular event, the less likely it is to occur. The sum of the probability of all possible events must equal 1.0. For example, if the probability of surviving is 0.70, the probability of dying must be 0.30.

The left side of Table 3-1 is called a contingency table. It presents information from a fictitious study of 1,000 cancer patients followed for 5 years postdiagnosis. Two "events" were assessed: the stage of cancer at diagnosis and survival status 5 years after diagnosis. From the table, you can see that 300 patients died within 5 years of diagnosis and that 700 patients survived at least 5 years following diagnosis. You can also see that 400 patients were in Stage I at diagnosis, 300 were in Stage II, 200 were in Stage III, and 100 were in Stage IV. You can convert the frequencies shown in the table on the left (in Table 3-1) into probabilities by dividing the number in each cell by the total sample size (i.e., 1,000). When you do this, you get the right-hand side of Table 3-1. There are a total of eight possible "outcomes" (e.g., being in Stage I and dying, being in Stage II and dying, etc.). The sum of these eight outcomes is 1.0, as it must be!

TABLE 3-1. Contingency Table

Frequency Table				Probability Table			
Stage	Die	Survive	Total	Stage	Die	Survive	Total
Stage I	80	320	400	Stage I	0.08	0.320	0.40
Stage II	75	225	300	Stage II	0.075	0.225	0.30
Stage III	80	120	200	Stage III	0.080	0.120	0.20
Stage IV	65	35	100	Stage IV	0.065	0.035	0.10
Total	300	700	1,000	Total	0.30	0.70	1.0

As highlighted in Table 3-2, there are two types of probabilities shown in the table, joint probabilities and marginal probabilities. Joint probabilities indicate the probability that two events will occur together. The joint probabilities are shown in the cells in the body of the table. For example, the probability of being in Stage II **and** dying is 0.075. Marginal probabilities are shown in the row and column labeled "Total." They indicate the probability that one of the events shown in the table will occur. (In this context, "Stage" and "Die"/"Survive" are called events.) As shown in the table, the probability of being in Stage I was 0.40; the probability of surviving was 0.70.

Multiplication Rule for Independent Events. Many statistical procedures deal with determining whether events are independent of one another. Events are independent if the occurrence of one event has no effect on the occurrence of the other event. That is, the events are unrelated (i.e., uncorrelated). In medicine, we often want to know if the probability of a patient's condition improving depends on the type of treatment we provide. As clinicians, we hope that illness outcomes are **not** independent of treatment. Rather, we hope that we can improve patients' chances of getting better, or getting better more quickly, by providing the most appropriate treatments available. So, the question becomes: "How can we tell if illness outcomes depend on (as opposed to being independent of) the type of treatment received?"

At the simplest level, a basic rule of probability helps us answer that question. This is the Multiplication Rule for Independent Events. If you have taken an introductory statistics course, you have probably heard of this rule. It states:

> If Outcome A and Outcome B are independent, the probability that they will occur together (i.e., their joint probability) will equal the product of their individual probabilities (i.e., their marginal probabilities).

TABLE 3-2. Joint Probabilities and Marginal Probabilities

	Probability Table				
	Stage	Die	Survive	Total	
Joint Probabilities	Stage I	0.08	0.320	0.40	Marginal Probabilities
	Stage II	0.075	0.225	0.30	
	Stage III	0.080	0.120	0.20	
	Stage IV	0.065	0.035	0.10	
	Total	0.30	0.70	1.0	

TABLE 3-3. Frequency Tables From Two Fictitious Studies

Study 1				Study 2			
	Frequencies				Frequencies		
Medication	Die	Survive	Total	Medication	Die	Survive	Total
A	125	125	250	A	125	125	250
B	125	125	250	B	125	125	250
C	125	125	250	M	50	200	250
D	125	125	250	N	200	50	250
Total	500	500	1,000	Total	500	500	1,000

Thus, if two events are independent:

$$P(Outcome\ A\ and\ Outcome\ B) = P(Outcome\ A) * P(Outcome\ B)$$

Table 3-3 presents data from two fictitious studies. In Study 1, patients were randomly assigned to receive one of four experimental medications: Medication A, Medication B, Medication C, or Medication D. In Study 2, patients were randomly assigned to receive either Medication A or Medication B or one of two other experimental medications (i.e., Medication M, Medication N). In both studies, an equal number of patients received each experimental medication, and 50% of the patients in the study died.

To determine if survival was independent of treatment, the frequencies shown in Table 3-3 can be converted into **joint probabilities** by dividing the number in each cell by the total sample size (i.e., 1,000), as shown in Table 3-4.

If the probability of surviving is independent of treatment, the product of the marginal probabilities for each cell will equal the joint probabilities shown in Table 3.4. For example, in the cell in Study 1 that corresponds to Medication A **and** Die, the marginal probability of receiving Medication A is 0.25 and the marginal probability of dying is 0.5. Thus, the expected probability of receiving Medication A and dying is $0.5 * 0.25 = 0.125$, which equals the joint probability shown in the table. If you do this for each cell in Study 1, you will see that the product of the marginals is equal to the joint probability shown in the table for all eight cells. This confirms that survival is independent of treatment in Study 1.

TABLE 3-4. Joint Probabilities

Study 1				Study 2			
	Probabilities				Probabilities		
Medication	Die	Survive	Total	Medication	Die	Survive	Total
A	0.125	0.125	0.25	A	0.125	0.125	0.25
B	0.125	0.125	0.25	B	0.125	0.125	0.25
C	0.125	0.125	0.25	M	0.05	0.20	0.25
D	0.125	0.125	0.25	N	0.20	0.05	0.25
Total	0.50	0.50	1.00	Total	0.50	0.50	1.00

The story is different in Study 2. In this study, the product of the marginals for receiving Medication M and dying is $0.5 * 0.25 = 0.125$. This is more than twice as high as the joint probability observed in the study (i.e., 0.05). Thus, in Study 2, one would conclude that survival rate is *not* independent of treatment. (Note: One concludes that the events are not independent if *any* of the cells differ from the product of the marginals.)

Conditional Probabilities. When two events are not independent, you can determine their conditional probabilities (i.e., the probability of one event occurring given that another event has already occurred). Conditional probabilities can be denoted as P(Y I X), which is read as the probability of Event Y given Event X. For example, one might ask: What is the probability of surviving given that a person receives Medication M? Conditional probabilities are calculated by computing the probabilities within each level of X. For example, using the data in Table 3-4 for Study 2, you can compute the probability of dying given that a person receives Medication M as: $P(\text{Die I Medication M}) = \frac{0.05}{0.25} = 0.2$. In contrast, the probability of dying for a person who receives Medication A in Study 2 is $P(\text{Die I Medication A}) = \frac{0.125}{0.25} = 0.5$. The difference between these two conditional probabilities is consistent with our previous conclusion. In Study 2, survival rate is **not** independent of treatment.

Addition Rule for Mutually Exclusive Events. Two or more events are mutually exclusive if they cannot occur at the same time (e.g., a person cannot both survive and die during a 1-year follow-up period). The addition rule for mutually exclusive events states that if Outcome A and Outcome B are mutually exclusive, the probability of observing either Outcome A or Outcome B is the sum of their individual probabilities. Thus,

$$P(\textit{Outcome A or Outcome B}) = P(A) + P(B)$$

Use caution in applying this rule. Not all events are mutually exclusive. For example, in a study, it is possible for some participants to have both diabetes and hypertension. Therefore, if you simply add the probability of having diabetes and the probability of having hypertension, you will overestimate the probability of having one or the other. For example, imagine that in a sample of 100 adults, 20 people have diabetes, 50 people have hypertension, and 40 people have neither. If you add the probability of having diabetes (0.20) and the probability of having hypertension (0.50) and the probability of having neither (0.40), you will see that it adds up to 1.1. Something has to be wrong. The events (i.e., having diabetes and having hypertension) must not be mutually exclusive because the sum of their individual probabilities does not equal 1.0. The answer must be that 10 people have both diabetes and hypertension. Thus, they are double counted. There are formulas for calculating probabilities associated with events that are not mutually exclusive, but it is usually sufficient to just think the problem through at an intuitive level. When you are reading the literature, be careful not to start adding probabilities without assuring yourself that the events are mutually exclusive.

Population Parameters and Sample Statistics

Once we go beyond simply using statistics to describe the characteristics of study participants, we enter the realm of inferential statistics. Inferential statistics involve using data from a sample to make inferences about a population. The remaining chapters in this book focus on different types of inferential statistical procedures.

Populations Versus Samples. To be able to interpret the results of inferential statistical procedures, you must understand the difference between a population and a sample (Figure 3-1).

1. **Sample.** In research, investigators collect data from a subset of the population of interest. For example, if an investigator wants to know if a certain medication is helpful in controlling

FIGURE 3-1. **Statistical Inference**

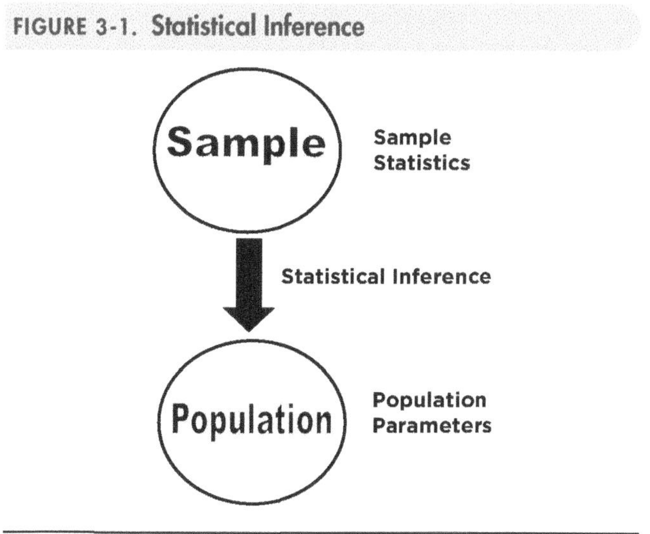

hypertension, she does not try to enroll every person in the world with hypertension in a study. That would be impossible and, even if it were possible, it would be incredibly expensive. Instead, she assembles a sample of people with hypertension.

2. **Population.** The population of interest in a study is comprised of those people to whom the investigators wish to generalize their findings. For example, if an investigator wanted to generalize her findings to all people with mild hypertension in the United States, she would need to assemble her sample in such a way that it is representative of that population. Obviously, she would not be able to generalize her findings to this population if her sample was limited to people with severe hypertension. A major issue that you will deal with as a clinician involves the population to which the results from a study may be generalized. More specifically, you will always want to know if they can be generalized to the patients you treat!

Population Parameters Versus Sample Statistics. As depicted in Figure 3-2, **sample statistics** such as the mean, standard deviation (SD), and percentages are calculated from the data collected in a study.

FIGURE 3-2. **Sample Statistics Versus Population Parameters**

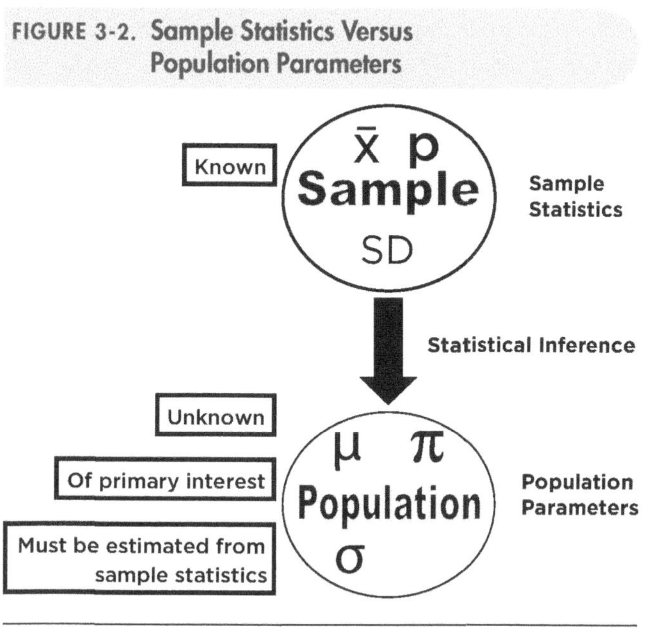

Thus, once data collection has been completed, all of the sample statistics are known (or can be computed from the data available). The sad thing is that, to a large extent, we are not interested in them. Our primary interest involves the population of interest. Don't get me wrong. It is great if the people who participate in studies benefit from the experimental treatments to which they are exposed. However, as clinicians, we really want to know if our patients will benefit from those treatments once they are marketed. Sample statistics only provide a vehicle for **estimating** the probability of treatment benefit (or harm) in the population of interest. This is one of the most important things for you to remember from this book!

Population parameters are values that correspond to sample statistics within the population as a whole. For example, μ is the population mean. It corresponds to the sample mean, $\bar{X}$. Unlike sample statistics, population parameters cannot be calculated. That would only be possible if data were collected from the entire population of interest. Thus, we are left being primarily interested in parameters that we cannot calculate. Our only option is to try to estimate these parameters from the sample statistics that are available. This estimation of population parameters from sample statistics is at the heart of statistical inference.

Theoretical Probability Distributions

Theoretical probability distributions are used to describe the distribution of a variable within a population of interest. Many of the statistical procedures used in the medical literature are based on three of these theoretical probability distributions: the binomial distribution, the Poisson distribution, and the Normal distribution. As described next, these three distributions make different assumptions about how the variable is distributed within the population.

1. **Binomial Distribution.** The binomial distribution is a discrete probability distribution dealing with dichotomous variables. It allows one to compute the probability of observing "X" specific outcomes in N trials assuming that the probability of the outcome in the population is π and that the outcome of each trial is independent of all other trials. The formula for computing these probabilities is $\frac{n!}{x!(n-x)!}\left[\pi^{x}(1-\pi)^{n-x}\right]$. As a simple example, imagine that one tossed a coin in the air 10 times and observed whether it showed a "head" or a "tail" when it landed. Here, n = 10 (the number of trials) and $\pi = 0.50$ because we know that (assuming a fair coin) the probability of observing a "head" is 0.50, as is the probability of observing a "tail." Using the formula above, it is possible to create a figure like Figure 3-3 that shows the probability of observing 0 heads in 10 tosses, 1 head in 10 tosses, 2 heads in 10 tosses, etc. From Figure 3-3, you can see that the probability

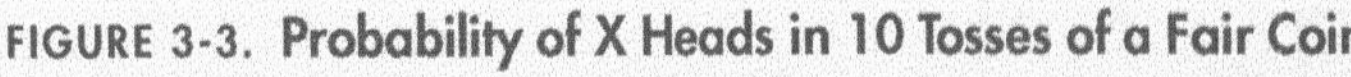

FIGURE 3-3. Probability of X Heads in 10 Tosses of a Fair Coin

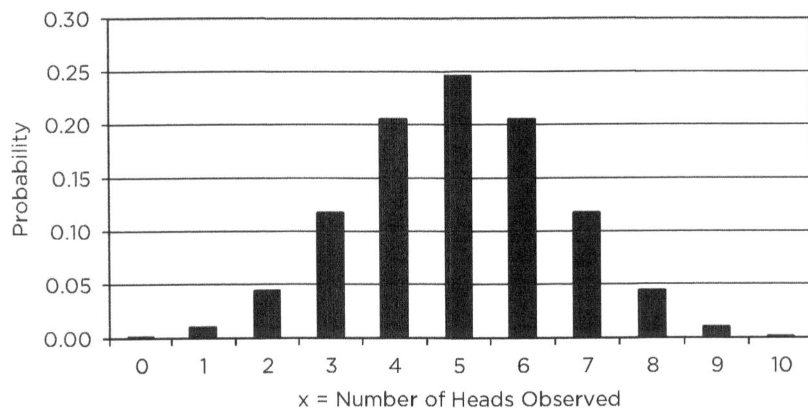

of observing exactly 5 heads in 10 tosses is only about 25%. There is about a 20% chance of observing 4 heads and about a 20% chance of observing 6 heads despite the fact that we know the true population proportion is $\pi = 0.50$. There is even a small possibility of observing no heads.

Health care providers usually do not care that much about the chances of different outcomes occurring when flipping a coin. However, the binomial formula can also help us solve more relevant problems like the following:

> Imagine that, without treatment, an illness kills 99% of those affected. An experimental treatment is tested on two patients. They both survive. What is the probability that both patients would have survived **if the treatment had no effect on the course of the illness?**

In this example, if the treatment has no effect on the course of the disease, the probability of survival (π) is 0.01 (i.e., 1.0–0.99). From the problem statement, we know that n = 2 because two patients were studied. We also know that x = 2 because two patients experienced the outcome of interest (survival in this case). When we plug these values into the binomial formula, we get: $\frac{2!}{2!(2-2)!}\left[.01^2(1-.01)^{2-2}\right] = .0001$. This value is the probability that both patients would have survived **if the treatment had no effect on the course of the illness**. Thus, *P* = 0.0001. Because this *P* value is so small, it suggests that both patients very likely would not have survived if the treatment had no effect on the course of the illness. However, from the problem statement, we know that both patients did survive. Therefore, it appears that the medication did have an effect on the course of the disease, improving the probability of surviving. (Note: In essence, we are rejecting the null hypothesis that the medication had no effect on the course of the disease. Hypothesis testing will be discussed in more detail later in this chapter.)

The shape of a binomial distribution is defined by two parameters, n and π. The mean of this theoretical probability distribution can be calculated by multiplying these two parameters such that: Mean = n(π). Thus, in the example where we flipped a fair coin 10 times, the mean of the distribution was: $n(\pi) = 10(0.5) = 5$. Looking at Figure 3-3, you can confirm that the distribution is centered on 5. The spread of the distribution around the mean (i.e., the SD of the mean) is also defined by n and π. It is calculated using the formula: $\sqrt{n\pi(1-\pi)}$. Thus, the SD of the mean, assuming n = 10 and $\pi = 0.50$, is 1.58.

As n increases, the binomial distribution is approximated by the normal distribution (discussed below), and the normal distribution can be used to calculate probabilities. As a general rule of thumb, when n is 30 or more, probabilities derived from the normal distribution will be very similar to those derived from the binomial formula. The charts in Figure 3-4 show how the shape of the binomial distribution changes as a function of π and n. Note that when π is 0.5, the shape of the binomial distribution is reasonably symmetrical and resembles the bell-shaped curve characteristic of the Normal distribution even for the smallest sample size shown (n = 10). As π moves away from 0.5, the shape of the distribution becomes more asymmetrical when n = 10. However, with the larger sample sizes shown, the shape of the distributions are reasonably symmetrical and resemble the normal distribution regardless of π, allowing probabilities associated with the normal distribution to be used to estimate probabilities derived from the binomial formula.

2. **Poisson Distribution.** The Poisson distribution is a discrete probability distribution, like the binomial distribution. However, it describes the probability of events that can occur multiple times to a single individual (e.g., being hospitalized). These are called "count" data. For example, the Poisson distribution might be used to assess the probability of a person being hospitalized a certain number of times given the number of expected hospitalizations per patient. The Poisson distribution is usually used within the context of events that are fairly rare. That is, the majority of individuals never experience the event, and only a few people experience the event more than

FIGURE 3-4. Shape of Binomial Distribution as a Function of π and n

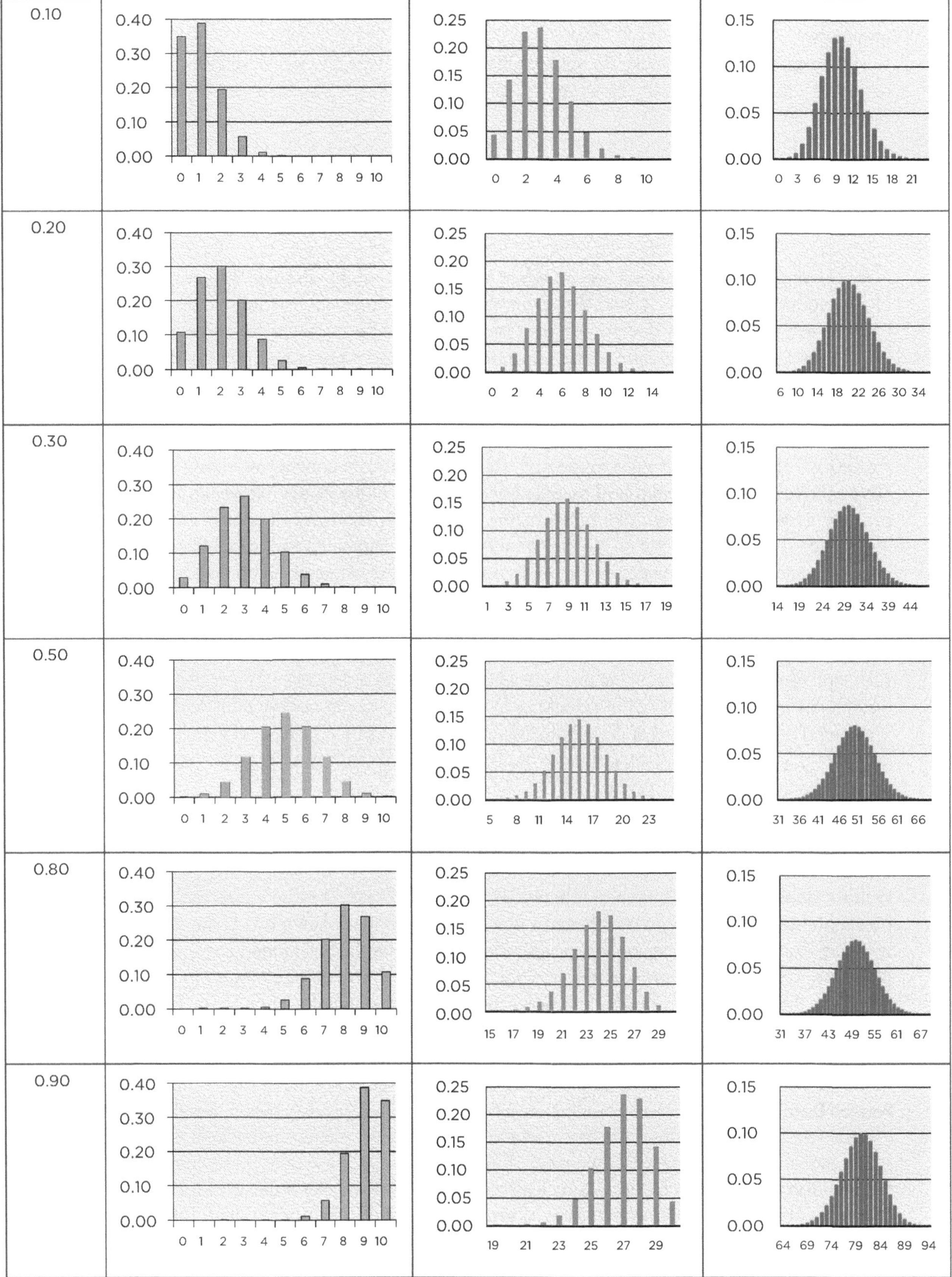

once within the time frame of interest. However, a few people may experience the event many times. Thus, the number of possible occurrences per person can range from 0 to infinity. For common events, the Poisson distribution is approximated by the Normal distribution and probabilities derived from the Normal distribution are used to approximate those that can be derived from the Poisson.

The formula for calculating probability using the Poisson distribution is $P(x) = \frac{\lambda^x e^{-\lambda}}{x!}$, where x is the number of events a specific individual experiences, λ is the mean number of events experienced, and *e* is the base of the natural logarithm (i.e., 2.718). (Note: In the Poisson distribution the SD of the variable is equal to the mean. Thus, only one parameter [i.e., λ] is needed to define a Poisson distribution.)

Imagine that a group of investigators would like to determine if the number of vertebral fractures experienced over a 10-year period is greater among women with osteoporosis taking a bisphosphonate compared with women with osteoporosis not taking a bisphosphonate. Also assume that from past studies, it is estimated that women with osteoporosis who are not taking a bisphosphonate experience an average of 4.2 vertebral fractures over a 10-year period. With this information, one can use the Poisson formula to calculate the probability that a woman with osteoporosis and **not** taking a bisphosphonate would experience a specific number of vertebral fractures over a 10-year period. Figure 3-5 presents the probability of a woman experiencing anywhere between 0 and 10 fractures during the 10-year time span. By comparing these probabilities to those observed in a sample of women with osteoporosis using a bisphosphonate, the investigators could calculate the probability that the distributions are the same (i.e., that bisphosphonate use does not affect the number of vertebral fractures experienced).

3. **Normal Distribution.** The normal distribution was introduced in Chapter 1. Therefore, only a few key characteristics of this distribution are reviewed here. Briefly, the normal distribution is a continuous probability distribution. The shape of this distribution is defined by two parameters: the population mean (μ) and the population SD (σ). The mean can have any value, and the SD can have any positive value. To facilitate the computation of probabilities, the normal distribution is usually converted to a standard normal distribution by performing a z transformation. The formula for performing a z transformation is $z = \frac{(x - \mu)}{\sigma}$. By definition, the mean of a standard normal distribution is 0 and the SD is 1.0.

The standard normal distribution is shown in Figure 3-6. Note that the figure is a solid color because it is used for continuous variables, where any value is possible. Note also that the mean is 0. The distribution is symmetrical and bell shaped. Approximately 2.5% of observations in the population have values less than 2 SDs below the mean, and 2.5% of the observations in the population have values greater than 2 SDs above the mean. The standard normal distribution

FIGURE 3-5. Poisson Distribution

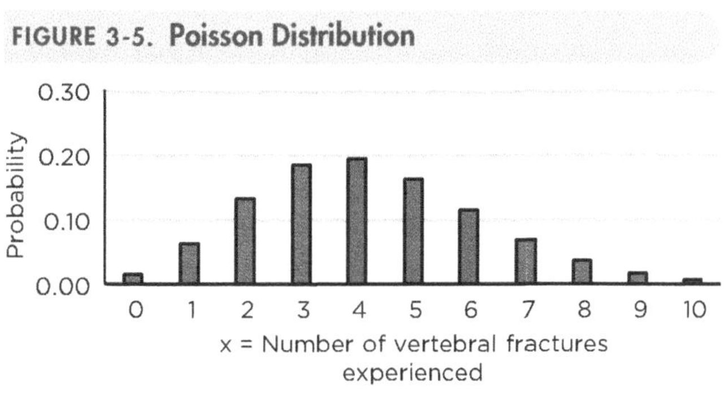

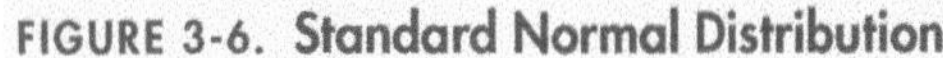

FIGURE 3-6. Standard Normal Distribution

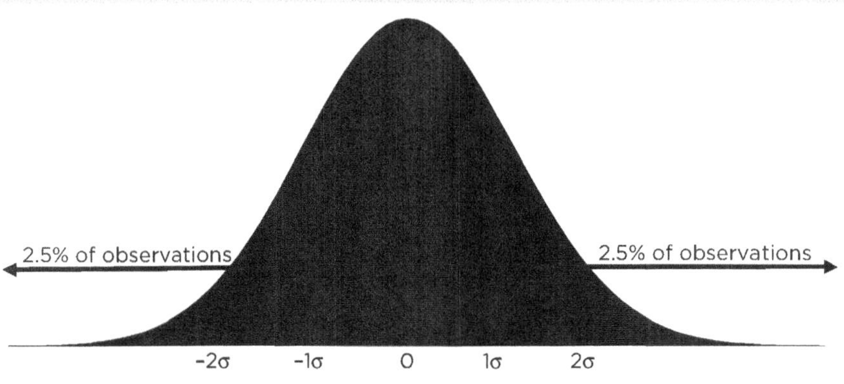

is used to calculate confidence intervals (CIs) and perform statistical tests involving continuous variables. Therefore, we will return to this distribution later in this chapter when we discuss those topics.

Sampling Distributions

The three probability distributions reviewed previously describe the theoretical distribution of variables (and, thus, observations) within a random sample. In contrast, sampling distributions describe how sample statistics (e.g., sample means, sample SDs) would be expected to vary **if multiple samples were available**. The essential idea is that, if you were to select multiple random samples from the same population and use each sample to estimate a population parameter, such as the population mean, you would get a slightly different answer each time, just because of sampling variability. For example, imagine that you wanted to estimate the average height of men in a population. Just by the luck of the draw, your first random sample might include a lot of relatively short men. If you were to draw a second random sample, it might include a lot of relatively tall men. Thus, the two sample means would differ. This is what we mean when we talk about "sampling variability."

Continuing with this example, remember that we are most interested in what the mean is in the population from which the two samples were drawn. (The purpose of collecting data from a sample and calculating the sample mean is to **estimate** the population mean.) However, if we were to draw two separate samples and get different sample means, we would have two different estimates of the population mean. Further, there would be no way that we could determine which sample mean provided the **best estimate** of the population mean without collecting data from the entire population, which we know is impossible. However, by understanding how sample statistics would vary, if multiple samples were available, we can develop estimates of population parameters that incorporate the uncertainty introduced by sampling variability.

With respect to the population mean, it can be shown that **if you were to draw an infinite number of samples of the same size from the same population:**

1. The mean of the sample means will equal the true population mean. Thus, the true population mean would be at the center of the sampling distribution.
2. The standard error (SE) of the mean will equal $\frac{\sigma}{\sqrt{n}}$, which is the SD of the sample means.
3. The sample means will be normally distributed as long as the sample size is reasonably large (e.g., 30 or more). Thus, based on probabilities associated with the normal distribution, 95% of the sample means will be within 2 SEs of the population mean.

These properties of the sampling distribution for the mean provide a solution for the problem described previously wherein each possible sample yields a slightly different estimate of the population mean. This solution involves the establishment of CIs around the estimate. In most studies, you only have one sample. For any numerical variable assessed in the study, the best estimate of the population mean (μ) is the sample mean ($\bar{X}$). The sample mean is called a "point estimate of the population mean." It is possible that the population mean is identical to the sample mean. But, that is unlikely. Fortunately, properties of the sampling distribution for the mean reviewed previously allow us to establish a CI around $\bar{X}$. Based on the probabilities associated with the normal distribution, if $n \geq 30$, the sample mean will be within 2 SEs of the true population mean 95% of the time. That is, if you collected data from all possible samples of sample size "n" in a given population, 95% of the sample means would be within 2 SEs of the true population mean.

These concepts can be translated into a formula to calculate CIs for the point estimate of the population mean. The formula for a 95% CI, assuming $n \geq 30$, is $\mu = \bar{X} \pm 2(SE)$.

For example, imagine that a study is conducted in which hip bone density is measured in 49 women. The mean bone density ($\bar{X}$) in the sample is 0.94 g/cm^2 with an SD of 0.15 g/cm^2. Based on these data, the best estimate of the population mean is 0.94 g/cm^2. However, it is unlikely that the population mean is exactly 0.94 g/cm^2. Therefore, investigators usually calculate CIs that they are pretty sure capture the true population mean. Often, they compute 95% CIs. This allows them to state with 95% confidence that the true population mean lies within the CI. Table 3-5 shows the calculations necessary to compute a 95% CI and uses the information in the example provided above to establish a 95% CI around the point estimate of 0.94 g/cm^2.

Given the CI calculated in Table 3-5, one can be 95% confident that the true population mean (μ) is somewhere between 0.90 and 0.98 g/cm^2. Further, you will be correct 95% of the time (i.e., the true population mean will be within that interval). But, the other 5% of the time, you will be wrong (i.e., the true population mean will be outside of the 95% CI). This highlights a key issue when performing statistical analyses. One can never be absolutely certain that one has drawn the correct conclusions. One can only reduce the probability of making errors. We will come back to this issue periodically throughout the remainder of this book.

SD Versus SE of the Mean. Two sample statistics are often confused, the SD and the SE. However, these 2 statistics are distinct and are used for different purposes.

1. **SD of a Variable.** The SD of a variable captures the amount of variation that exists among observations in a sample. The greater the variation among study participants, the greater the SD will be. The SD is used primarily when an investigator wants to describe study participants. It can also be used to determine where individual study participants fall in the distribution of observations (e.g., whether an individual is tall or short relative to other study participants). Thus, the SD is used primarily within the realm of descriptive statistics.
2. **SE of the Mean.** The SE of the mean indexes the amount of error associated with estimating a population mean from a sample mean (i.e., error due to sampling variability). The SE is used when making inferences concerning the population mean based on data collected from a sample. Investigators use the SE when they calculate CIs and perform statistical tests. Thus, the SE is used primarily within the realm of inferential statistics, the focus of this chapter.

TABLE 3-5. Calculation of Confidence Interval

Step	Calculations Required	Solved for Data in Example
1.	$SE = \frac{SD}{\sqrt{n}}$	$SE = \frac{0.15}{\sqrt{49}} = 0.02$
2.	$95\%\ CI = \bar{X} \pm 2SE$	$0.94 \pm 2(0.02) =$ 0.90 *to* 0.98 *g/cm*^{2}

Making Inferences Concerning the Population Mean

In medicine, investigators sometimes want to know if the mean in a specific population of interest is equal to some more general population mean. For example, an investigator might want to know if the mean bone density of women who are on long-term, low-dose oral prednisone therapy (the specific population of interest in this example) is the same as the mean bone density among women in the general public (the more general population in this example). Two approaches may be used to address this type of question: calculation of CIs and hypothesis testing. Each approach is reviewed below.

Calculation of CIs. CIs were introduced previously. Now, we will use them to answer the following research question.

Research Question: Is the bone density of women between the ages of 20 and 29 who are on long-term, low-dose oral prednisone therapy the same as the mean bone density of women in this age group in the general public?

Note that the population of interest in this research question is women between the ages of 20 and 29 who are on long-term, low-dose oral prednisone therapy. It would be impossible to measure the bone density of everyone in this population. Therefore, to answer the question, imagine that an investigator performs bone density exams on a sample of 49 women drawn from this population (i.e., women between the ages of 20 and 29 who are on long-term, low-dose oral prednisone therapy). Also imagine that the investigator knows from past studies that the mean bone density among women in this age group in the general public, most of whom do *not* use prednisone, is 0.99 g/cm^2. This is the established population norm for women in the general public.

The investigator finds that the mean bone density in the sample of 49 women using long-term, low-dose oral prednisone is 0.95 g/cm^2 (SD = 0.12). This information can be used to calculate the 95% CI for the sample mean as shown in Table 3-6.

The investigator can conclude from the CI that there is a 95% chance that the mean bone density for the population of women between the ages of 20 and 29 who are on long-term, low-dose oral prednisone therapy is somewhere between 0.92 and 0.98 g/cm^2. Further, because the value of 0.99 g/cm^2, which is the mean bone density among women aged 20 to 29 in the general public, does **not** lie within the CI, the investigator can also conclude with 95% confidence that the mean bone density of women aged 20 to 29 who are on long-term, low-dose oral prednisone therapy is **not the same** as similarly aged women in the general public.

Note that the conclusions reached previously do not mention the 49 women in the study. As stated previously, we are not primarily interested in the bone density of the 49 women in the sample. We are interested in the mean bone density in the population from which they were drawn (i.e., women aged 20 to 29 who are on long-term, low-dose oral prednisone therapy). The sample mean is simply an estimate of the mean bone density in that population. The 95% CI identifies the range of plausible values for the population mean and allows investigators to conclude with 95% confidence that the population mean does not lie outside of that range.

TABLE 3-6. Calculation of Confidence Interval (SD = 0.12)

$$95\%\ \text{CI: } 0.95 \pm 2.0\left(\frac{0.12}{\sqrt{49}}\right)$$

$$95\%\ \text{CI: } 0.95 \pm 0.03$$

$$95\%\ \text{CI: } 0.92 \text{ to } 0.98$$

CI, confidence interval.

TABLE 3-7. Calculation of Confidence Interval (SD = 0.21)

$$95\%\ \text{CI: } 0.95 \pm 2.0\left(\frac{0.21}{\sqrt{49}}\right)$$

95% CI: 0.95 ± 0.06

95% CI: 0.89 to 1.01

CI, confidence interval.

To give another example, we will change the data from the previous example just a little. Imagine that the investigator collected data from a different sample of 49 women using long-term, low-dose oral prednisone. This time the sample mean and SD were 0.95 g/cm^2 (SD = 0.21). Note that only the SD has changed. This information is again used to calculate the 95% CI for the sample mean as shown in Table 3-7.

Note that the increase in the SD from the first example has the effect of increasing the SE and widening the CI. Given these data, the investigator would conclude from the CI that there is a 95% chance that the mean bone density for the population of women between the ages of 20 and 29 who are on long-term, low-dose oral prednisone therapy is somewhere between 0.89 and 1.01 g/cm^2. Further, because the value of 0.99 g/cm^2, which is the mean bone density among women aged 20 to 29 in the general public, lies within the CI, the investigator would also conclude that the mean bone density of women aged 20 to 29 who are on long-term, low-dose oral prednisone therapy **may be the same** as similarly aged women in the general public. In other words, there is insufficient evidence to conclude that the mean bone density of women in this age range taking long-term, low-dose oral prednisone differs from the general public.

Note that, in this second example, we are not saying that we are 95% confident that the means are the same. We are simply saying that there is insufficient evidence to conclude that they differ. This conclusion is similar to one that might be reached when serving on a jury. A jury might find a person "not guilty" not because they are convinced of the person's innocence but only because there is insufficient evidence to find the person guilty. This issue will be discussed again later in this chapter within the context of hypothesis testing.

Thus far, only the 95% CI has been introduced. However, probabilities associated with the Standard Normal distribution allow one to calculate CIs for any level of confidence an investigator desires. In the medical literature, the 95% CI is used most often. However, you will also see 90% and 99% CIs used.

The general formula for a CI for a sample mean is $\bar{X} \pm CV(SE)$. In this formula, CV stands for "critical value." The CV is determined by the level of confidence you want and the sample size. The precise values are based on probabilities associated with the Standard Normal distribution. For example, as shown in the figure to the left in Figure 3-7, assuming that the sample size is 30 or more, the CV for a 90% CI

FIGURE 3-7. Critical Values for Standard Normal Distribution

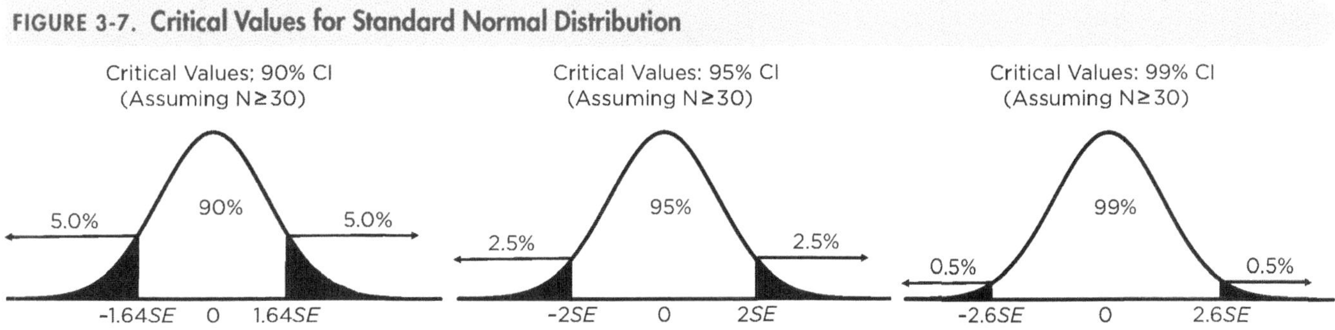

CI, confidence interval; SE, standard error.

is 1.64. Thus, the true population mean will lie within 1.64 SEs of the sample mean 90% of the time. Under the same assumptions, the CV for a 95% CI is 1.96 (always rounded to 2.0 in this book) and the CV for a 99% CI is 2.6.

Notice that as the level of desired confidence increases from 90% to 95% to 99%, the CV increases. This increases the width of the CI. Thus, the more confident investigators want to be that they have captured the true population mean within the CI, the wider they must make the CI.

Width of CIs. In general, investigators would like CIs to be narrow. The narrower the CI, the more precise the estimate of the population mean. As just stated, increasing the desired level of confidence increases the width of the CI. The width of the CI is also affected by the SE of the mean. Remember that the formula used to compute CIs is $\overline{X} \pm CV(SE)$. From this formula, you can see that as the SE of the mean increases, the width of the CI increases as well.

Going a step further, the formula used to compute the SE is $\frac{SD}{\sqrt{n}}$. From this formula, you can see that SE becomes larger (and CIs become wider and less precise) as the SD increases. In contrast, the SE becomes smaller (and CIs become narrower and more precise) as sample size (n) increases.

When designing a study, investigators may use inclusion and exclusion criteria to achieve a relatively homogeneous sample. One consequence of these procedures is to minimize variability among study participants and, thus, the SD of observed variables. In addition, investigators will usually attempt to enroll a sufficient number of study participants so that CIs reach a desired level of precision.

The T-Distribution. Before turning to hypothesis testing, I need to introduce another distribution, the t-distribution. You probably noticed that when discussing the CVs used to compute CIs, I kept repeating that you had to assume that the sample size was 30 or more. This is because, for simplicity, I wanted to use probabilities associated with the z-distribution. With smaller sample sizes, life is a bit more complex.

As long as $n \geq 30$, the sampling distribution of the mean approximates the Standard Normal (z) distribution. However, as sample size decreases, the sampling distribution becomes flatter and the tails get "heavier" (i.e., they contain more area). This new distribution is called a t-distribution. This is shown graphically in Figure 3-8.

As a consequence of this flattening of the distribution, the CVs associated with any CI become larger. The end result of this increase in the CVs is that CIs become wider (and, thus, less precise). Table 3-8 presents CVs for the t-distribution given different sample sizes.

Hypothesis Testing. Hypothesis testing is the second approach that can be used to determine if the mean in a specific population of interest is equal to some more general population mean. In this section, I first review the steps involved in hypothesis testing. I then work through the bone density example introduced

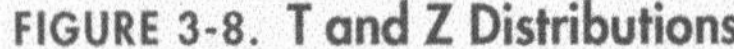
FIGURE 3-8. T and Z Distributions

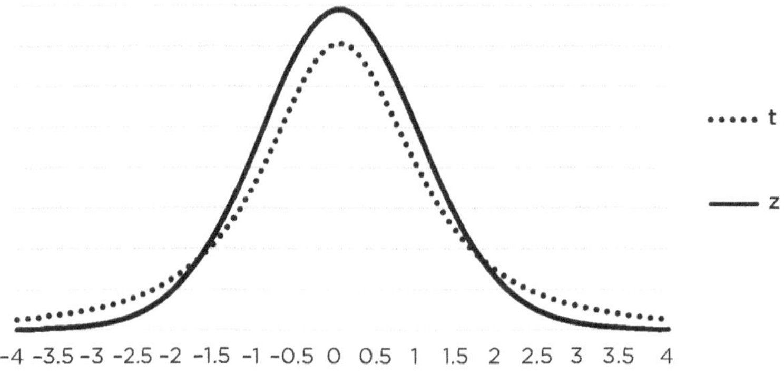

TABLE 3-8. Critical Values for Calculation of Confidence Intervals

Distribution (df)	90% CI	95% CI	99% CI
Z (standard normal)	1.64	1.96	2.576
t (30)	1.70	2.04	2.75
t (20)	1.73	2.09	2.85
t (10)	1.81	2.23	3.17
t (5)	2.02	2.57	4.03

Note: In the context of the t-distribution, the term "df" is equal to the sample size minus the number of means being estimated. One mean is estimated when computing a CI and when performing 1-sample t-tests and paired t-tests. Two means are estimated when performing independent groups t-tests.
CI, confidence interval; df, degrees of freedom.

previously, this time by testing the null hypothesis that the mean bone density of women who are on long-term, low-dose oral prednisone therapy is the same as the mean bone density of women in the general public.

Steps in Hypothesis Testing. Hypothesis testing involves five steps.

1. **Specify the Null and Alternative Hypotheses.** Under the null hypothesis (H_0), the population means are assumed to be equal. Under the alternative hypothesis (H_A), the population means are assumed to differ. Alternative hypotheses can either be 1-tailed or 2-tailed. Two-tailed alternative hypotheses, like the one shown below, simply assume that the means are not the same, whereas 1-tailed alternative hypotheses specify the assumed direction of the difference. For example, a 1-tailed alternative hypothesis might state that the mean in the general population is greater than the mean in the population interest.

$$H_0: \mu_{GeneralPopulation} = \mu_{PopulationOfInterest}$$

$$H_A: \mu_{GeneralPopulation} \neq \mu_{PopulationOfInterest}$$

2. **Determine the Appropriate Test Statistic.** Because the hypotheses stated previously require collecting data from only 1 sample (we are assuming that the mean in the general population is known) and because we are interested in differences in means, a 1-sample t-test is the appropriate test statistic, assuming that n ≥ 30.

   The formula for a 1-sample t-test is $t = \frac{\bar{X} - \mu_{GP}}{SE_{\bar{X}}}$. In this formula, "t" is the test statistic, $\bar{X}$ is the sample mean, μ_{GP} is the mean in the general population, and $SE_{\bar{X}}$ is the sample SE.

   Under the null hypothesis, the numerator in this formula is expected to be "0." Thus, one can say that "0" is the expected value of "t" under the null hypothesis. If the null hypothesis is true, you expect the numerator in this formula to be close to "0."

   Note that, if the sample mean ($\bar{X}$) is identical to the general population mean (μ_{GP}), the value of the test statistic (t) will be "0." As the difference between the sample mean and the general population mean increases, the t-statistic becomes larger. Dividing the observed difference by the SE of the mean ($SE_{\bar{X}}$) has the effect of converting the observed difference into SE units. Thus, if t = 1.5, the observed difference is 1.5 SEs away from "0" (the expected value under the null hypothesis). The advantage of converting the difference in means into SE units is that they then can be related to the probability values (i.e., *P* values) associated with the t-distribution.

The *P* values reflect the probability that the observed difference or any difference more extreme (larger) would have occurred if the population means were the same. Put another way, the *P* values reflect the probability that the observed differences would have occurred **if** the null hypothesis was true.

3. **Set Alpha.** The value at which alpha is set determines the likelihood that the null hypothesis will be rejected when it is actually true (i.e., the likelihood of concluding that the mean in the population of interest differs from the general population mean when it actually does **not** differ). If an investigator sets alpha at 0.05, it means that he is willing to accept a 5% chance of incorrectly concluding that a difference in population means exists when, in reality, the population means are the same. This is called an alpha or Type I error. (Note: Performing a 2-tailed hypothesis test with alpha set at 0.05 would result in the same conclusions one would reach by calculating a 95% CI. Similarly, performing a hypothesis test with alpha set at 0.10 would result in the same conclusions one would reach by calculating a 90% CI, and setting alpha at 0.01 would result in the same conclusions one would reach by calculating a 99% CI.).

   Setting alpha allows one to determine the CV associated with the test statistic (t). This is the same CV discussed previously within the context of CIs. Thus, assuming that a 2-tailed alternative hypothesis was stated and $n \geq 30$, if alpha is set at 0.05, the CV is 2.0, just like for a 95% CI. (Note: If a 1-tailed alternative hypothesis is specified in Step 1, the CV will be smaller. This increases the chances of rejecting the null hypothesis, assuming that any differences observed are in the direction hypothesized.)
4. **Calculate Test Statistic.** In this step, data collected from the sample of study participants are plugged into the formula for the test statistic as determined in Step 2, and the necessary computations are performed to calculate the test statistic.
5. **Interpret Results.** In this step, the *P* value associated with the test statistic ("t" in this case) is determined. In general, the larger the test statistic is, the smaller the *P* value will be. Remember that the *P* value reflects the probability that the observed difference or any difference more extreme (larger) would have occurred if the population means were the same. Thus, the smaller the *P* value is, the less likely it is that the null hypothesis is true.

   If the *P* value is less than or equal to alpha (see Step 3), you reject the null hypothesis and conclude that the mean in the population of interest differs from the general population mean. If the *P* value is greater that alpha, you do **not** reject the null hypothesis. In this case, you would conclude that there is insufficient evidence to conclude that the mean in the population of interest differs from the general population mean. Box 3-1 illustrates these steps.

Potential Errors in Hypothesis Testing. When investigators are testing hypotheses, they can never be certain that their conclusions are correct. As a reader of the medical literature, you can never be certain either! Table 3-9 shows the four possible outcomes that can occur when testing a hypothesis. The rows indicate what the investigators in the study concluded based on the data from their sample. In the top row, the investigators concluded that a difference in population parameters exists and rejected the null hypothesis. In the bottom row, the investigators find that there is insufficient evidence to conclude that a difference in population parameters exists and, therefore do **not** reject the null hypothesis.

The columns in the table indicate whether, in reality, a difference in **population** parameters (e.g., population means) really exists. In the first column, a difference in population parameters does exist. In the second column, no difference exists. In case you have forgotten, we never know which column we are in because that would require knowledge of the population parameters. Again, the only way to know the true population parameters would be to collect data from the entire population, which is impossible.

The cells in the table indicate the 4 different outcomes that can occur when an investigator performs a hypothesis test. **If the investigator rejects the H_0**, he could be correct. That is, a true difference in population parameters does exist. However, he could be wrong. That is, the population parameters are the same. This outcome is called a Type I (alpha) error and is depicted by the shaded box on the top row of the table. **If the investigator does not reject the H_0**, he could be right. That is, the population parameters are the same.

BOX 3-1. Hypothesis Testing Example

Research Question	Is the bone density of women, aged 20 to 29, on long-term, low-dose oral prednisone therapy different than the norm established for women in that age group in the general population?
Study Design	Perform bone density examinations on 49 women between the ages of 20 and 29 on long-term, low-dose oral prednisone therapy. Compare the sample mean obtained to an established norm for women in that age group in the general population.
Results	Mean bone density in the sample is 0.95 g/cm^2 (SD = 0.12). The norm established for women aged 20 to 29 in the general population is 0.99 g/cm^2.

Step	Application to Example
1. Specify the null and alternative hypotheses	$H_0{:}\mu_{WomenInGeneralPopulation} = \mu_{WomenTakingPrednisone}$ $H_A{:}\mu_{WomenInGeneralPopulation} \neq \mu_{WomenTakingPrednisone}$
2. Determine the appropriate test statistic	Because data were collected from only 1 sample and the mean in the general population is assumed to be known, the appropriate test is a 1-sample t-test.
3. Set alpha	Set alpha at $P < 0.05$.
4. Calculate test statistic	$t = \frac{X - {}_{GP}}{SE_{\bar{X}}}; t = \frac{0.95 - 0.99}{0.12/\sqrt{49}} = -2.33$
5. Interpret results	The *P* value associated with the test statistic (−2.33), assuming a 2-tailed test, is <0.02. (*P* values are generated automatically by most statistical software and can also be found in t-tables, which are widely available on the internet.) Because 0.02 is less than alpha (which we set at 0.05 in Step 3), we would reject the null hypothesis. In a paper reporting study findings, an investigator might state, "Our findings indicate that the mean bone density of women aged 20 to 29 on long-term, low-dose oral prednisone therapy is lower than that observed in the general population ($P < 0.02$)."

However, he could be wrong. That is, the true population parameters are not the same. This outcome is called a Type II (beta) error and is depicted by the shaded box on the bottom row of the table.

Investigators attempt to design studies in a manner that minimizes making both Type I and Type II errors. Each type of error is discussed in more detail.

1. **Type I Error (α Error).** A Type I or alpha error occurs when an investigator rejects the null hypothesis when the population parameters are really the same. Put another way, *"The investigator concludes that there is a difference when, in reality, there is not."* (In a study evaluating the effectiveness of

TABLE 3-9. Possible Outcomes of Hypothesis Testing

	True Difference?	
Conclusion	**Yes**	**No**
Difference (Reject H_0)	Correct! Power	Type I (alpha) error
No difference (do **not** reject H_0)	Type II (beta) error	Correct!

a medication, this is equivalent to an investigator concluding that the medication is effective when, in reality, it is not.) When performing hypothesis tests, investigators control Type I errors when they set alpha. By convention, alpha is usually set at 0.05 or 0.01. With alpha set at 0.05, if an investigator conducted 100 studies **and the population parameters were really the same**, the investigator would make a Type I error (concluding that the population populations differ) in 5 of the studies.

2. **Type II Error (β Error).** A Type II or beta error occurs when investigators conclude that there is no difference in population parameters when, in reality, there is a difference. Put another way, *"The investigators miss a true difference."* (In a study evaluating the effectiveness of a medication, this is equivalent to an investigator concluding that the medication is not effective when, in reality, it is effective.) Investigators control Type II errors when they design a study by ensuring that they enroll a sufficient number of study participants to be able to compute precise estimates of population parameters. By convention, investigators attempt to keep the probability of making a Type II or beta error at or below 0.20. In a study in which the probability of making a beta error is 0.20 and **the true population parameters are different**, the investigators have a 20% chance of failing to detect this difference.

Detecting True Differences: Power. In most cases, when investigators conduct a study, they expect to reject the null hypothesis. For example, investigators might compare two medications because they believe that one is safer or more effective than the other. Therefore, they want to design their studies in a way that gives them a good chance of detecting any differences that exist. This ability to detect a true difference is called **power**.

As shown in Table 3-9, power is the opposite of a Type II (β) error. Both are based on the assumption that a true difference in population parameters exists. **If** a true difference in population parameters exists, power = 1 − β. Thus, if Type II (β) error is 0.20, power is 0.80. Investigators usually attempt to design studies so that power is at least 0.80.

Power is influenced by several factors. These include the level at which alpha error is set, the hypothesized difference between population parameters, and the SE of the sample mean (which, in turn, is affected by the SD of the variable under consideration and the sample size). To understand how these factors influence power, it is helpful to consider Figure 3-9. The top figure on the left depicts the sampling distribution for the mean under the **null hypothesis**. This sampling distribution is based on the assumption that the null hypothesis is true. The distribution centers on the population mean hypothesized under the null hypothesis. The CV shows the point at which sample statistics further from the center of this distribution would lead to rejection of the null hypothesis.

The next figure adds the sampling distribution for the mean under the **alternative hypothesis**. This sampling distribution is based on the assumption that the alternative hypothesis is true. It centers on the population mean hypothesized under the alternative hypothesis. Notice that most of the sampling distribution for the mean under the alternative hypothesis lies to the right of the CV, the area in which the null hypothesis would be rejected. However, a portion of the sampling distribution for the mean under the alternative hypothesis lies to the left of the CV. This overlap in the two sampling distributions is what creates the possibility of both Type I and Type II errors.

The three lower figures identify the areas in the sampling distributions that correspond to power, Type II error, and Type I error, respectively. In the first figure, power corresponds to the area in the sampling distribution under the **alternative** hypothesis that lies to the right of the CV. This area reflects the probability that **if** the alternative hypothesis is true, the sample mean will be far enough away from the mean under the null hypothesis that the null hypothesis will be rejected. As the size of this area increases, power increases.

In the second figure, Type II error corresponds to the area in the sampling distribution under the **alternative** hypothesis that lies to the left of the CV. This area reflects the probability that even though the alternative hypothesis is true, the sample mean will be close enough to the mean under the null hypothesis that it is not possible to reject the null hypothesis. As the size of this area increases, Type II error increases.

FIGURE 3-9. Factors That Influence Power

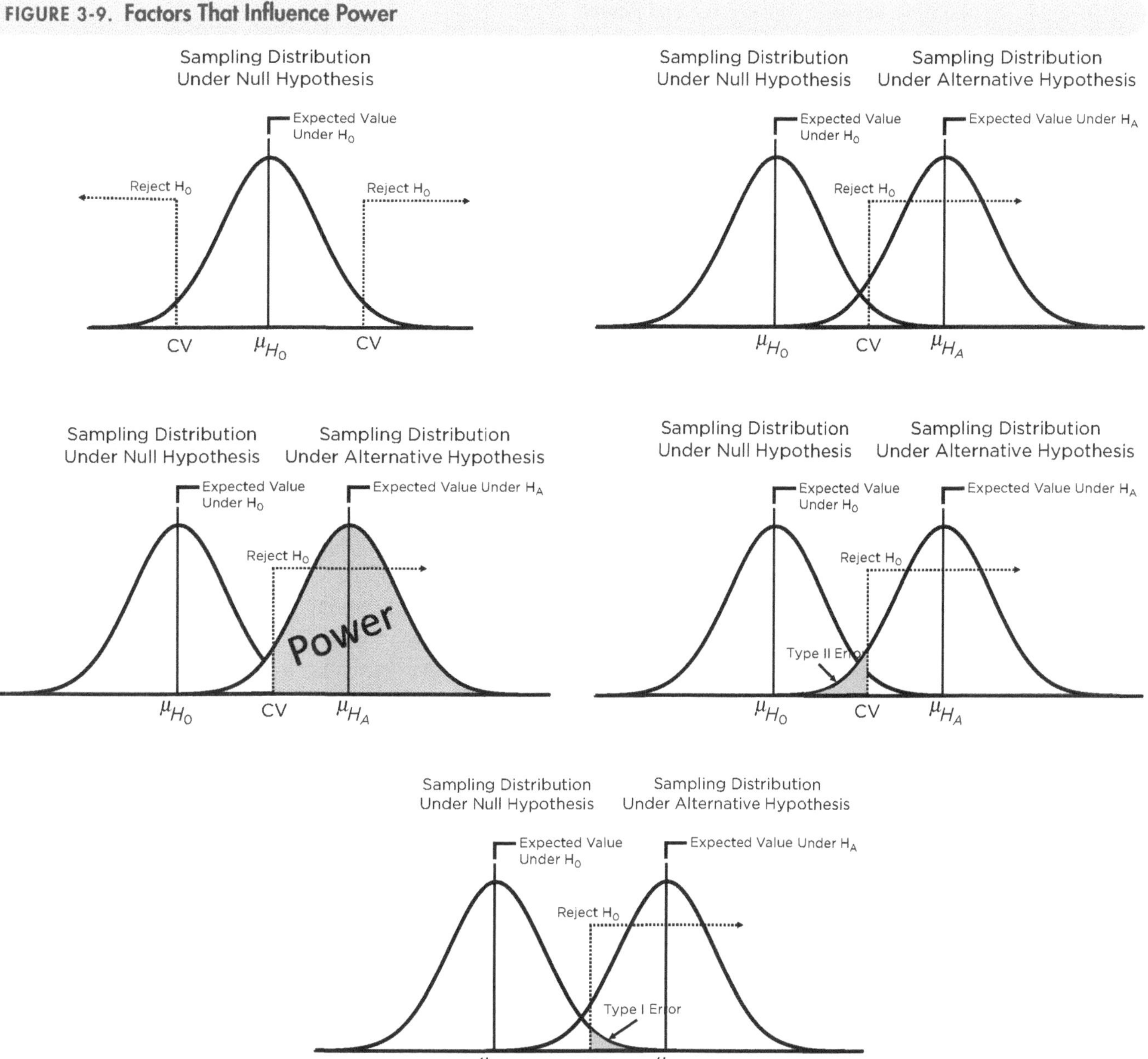

In the third figure, Type I error corresponds to the area in the sampling distribution under the **null** hypothesis that lies to the right of the CV. This area reflects the probability that even though the null hypothesis is true, the sample mean will be so far away from the mean under the null hypothesis that the null hypothesis will be rejected. As the size of this area increases, Type I error increases.

With this background, we now turn to how power is affected by the level at which alpha is set, the hypothesized difference between population parameters, and the SE of the sample mean. For illustration, we begin with a fictitious variable that has a mean of 100 under the null hypothesis and 140 under the alternative hypothesis. We also begin with the assumption that the SE of the variable is 10.

Alpha Level. Consider what happens when you decrease alpha error (e.g., set alpha error at 0.01 rather than 0.05). As you know, to decrease alpha, the CV must be increased. The effect of this change is shown in Figure 3-10. When alpha is set at 0.05, as it is in the figure on the left, the CV is 2.0. Thus,

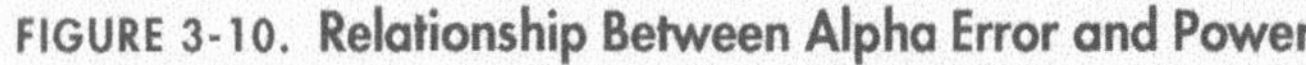

FIGURE 3-10. Relationship Between Alpha Error and Power

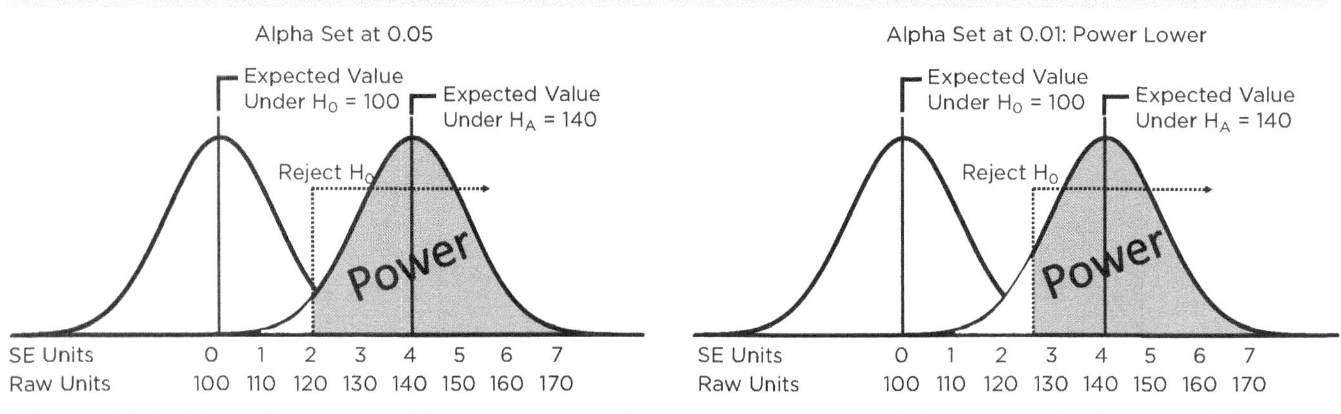

SE, standard error.

if the sample mean is more than 2 SEs away from the mean under the null hypothesis, the null hypothesis will be rejected.

In contrast, when alpha is set at 0.01, the CV is 2.6, as shown in the figure on the right. This moves the CV closer to the mean hypothesized under the alternative hypothesis, reducing the area of the sampling distribution under the alternative hypothesis that lies to the right of CV (i.e., the area that corresponds to power). Thus, decreasing Type I (α) error, decreases power. Remember also that decreasing power, increases Type II (β) error. Thus, investigators must make trade-offs between Type I and Type II error. To increase power (and decrease Type II) error, it may be necessary to accept a higher risk of making a Type I error.

Hypothesized Difference Between Population Parameters. Now, consider what happens if an investigator believes the difference between the mean under the alternative hypothesis and the mean under the null hypothesis is smaller than originally hypothesized. (The difference between parameters hypothesized under the null versus alternative hypothesis is called the **effect size**.) As shown in the figure on the left in Figure 3-11, we began by assuming that the mean under the alternative hypothesis was 140. The figure on the right shows what would happen if we hypothesized that the mean under the alternative hypothesis was 130. As you can see from the figures, this has the effect of shifting the distribution for the mean under the alternative hypothesis to the left, increasing the amount of overlap between the two distributions.

FIGURE 3-11. Relationship Between Effect Size and Power

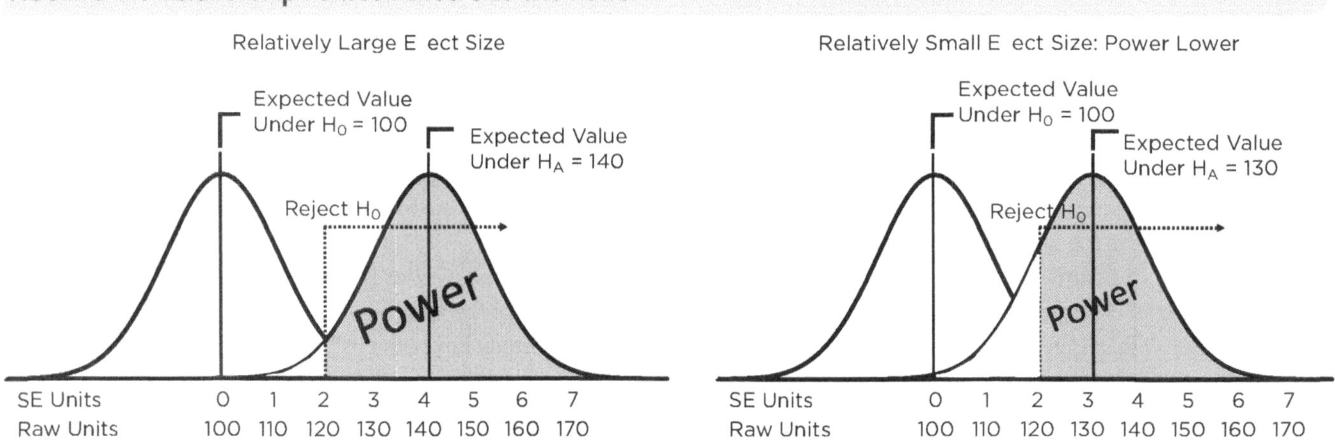

SE, standard error.

FIGURE 3-12. **Relationship Between Standard Error and Power**

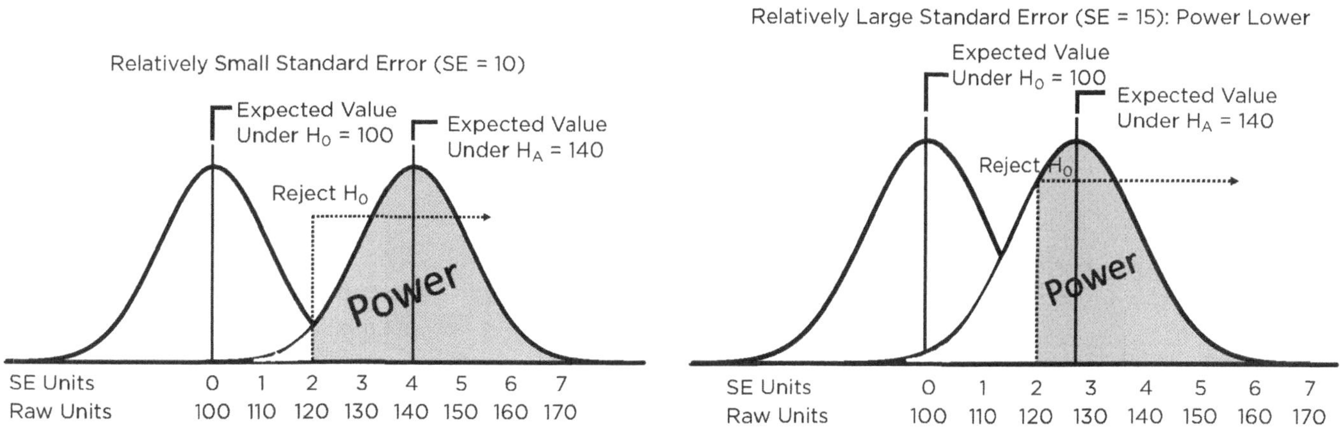

SE, standard error.

This results in a decrease in power as can be seen by the smaller area to the right of the CV (CV = 2.0 if alpha = 0.05). In general, all other things held constant, as the hypothesized effect size becomes smaller, power is reduced.

SE of the Mean. Finally, consider what happens as the SE of the mean increases. As shown in the figure on the left in Figure 3-12, we began by assuming that the SE was 10. The figure on the right shows what would happen if the SE was 15. As before, this has the effect of shifting the distribution for the mean under the alternative hypothesis to the left, increasing the amount of overlap between the two distributions. This is because, if the SE is 15, the difference between the means hypothesized under the null and alternative hypotheses are 2.67 SE units apart (i.e., $\frac{140-100}{15} = 2.67$). In contrast, the two means were separated by 4.0 SE units when the SE was assumed to be 10 (i.e., $\frac{140-100}{10} = 4.0$). The shift in the sampling distribution for the mean under the alternative hypothesis results in a decrease in power as can be seen by the smaller area to the right of the CV (CV = 2.0 if alpha = 0.05). In general, all other things held constant, as the SE of the mean increases, power decreases.

Remember that two factors affect the SE of the mean: the SD of the variable of interest and sample size. As discussed previously, increases in the sample size decrease the SE. This provides a mechanism for investigators to wield considerable control over the level of power they achieve in their studies. Prior to conducting a study, investigators should perform a power analysis. The results of this analysis tell the investigator approximately how many study participants are needed to achieve a desired level of power. When reading published papers, you should check to see if the investigators performed a power analysis. Additional questions to consider when evaluating power analyses reported include the following: (1) Are the effect sizes hypothesized reasonable? (2) Would smaller effect sizes be clinically meaningful? and (3) Did the investigators achieve their targeted sample size?

Final Thoughts

In this chapter, we introduced two approaches to determine whether the mean in a specific population of interest differs from a general population mean: estimation of CIs and hypotheses testing. Both approaches will always lead to exactly the same conclusions. Hypothesis testing has been the more traditional approach. However, estimation of confidence has become the preferred approach in medicine because CIs provide somewhat more information than hypothesis tests. That is, when creating CIs, it is easy to see how close the sample mean is to the mean under the null hypothesis.

Finally, this chapter has focused on **statistical significance**. However, very small differences between sample means may be statistically significant, especially in studies involving large samples. Just because a difference is statistically significant does not mean that it is **clinically meaningful**. Making this decision requires the application of clinical expertise. When reading a paper that presents statistically significant findings, readers should always ask themselves whether the differences are clinically meaningful.

Self-Study Questions

1. Imagine that a new drug is available to treat a rare and aggressive form of cancer. A study is conducted. A total of 500 people receive the new medication. A total of 1,500 people receive standard care. All patients are followed for 1 year. Among the people receiving the new medication, 200 die before the end of the follow-up period. Among the people receiving standard care, 200 die before the end of the follow-up period.

   A. In this example, is survival independent of the medication taken?
   B. What is the conditional probability of surviving if a person receives the new medication?
   C. What is the conditional probability of surviving if a person receives standard care?

2. Imagine that it is thought that Medication A causes birth defects when women take it during pregnancy. Data from a cohort of 100,000 women are available. Among these women, 10,000 took Medication A during pregnancy, and 10 of these women gave birth to babies with one or more birth defects. Among the 90,000 women who did **not** take the medication during pregnancy, 90 gave birth to babies with one or more birth defects.

   A. In this example, are birth defects independent of whether Medication A was taken during pregnancy?
   B. What is the conditional probability of having a baby with a birth defect among women who took Medication A during pregnancy?
   C. What is the conditional probability of having a baby with a birth defect among women who did **not** take Medication A during pregnancy?

3. Imagine that you collected data concerning weight in a sample of 36 people. The mean weight in the sample is 180 pounds with an SD of 20 pounds.

   A. Assuming that the variable is normally distributed, about how many people in the sample weigh between 160 and 200 pounds? About how many weigh between 140 and 220 pounds?
   B. Using the data provided, calculate the standard error (SE) of the mean for weight.
   C. Calculate a 95% confidence interval (CI) for the mean.
   D. What would you tell someone who asked, "What is the average weight in the population from which this sample was drawn?"
   E. Calculate a 99% CI for the mean. Why is the 99% CI wider than the 95% CI?
   F. Now, what would you tell someone who asked, "What is the average weight in the population from which this sample was drawn?"
   G. Imagine that data had been available for 400 people but that the mean weight was still 180 pounds and the SD was still 20 pounds. Do you think the CIs for weight would become wider or narrower? Why? Compute the 95% CI using these data to check your answer.
   H. Imagine that you want to determine whether the mean weight in the population from which this sample was drawn was 175 pounds. Further, you only want to conclude that the mean weight is different than 175 pounds if you are at least 95% certain that it is different.
      i. Based on the data from the sample where N = 36, what would you conclude?
      ii. Based on the data from the sample where N = 400, what would you conclude?

I. In the sample of 400 people, imagine that the mean weight was still 180 pounds but that the SD was 40 pounds. Compute the 95% and 99% CIs for weight using these data.
   i. Based on the 95% CI, would your conclusion be the same as in part h (ii)?
   ii. What if you only wanted to conclude that the mean weight is different than 175 pounds, if you were at least 99% certain that it is different? What would you conclude?
   iii. If the SD had been 20 pounds, would your conclusion have been different?

J. Assume that the mean in the population from which the sample was drawn was **not** 175. Based on all of the above, what set of conditions (i.e., sample size, SD, type of CI) provided the greatest power to rule out the possibility that the true population mean could be 175?

4. Imagine that you collected data concerning weight in a sample of 36 people. The mean weight in the sample is 180 pounds with an SD of 20 pounds. Now, imagine that you want to test the hypothesis that the mean in the population from which this sample was drawn is different from 175 pounds.

   A. What is the null hypothesis?
   B. What is the alternative hypothesis?
   C. Compute a z-score to determine whether you should reject the null hypothesis.
   D. What do you conclude?
   E. If the sample size had been 400, would that have changed your conclusion?

5. Is the following statement true or false? Population parameters can be calculated from the data collected in a study. (True/False)

6. The SE of a variable

   A. Indexes the amount of variance among observations in a sample
   B. Indexes the amount of variance that would be observed in the means of different random samples (of a fixed sample size) that are drawn from the same population
   C. Decreases as sample size decreases
   D. A and B
   E. A and C

7. Probabilities can:

   A. Range from −1 to +1
   B. Range from 0 to infinity
   C. Range from 0 to +1
   D. Take any value

8. If the probability that an event will happen is 0.8, the probability that it will **not** happen is:

   A. −0.2
   B. 0.2
   C. 0.5
   D. 0.7
   E. 1.0

9. Which of the following statements is true with respect to the binomial distribution?

   A. It is appropriate to use when analyzing proportions.
   B. It can only be used with dichotomous variables.
   C. The value calculated by the binomial formula is a probability.
   D. It can be used to analyze problems even if the sample size is quite small.
   E. All of the above

10. Imagine that 40% of patients who begin therapy with lipid-lowering drugs discontinue therapy (without the knowledge of their physician) within 1 year of therapy initiation. A pilot study is conducted to determine if a pharmacist-directed lipid management program can improve medication adherence. Ten patients are enrolled into the pilot study. At the end of a 1-year follow-up period, all 10 patients are still taking their medication as prescribed by their physician. What is the probability that all 10 patients would still be complying with their lipid medications if the disease management program had no effect on compliance?

   A. 0.05
   B. 0.01
   C. 0.006
   D. 0.0001

11. Imagine that 20% of patients who begin therapy with lipid-lowering drugs discontinue therapy (without the knowledge of their physician) within 1 year of therapy initiation. A pilot study is conducted to determine if a pharmacist-directed lipid management program can improve medication adherence. Ten patients are enrolled into the pilot study. At the end of a 1-year follow-up period, all 10 patients are still taking their medication as prescribed by their physician. What is the probability that all 10 patients would still be complying with their lipid medications if the disease management program had no effect on compliance?

   A. 0.01
   B. 0.05
   C. 0.11
   D. 0.20
   E. 0.0001

12. The SE of the mean of a variable is affected by:

   A. The SD of the variable
   B. The number of people in the sample from which the mean was calculated
   C. A and B

13. The SE of the mean is:

   A. The average distance of individual observations in a sample from the sample mean
   B. Given a specific sample size, the average distance of all possible sample means from the true population mean
   C. The probability of incorrectly rejecting the null hypothesis
   D. The probability of incorrectly accepting the null hypothesis
   E. The probability of incorrectly rejecting the alternative hypothesis

14. Two events are independent if:

   A. They cannot occur at the same time
   B. The probability of one event does not alter the probability of the other event
   C. The probability of each event is 0.5
   D. The probabilities of all possible outcomes are equal
   E. None of the above

15. You are reading a study that involves 1,000 patients with diabetes. In total, 250 of these patients receive a new experimental medication thought be superior to existing therapy in achieving long-term glycemic control. The remaining 750 patients receive an existing medication. All patients are evaluated bimonthly. Among the patients receiving the experimental medication, 150 are consistently rated as being within guidelines for glycemic control. Among patients receiving the existing medication, 300 are consistently rated as being within guidelines for glycemic control. Based on the multiplication rule for independent events, does glycemic control appear to be independent of the type of medication the person is taking?

   A. Yes, glycemic control appears to be independent of the type of medication taken.
   B. No, glycemic control does **not** appear to be independent of the type of medication taken.

16. You are reading an article in a journal. The article reports that patients receiving an experimental medication were more likely to report gastrointestinal distress compared to patients receiving a placebo ($P = .08$). If alpha was set at $P < 0.05$, what would you conclude from this information?

   A. The difference between patients taking the experimental medication versus placebo was statistically significant.
   B. The difference between patients taking the experimental medication versus placebo was **not** statistically significant.

17. In a sample of 2,000 people, 100 people were taking Drug A. Of these people, 10 died. In this sample, what is the **joint probability** of taking Drug A and dying?

   A. 0.005
   B. 0.05
   C. 0.10
   D. 0.20
   E. 0.30

18. In a recent paper, investigators report that participants in a study who were given a new drug for weight control lost an average of 3 pounds over a 1-month period. The 95% CI for this mean estimate was 0.8 to 5.2 pounds. Based on this information only, what would you conclude?

A. The reported results are statistically significant.
B. The reported results are **not** statistically significant.
C. A conclusion cannot be reached because no *P* value is given.
D. A conclusion cannot be reached because no information about power is provided.
E. C and D

19. If all other things are held constant, when sample size increases, the SE of estimates based on data from the sample will:

A. Decrease
B. Stay the same
C. Increase

20. Suppose there is a study showing that the mean bone density of women is 1.00 ± 0.15 g/cm^2, and the mean bone density of men is 1.07 ± 0.09 g/cm^2. The 95% confidence level for the difference between these means is 0.02 to 0.14 g/cm^2. How is this information interpreted?

A. The true difference in the mean bone density of men and women is 0.07 g/cm^2.
B. Because the 95% CI does not include "1," the difference is statistically significant.
C. There is 95% chance that the true difference in the mean bone density of men and women is between 0.02 and 0.14 g/cm^2.
D. A *P* value is needed to determine whether the difference is statistically significant.

21. If an investigator sets alpha at 0.05, we know that:

A. The chance that the investigator will make a Type I error is 5%
B. The chance the investigator will make a Type II error is 5%
C. Power is 0.95
D. Power is 0.05

22. Imagine that you are reading a paper that reports the mean bone mineral density in a sample and the 95% CI for the point estimate of the mean. What percentage of the time would you expect the true population mean bone density to be captured within the 95% CI?

A. 5% of the time
B. 95% of the time
C. 99% of the time
D. 100% of the time

23. Is the following statement true or false? A 95% CI will always be narrower than a 99% CI. (True/False)

24. When one performs a hypothesis test, the null hypothesis is:

A. The means in the samples being compared are the same
B. The means in the populations from which the samples were drawn are the same
C. The means in the samples being compared are different
D. The means in the populations from which the samples were drawn are different

25. When an investigator writes in a paper that one treatment is more effective than another ($P < 0.05$), this indicates that:

A. He is absolutely certain that the treatment is more effective than the other
B. The chance that the treatments are equally effective is less than 5%
C. He cannot completely rule out the possibility that the treatments are equally effective
D. A and B
E. B and C

26. If a team of scientists concludes that there is no evidence that either of 2 treatments is superior to the other, what type of error might they be making?

A. Alpha (Type I) error
B. Beta (Type II) error
C. They could be making either an alpha or beta error.
D. This is a trick question; scientists don't make mistakes . . . especially when they are working in a team.

27. Imagine that a study is conducted among 3,000 people with flu-like symptoms. In total, 1,000 people receive penicillin. The remainder receive placebo. Among the people who receive penicillin, 800 report feeling better within 2 days of the initiation of therapy. Among the people who receive placebo, 1,000 report feeling better within 2 days of therapy initiation. Based on this information, what is the conditional probability of feeling better within 2 days of the initiation of therapy given that the patient received penicillin?

A. 0.40
B. 0.50
C. 0.80
D. 1.0
E. The probability cannot be determined from the information provided.

28. Based on the information in Question 27, does recovery (i.e., feeling better within 2 days of the initiation of therapy) appear to be independent of treatment?

A. Yes, recovery appears to be independent of treatment.
B. No, recovery appears to depend on the type of treatment received. People who take penicillin appear to recover more quickly.

T-Tests and Analysis of Variance

4

When an outcome variable is assessed on a numerical scale and observations are normally distributed, investigators use t-tests and analysis of variance (ANOVA) to answer questions that involve differences in population means across groups (e.g., whether the mean bone density of women taking prednisone is the same as women not taking prednisone). T-tests are used when there are only two groups of interest. ANOVA is used when there are more than two groups. T-tests and ANOVA can be used even if the outcome variable is not normally distributed, as long as the distribution of the outcome variable is not strongly skewed and each mean estimate is based on a sample size of 30 or more. In studies of this size, the sampling distribution of the means can be assumed to be normal, even if the observations in the sample are not.

After reading this chapter, you should be able to do the following:

1. Describe the relationship between hypothesis testing and estimation of confidence intervals (CIs).
2. Describe situations in which the following statistical tests would be used: 1-sample t-test, paired t-test, independent groups t-test, 1-way analysis of variance (ANOVA), factorial ANOVA, and ANOVA with repeated measures.
3. State the assumptions upon which t-tests and ANOVA are based.
4. Explain why multiple comparisons create a problem in the interpretation of t-tests and ANOVA.
5. Describe the post hoc comparison process and explain how post hoc comparisons attempt to minimize problems caused by multiple comparisons.
6. Given the results of analyses involving t-tests or ANOVA, determine whether an observed difference is statistically significant, the likelihood that any observed differences were due to chance, and the likelihood that any statistically nonsignificant differences were due to a lack of power.
7. Given the results of a t-test or ANOVA in the form of a table or text, identify and interpret observed relationships.
8. Given the results of a t-test or ANOVA in the form of a graph, interpret both main effects and interactions.

T-Tests

There are three different types of t-tests, each of which is used in a specific situation. The three types of t-tests are as follows:

1. **1-Sample T-Test.** An investigator collects data from only one sample and compares the sample mean to the mean in a more general population that is assumed to be known.
2. **Paired T-Test.** An investigator collects data from only one sample and measures each subject at two different points in time (Time 1 and Time 2) or under two different conditions and compares the sample means obtained at the two different time points (under the two different conditions) to one another.
3. **Independent Groups T-Test.** An investigator collects data from two independent samples and compares the sample means to one another. Each type of t-test is reviewed.

1-Sample T-Tests

1-Sample t-tests are used to determine if the mean in the specific population from which a sample was drawn (e.g., women aged 20–29 on long-term, low-dose prednisone therapy) is equal to the mean in a more general population (e.g., women aged 20–29 in the general public) that is assumed to be known. These tests are used in situations where there is only one sample and data are collected from the sample only one time. The example of hypothesis testing detailed in Chapter 3 of this book was an example of a 1-sample t-test.

Paired T-Tests

Paired t-tests are usually used in situations where there is only one sample but data are collected from each subject in the sample at two different points in time. Paired t-tests can also be used in situations that involve two samples but where each observation in one sample is **matched** with an observation in the other sample. In this case, the observations in the two samples are "paired."

Table 4-1 provides an example of the structure of the data from this type of study design. In this example, there are only five people in the study. However, there are a total of 10 observations, because each person was assessed two times. One could analyze these data by comparing the mean of the five observations made at Time 1 to the mean of the five observations made at Time 2. However, that would not be correct because it would require the assumption that the observations made at Time 1 were independent of the observations made at Time 2. In this case, it is obvious that the observations made at the two time points are not independent because the same people were assessed at both times. Thus, there is likely to be a correlation between the Time 1 and Time 2 assessments. Instead, to perform a paired t-test, a **difference score** must be computed for each person in the study by subtracting each person's Time 1 score from their Time 2 score. This difference is sometimes called the **change score**. (Note: You could just as easily subtract Time 2 from Time 1.) If there was no change between the two time points (i.e., the null hypothesis is true), the mean difference between Time 1 and Time 2 would be expected to be "0" (i.e., the expected value under the null hypothesis). The further the observed mean difference is from this expected value, the more likely that a "true" change occurred between the two assessments.

The formula for a paired t-test is $t = \frac{\bar{D}}{SE_D}$, where $\bar{D}$ is the mean of the observed differences and SE_D is the standard error (SE) of the difference score. SE_D is determined by computing the standard deviation (SD) of the difference score and dividing it by the square root of the sample size (i.e., $\frac{SD_D}{\sqrt{N}}$). In Table 4-2, $\bar{D}$ is –0.024 and SE_D is 0.003. If the pairs of observations are highly correlated, paired designs can be quite powerful. This can be seen in the data presented in Table 4-2. Notice how much smaller the SE_D is

TABLE 4-1. Paired T-Test Data Example

Subject	Time		Change Over Time
	Time 1	Time 2	
Person 1	X_{11}	X_{12}	D_1
Person 2	X_{21}	X_{22}	D_2
Person 3	X_{31}	X_{32}	D_3
Person 4	X_{41}	X_{42}	D_4
Person 5	X_{51}	X_{52}	D_5

TABLE 4-2. Example of Paired T-Test Calculations

Subject	Time: Baseline	Time: Follow-Up	Change Over Time
Person 1	0.66	0.64	–0.02
Person 2	0.75	0.72	–0.03
Person 3	0.80	0.76	–0.04
Person 4	0.88	0.85	–0.03
Person 5	0.93	0.91	–0.02
Person 6	0.98	0.95	–0.03
Person 7	1.00	0.98	–0.02
Person 8	1.01	0.99	–0.02
Person 9	1.02	1.01	–0.01
Mean	0.892	0.868	–0.024
SD	0.129	0.133	0.009
SE	0.043	0.044	0.003

SD, standard deviation; SE, standard error

(0.003) compared to the SE of the observations at either baseline (0.043) or follow-up (0.044). Remember that if all other things are held constant, as the SE decreases, power increases.

Differences between paired means can also be assessed by computing a confidence interval (CI) for the change score. The formula to calculate a CI for the mean change score observed is $\bar{D} \pm CV(SE_D)$. Notice the similarity between this formula and the formula for a paired t-test, $t = \frac{\bar{D}}{SE_D}$.

For the data shown in Table 4-2, $t = -\frac{0.024}{0.003} = -8$. This value exceeds the critical value (CV) of 2.0 (assuming alpha error set at 0.05), leading to rejection of the null hypothesis. Based on this, one would not expect the 95% CI for the mean change score to include 0, the expected value if the null hypothesis were true. You can confirm this by plugging the values from the table into the CI formula as follows: $-0.024 \pm 2(0.003) = -0.018$ *to* -0.03. Another example is provided in Box 4-1.

Independent Groups T-Tests

Independent groups t-tests are used in situations where there are two samples and data have been collected from each sample at only one point in time. Remember that the research question of interest in these situations is not whether the **sample** means are the same; the research question of interest is whether the means are the same in the **populations** from which the samples were drawn.

The formula for an independent groups t-test is $t = -\frac{\bar{X}_1 - \bar{X}_2}{SE_{Difference}}$, where $\bar{X}_1$ is the mean in one sample and $\bar{X}_2$ is the mean in the other sample. $SE_{Difference}$ reflects the SD of observations within each sample and the size of each sample. The formulas for calculating the $SE_{Difference}$ can get very ugly when the sample sizes differ in the two groups and when the SDs are not approximately equal across groups. At an intuitive level, just keep in mind the following two general rules: (1) as the sample size increases, the $SE_{Difference}$ decreases, and (2) as the SD of observations increases, the $SE_{Difference}$ increases.

Differences between means in two independent groups can also be assessed by computing CIs. The formula to calculate a CI for the difference between the means in two independent samples is

BOX 4-1. Paired T-Test Example

Imagine that a team of investigators wants to know if bone density decreases following the initiation of prednisone therapy. They perform bone density examinations on 49 women between the ages of 20 and 29 at the initiation of prednisone therapy and reassess bone density 1 year later. The mean bone density in the sample at baseline was 0.98 g/cm². At the 1-year follow-up, the mean bone density in the sample was 0.96 g/cm². The mean change score was –0.02, and the SD of the change score was 0.095.

Calculations

$$t = \frac{\bar{D}}{SE_D} = -\frac{.02}{\frac{0.095}{\sqrt{49}}}, t = \frac{\bar{D}}{SE_D} = -\frac{0.02}{0.0136} = -1.47\ (P = 0.15)$$

$$\begin{aligned} 95\%\ CI &= \bar{D} \pm CV(SE_D) \\ &= -0.02 \pm 2(0.0136) \\ &= -0.02 \pm 0.0272 \\ &= -0.472\ to\ 0.0072 \end{aligned}$$

Interpretation: Assuming that alpha for the t-test was set at 0.05, the investigators would conclude that the study provides no evidence that prednisone decreases bone density during the first year following the initiation of therapy. Thus, they would **not** reject the null hypothesis. This is because (1) the *P* value associated with the test statistic is 0.15, which is greater than alpha, and (2) "0," which is the expected value of the difference in means under the null hypothesis, is contained within the 95% CI.

Possible Error: Whenever investigators fail to reject the null hypothesis, the type of error that they might have made (and we can never be sure whether they did or not) is a Type II (β) error. That is, they may have missed a true difference. In this example, prednisone may decrease bone density, but the study may have been insufficiently powered to detect this effect. Investigators can control the amount of power that they have by enrolling a sufficient number of people in a study. Power of 80% or above is usually considered adequate. Even with this amount of power, investigators run a 20% chance of missing a true difference. In published papers, investigators should **always** tell you how much power they had to detect differences in the primary end points of interest.

$(\bar{X}_1 - \bar{X}_2) \pm CV(SE_{Difference})$. Again, notice how similar this is to the other CIs we have been computing. All we are doing is substituting the appropriate means of interest in the first part of the equation and the appropriate SE in the second part. The basic structure of the formula remains the same.

Box 4-2 is an example of a scenario involving an independent groups t-test. The example includes the calculation of an appropriate CI for this scenario.

T-Test Recap

Regardless of the type of t-test, the t-statistic tells you how many SEs the observed difference is from the expected value under the null hypothesis, which is "0" when differences in means are being examined. The larger "t" is, the less likely it is that the null hypothesis is true. As "t" increases, the *P* value associated with "t" decreases. (Remember: The *P* value associated with "t" indexes the probability that a difference as large, or larger, than the one observed would have occurred **if the null hypothesis were true**.)

Table 4-3 summarizes the formulas for 1-sample t-tests, paired t-tests, and independent groups t-tests. The table also shows the formulas for the CI that might be used in the same situations in which the t-test is used.

T-tests are used when (1) investigators want to test a hypothesis, (2) the dependent variable (i.e., outcome variable) is measured on a numerical scale, (3) the dependent variable is normally distributed **or** the sample size in each group is 30 or more, and (4) investigators want to examine mean differences

BOX 4-2. Independent Groups T-Test Example

Imagine that a team of investigators want to know whether, among women on long-term prednisone therapy, bone density is greater among those taking a vitamin D supplement compared to those not taking a supplement. To answer this research question, they enroll a sample of 100 women on long-term prednisone therapy. Upon enrollment in the study, the women are asked whether they are currently using a vitamin D supplement on a regular basis. Investigators also assess the bone density of all study participants. In the sample, 55 women used a vitamin D supplement. The mean bone density among these women was 0.99 g/cm^2 (SD = 0.16). The other 45 women did not use a vitamin D supplement. The mean bone density among these women was 0.92 g/cm^2 (SD = 0.12). The standard error of the difference was 0.028.

Calculations

$$t = \frac{\bar{X}_1 - \bar{X}_2}{SE_{Difference}} = \frac{0.99 - 0.92}{0.028} = 2.5\ (P = 0.014)$$

$$\begin{aligned} 95\%\ CI &= (\bar{X}_1 - \bar{X}_2) \pm CV(SE_{Difference}) \\ &= (0.99 - 0.92) \pm 2(0.028) \\ &= 0.07 \pm 0.056 \\ &= 0.014\ \textit{to}\ 0.126 \end{aligned}$$

Interpretation: Assuming that alpha for the t-test is set at 0.05, the investigators would conclude that the bone density of women using prednisone who are on concomitant therapy with Vitamin D have greater bone density than women using prednisone who do not also use Vitamin D. Thus, they would reject the null hypothesis. This is because (1) the *P* value associated with the test statistic is 0.014, which is less than alpha, and (2) "0," which is the expected value of the difference in means under the null hypothesis, is **not** contained within the 95% CI.

Possible Error: Whenever investigators reject the null hypothesis, the type of error that they might have made (and we can never be sure whether they did or not) is a Type I or alpha error. That is, they said that something made a difference when in fact it did not. Type I or alpha error is determined by the level at which alpha is set or the type of CI calculated. If alpha is set at 0.05 (or a 95% CI is calculated), the investigators run a 5% chance of concluding that something made a difference when in fact it did not. If alpha is set at 0.01 (or a 99% CI is calculated), the investigators run a 1% chance of concluding that something made a difference when in fact it did not. And so on . . .

TABLE 4-3.

Type of T-Test	Formula	Corresponding Confidence Interval
1-Sample t-test	$t = \frac{\bar{X} - \mu_{GP}}{SE_{\bar{X}}}$	$\bar{X} \pm CV(SE_{\bar{X}})$
Paired t-test	$t = \frac{\bar{D}}{SE_D}$	$\bar{D} \pm CV(SE_D)$
Independent groups t-test	$t = \frac{\bar{X}_1 - \bar{X}_2}{SE_{Difference}}$	$(\bar{X}_1 - \bar{X}_2) \pm CV(SE_{Difference})$

across groups or across time and no more than two groups are of interest. All three types of t-tests assume the following:

1. The dependent (i.e., outcome) variable is measured on a numerical scale.
2. The outcome variable is normally distributed **or** the sample size in each group is 30 or more.
3. There are no more than two groups.

Each type of t-test also has specific assumptions. **1-Sample t-tests** assume that the mean in the reference population (e.g., general public) is known. **Paired t-tests** assume that pairs of observations are analyzed. **Independent groups t-tests** assume (1) there are exactly two samples, (2) the samples are independent (i.e., knowing something about individuals in one sample provides **no** information about the individuals in the other sample), and (3) either (a) an equal number of people are in each sample **or** (2) the SD of the outcome variable is equal in the samples. This last requirement is called the assumption of homogeneity. Investigators can correct for violations of this assumption. When reading the literature, look to see if the sample sizes and SDs are approximately equal in the groups being compared. (Small differences are usually acceptable. However, if you see differences of twofold or greater, you should start to be concerned.) If you observe differences, check to see if the investigators corrected for violating the assumption of homogeneity. (Note: Correcting for a lack of homogeneity usually results in a loss of power and, consequently, an increase in Type II [β] error.)

Multiple Comparisons and Alpha Error

As shown in Table 4-4, when investigators set alpha at 0.05, it means that for each hypothesis they test, **if the null hypothesis is actually true** (i.e., there is no difference in population means), they have a 5% chance of rejecting it (resulting in an Type I [α] error) and a 95% chance of (correctly) **not** rejecting it.

Now consider what happens when an investigator performs multiple hypothesis tests. **If the null hypothesis is really true for each hypothesis of interest**, then the investigator has a 95% chance of drawing the correct conclusion for each test. However, the more hypotheses he tests, the more likely it becomes that he will make an alpha error at least once. Thus, Type I (α) error is inflated by performing multiple hypothesis tests, as demonstrated in Box 4-3.

There are two primary strategies that investigators can use to minimize the inflation of Type I (α) errors when performing hypothesis tests. First, investigators can limit the number of hypotheses they test. One way this might be accomplished is for the investigators to declare one or two "primary endpoints" (i.e., outcomes) prior to conducting a study. Readers then can feel fairly comfortable that the *P* values associated with these endpoints reflect the true probability of Type I (α) errors. *P* values associated with other end points reported in the study will be less trustworthy and should be interpreted with awareness of the potential for inflation of Type I (α) errors when many hypothesis tests are performed.

TABLE 4-4. Conventional Levels for Type I and Type II Error

	True Difference?	
Conclusion	**Yes**	**No**
Difference (Reject H_0)	0.80	0.05 Type I (α) error
No difference (do **not** reject H_0)	0.20 Type II (β) error	0.95

BOX 4-3. Example of Inflation of Type I (α) Error

Imagine you are reading a study in which the investigators examined the effect of an experimental medication on three outcome variables. Half of the people in the study were randomly assigned to take the experimental medication. The other half took a placebo. The investigators performed three t-tests, each test examining differences between the two groups on one of the outcome variables. For each test, statistical significance was evaluated with alpha set at 0.05. **Assuming that the medication has no effect on any of the outcome variables**, what is the probability of concluding that the medication does have an effect on at least one of the outcomes (i.e., make at least one alpha error)?

This problem can be answered by referring to the multiplication rule for independent events. If the probability of correctly not rejecting the null hypothesis is 0.95 for each test, the probability of correctly not rejecting the null hypothesis for all three tests can be computed as

$$0.95 * 0.95 * 0.95 = 0.857$$

It follows that the probability of making at least one Type I (α) error is

$$1 - 0.857 = 0.143$$

Thus, Type I (α) error is inflated by performing multiple hypothesis tests.

Now, assume that four outcomes are examined and that the medication has no effect on any of the outcome variables. The probability of correctly not rejecting the null hypothesis for all four outcomes is

$$0.95 * 0.95 * 0.95 * 0.95 = 0.815$$

It follows that the probability of making at least one Type I (α) error is

$$1 - 0.815 = 0.185$$

Now, assume that five outcomes are examined and that the medication has no effect on any of the outcome variables. The probability of correctly not rejecting the null hypothesis for all five outcomes is

$$0.95 * 0.95 * 0.95 * 0.95 * 0.95 = 0.774$$

It follows that the probability of making at least one Type I (α) error is

$$1 - 0.774 = 0.226$$

Thus, the more tests performed, the greater the inflation of Type I (α) errors.

Alternatively, investigators can control for the problem of multiple comparisons statistically. There are a wide variety of statistical approaches that can be used to accomplish this task. Most involve testing individual hypotheses with alpha set lower than 0.05. The easiest approach to understand at a conceptual level is called the Bonferroni correction. It involves dividing alpha by the number of tests performed. In the previous example, if an investigator examined three outcomes and wanted the overall alpha level to be 0.05, the investigator would divide 0.05 by 3 (i.e., the number of hypotheses to be tested). Each hypothesis test would then be evaluated with alpha set at 0.0167. (Note: You can work this problem backward to see that it accomplishes the desired mission. With alpha set at 0.0167, **if the null hypothesis is really true for each hypothesis of interest**, then the investigator has a 98.33% [i.e., 1 – 0.0167] chance of drawing the correct conclusion for each test. The probability of correctly failing to reject the null hypothesis for all three tests can be computed as $0.9833 * 0.9833 * 0.9833 = 0.951$. Thus, the probability of making at least one Type I [α] error when performing the three tests is 0.049 [i.e., 1 – 0.951], very close to the value of 0.05 at which alpha is usually set.)

ANOVA

ANOVA extends the basic principles that underlie t-tests. Investigators turn to ANOVA when they are interested in an outcome variable that is assessed on a numerical scale and they are interested in differences in means across groups but where there are more than two groups of interest.

When discussing t-tests, I didn't use the term "independent variable." However, it may be helpful to note that when performing t-tests or ANOVA, the factor that distinguishes the groups of interest is the independent variable. For example, in the hypothetical study described in the section on independent groups t-tests in which we compared the mean bone density of women on long-term prednisone therapy who either (1) were taking a vitamin D supplement or (2) were not taking a vitamin D supplement, the independent variable of interest was "use of vitamin D supplementation." In ANOVA, the number of groups is often referred to as "levels." Thus, in the previous study, there was one independent variable (i.e., "use of vitamin D supplementation") with two levels (i.e., using a vitamin D supplement versus not using a vitamin D supplement).

In addition to the fact that ANOVA can handle independent variables with more than two levels (i.e., groups), it can also handle situations where investigators are interested in more than one independent variable. For example, if the previous study had included men as well as women, sex might have been another independent variable of interest. In this section, we will start with the simplest type of ANOVA, 1-way ANOVA, where there is only one independent variable of interest. We will then move to the more complex designs.

One-Way Analysis of Variance (1-Way ANOVA)

1-Way ANOVA is a very simple extension of an independent groups t-test. In fact, if the independent variable of interest only has two levels (i.e., two groups of interest), an investigator can use either a t-test or ANOVA to examine mean differences. The same conclusions will be reached with both procedures.

All ANOVA procedures involve **partitioning** (i.e., dividing) the variance of the dependent (outcome) variable into separate portions. The total variance of the outcome variable is indexed by a term called the **total sums of squares (SS).** It is computed by (1) calculating the difference between each observed value in the sample and the overall sample mean, (2) squaring each difference, and (3) summing all of the squared differences. This can be summarized by the formula $\Sigma(X_i - \bar{X})^2$, where X_i denotes an observed value and $\bar{X}$ denotes the overall sample mean. (Note: Total SS is a good name for this quantity because it is calculated by summing a bunch of squared differences.) In essence, the total SS reflects the variability of the outcome variable among individuals in a sample relative to the overall sample mean. If everyone in the sample is close to the mean, the total SS will be small. If there is a wide spread of people on both sides of the mean, the total SS will be large. The total SS also reflects the extent to which the values of individuals in the sample **cannot** be predicted by the overall sample mean. Box 4-4 provides an example of calculating the total SS for a fictitious study involving eight participants.

In 1-way ANOVA, the total SS is partitioned into two portions: (1) the portion that can be explained by the independent variable of interest and (2) the portion that cannot be explained by the independent variable.

1. **Between Groups SS**: The between groups SS reflects the portion of the variance in the outcome variable that can be explained by the independent variable. If the independent variable explains a lot of the variance in the outcome variable, the between groups SS will be large. Remember that in 1-way ANOVA, there is only one independent variable. It will always be a nominal variable with two or more levels (i.e., groups). For example, an investigator might want to examine differences in the effectiveness of four different drugs used to treat hypertension. In this study, the independent variable would be "drug," and this variable would have four different levels, with each level corresponding to one of the drugs being investigated (e.g., Drug A, Drug B, Drug C,

BOX 4-4. Calculating Total Sums of Squares (SS)

Imagine that a study was conducted in which eight people were weighed. The table shows the weight of each of the eight study participants and the overall sample mean weight.

Person 1	Person 2	Person 3	Person 4	Person 5	Person 6	Person 7	Person 8	Mean
180	170	160	150	140	130	120	110	145

If you were asked to estimate the weight of one of the eight people in the sample, without any other information, you would be best off estimating the person's weight as 145 pounds (i.e., the overall sample mean). Your estimate would never be off by more than 35 pounds. Further, it can be shown that, over multiple trials, this strategy would result in more accurate estimates than any other strategy you could use—if you had no information about the people whose weight you were being asked to estimate other than that they were participants in this study.

If you used this strategy to estimate the weight of each participant in this study, the differences between your estimates and the actual observations would correspond to the total SS. Thus, the total SS reflects the extent to which the values of individuals in a sample **cannot** be predicted by the overall sample mean.

The figure to the right depicts calculation of the total SS for this example, and the actual computations are provided below.

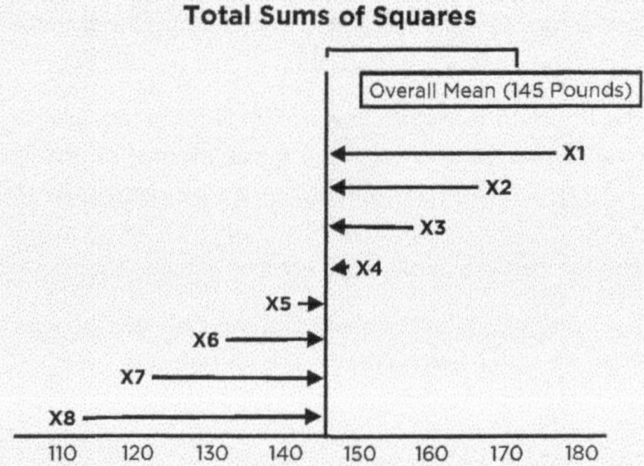

$$\text{Total SS} = (180-145)^2 + (170-145)^2 + (160-145)^2 + (150-145)^2 + (140-145)^2 + (130-145)^2 + (120-145)^2 + (110-145)^2 = 4{,}200$$

Drug D). The formula for calculating the between groups SS is $\sum n_{Group} (\bar{X}_{Group} - \bar{X}_{Overall})^2$, as illustrated in Box 4-5. The most important thing to recognize in this formula is that as the difference between the group means and the overall sample mean increases, the between groups SS also increases. In contrast, if the group means differ little from the overall sample mean, the between groups SS would be close to "0." Conceptually, if the between groups SS is "0," the independent variable does **not** explain any of the variance in the outcome variable.

2. **Error SS:** The error SS reflects the variation in the outcome variable that **cannot** be explained by the independent variable. It can be calculated in different ways. However, it can be derived most easily by simply subtracting the between groups SS from the total SS. As indicated previously, 1-way ANOVA involves partitioning the variance in the outcome variable into two portions. The between groups SS reflects the portion that can be explained by the independent variable. The error SS reflects the portion that cannot be explained by the independent variable. Thus, total SS = between groups SS + error SS. Once you know two of the three SS in this formula, it is pretty easy to figure out the remaining one. Thus, error SS = total SS – between groups SS.

BOX 4-5. Calculating Between Groups Sums of Squares (SS)

In the study introduced in Box 4-4, we began by assuming that we did not know anything about the eight study participants except their weight. However, as you can see in the table below, some of the people in the study were men and some were women. Thus, "sex" might be used as an independent variable to see if it can explain some of the variation in weight that we calculated previously.

In the table, you can see that the mean weight for males in the sample was 165 pounds and that the mean weight for females in the sample was 125 pounds.

Person 1	Person 2	Person 3	Person 4	Person 5	Person 6	Person 7	Person 8	Mean
180	170	160	150	140	130	120	110	145
M	M	M	M	F	F	F	F	
							Males	165
							Females	125

F, female; M, male.

Remember that the formula for calculating the between groups SS is $\Sigma n_{Group} (\bar{X}_{Group} - \bar{X}_{Overall})^2$

The figure to the right shows all of the relevant means (i.e., the overall sample mean and the group means) diagrammatically. This figure helps illustrate that as the distance between the group means increases, the between groups SS increases. If the group means were identical, the between groups SS would be 0.

The computations for calculating the between groups SS from the data in this example are shown below.

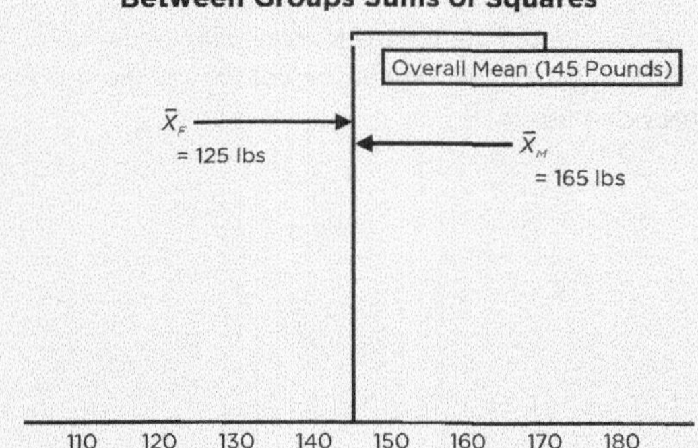

$$\text{Between Groups SS} = 4(125-145)^2 + 4(165-145)^2 = 3{,}200$$

Quantifying the Proportion of Variance Explained

The between groups SS and total SS can be used to compute the R^2 statistic. R^2 indicates the proportion of variance in the outcome variable that is explained by the independent variable as illustrated in Box 4-6. The formula for R^2 is $\frac{\textit{Between Groups SS}}{\textit{Total SS}}$. R^2 can range from 0 to 1.0. If the independent variable explains none of the variance in the outcome variable, R^2 will be 0. In contrast, if the independent variable explains all of the variance in the outcome variable, R^2 will be 1.0. More generally, as the proportion of variance in the outcome variable that is explained by the independent variable increases, R^2 increases (to the maximum value of 1.0).

Evaluating Statistical Significance

The F-statistic is used test the null hypothesis that **all** of the group means are equal to one another. The alternative hypothesis is that all of the group means are not equal to one another. Thus, if there are four groups of interest and three of the group means are identical to one another, but the fourth mean differs from the others, the null hypothesis would be rejected. After rejecting the null hypothesis, investigators would still need to determine which specific means differ from one another.

BOX 4-6. Proportion of Variance Explained R^2

From the data presented in Boxes 4-4 and 4-5, we know that the total SS was 4,200 and that the between groups SS was 3,200. From this, we can calculate the proportion of variance in weight that is explained by sex using the formula $R^2 = \frac{\textit{Between Groups SS}}{\textit{Total SS}}$.

Plugging the values from the example into this formula gives us $\frac{3{,}200}{4{,}200} = 0.76$.

Thus, based on the data provided in Box 4-5, 76% of the variation in weight can be explained by sex.

Let's imagine that the data from the study had been a little bit different. As shown below, imagine that all the men in the study had weighed 165 pounds and that all the women in the study had weighed 125 pounds. The overall sample mean is still 145 and the group means remain the same (i.e., 165 for men and 125 for women). Therefore, the between groups SS has to remain the same as well.

Person 1	Person 2	Person 3	Person 4	Person 5	Person 6	Person 7	Person 8	Mean
165	165	165	165	125	125	125	125	145
M	M	M	M	F	F	F	F	
							Males	165
							Females	125

F, female; M, male.

However, the total SS has changed. The new computations for the total SS are

$$\begin{aligned} \textit{Total SS} &= (165-145)^2+(165-145)^2+(165-145)^2 \\ &+(165-145)^2+(125-145)^2+(125-145)^2 \\ &+(125-145)^2+(125-145)^2 = 3{,}200 \end{aligned}$$

This is depicted diagrammatically in the figure to the right. From the figure, it should be clear that all of the variation in weight (given these new data) is explained by sex. Therefore, it should come as no surprise that

$$R^2 = \frac{3{,}200}{3{,}200} = 1.0$$

Total Sums of Squares

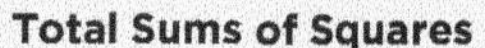

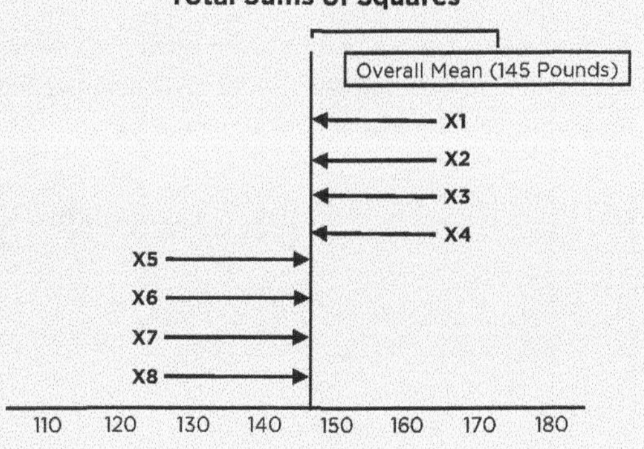

The formula for an F-test is $F(df_{Numerator}, df_{Denominator}) = \frac{SS_{Between}/df}{SS_{Error}/df}$. The term "df" in this formula stands for degrees of freedom. Within the context of 1-way ANOVA, the numerator df is equal to the number of groups being compared minus 1, and the denominator df is equal to the number of people in the study minus the number of groups being compared.

The F-statistic shares many similarities with the t-statistic discussed previously in the section on t-tests. Note that the numerator for the F-test indexes the differences among group means (just like the numerator did in the formulas for t-tests) and the denominator indexes error (just like the denominator did in the formulas for t-tests). When there are only two groups in a 1-way ANOVA, the F-statistic will equal the t-statistic squared (i.e., $F = t^2$). Thus, investigators could analyze the data using either a t-test or an F-test, and they would draw the exact same conclusion. Assuming that error variance is held constant, both the t- and F-statistics increase as the difference between group means increases. The expected value for both the t- and F-statistic **if the null hypothesis is true** is "0." Remember that the CV for a t-test, assuming each group has 30 or more subjects and alpha is set at 0.05, is approximately 2.0. Under these same assumptions, if only two groups are being compared, the CV for the F-test in 1-way ANOVA is about 4.0 (i.e., 2.0^2). See Box 4-7 for an example of using the F-statistic to evaluate statistical significance in a 1-way ANOVA involving only two groups.

Determining Which Specific Means Differ From One Another

In studies that involve more than two groups, if the F-test is **not** statistically significant, that is the end of the story. That is, there is insufficient evidence to conclude that any of the group means differ from one another.

However, if the F-test is statistically significant, one still needs to determine which specific means differ from one another. This is accomplished by performing pairwise comparisons (e.g., comparing $\bar{X}_1$ to $\bar{X}_2$, $\bar{X}_1$ to $\bar{X}_3$, $\bar{X}_2$ to $\bar{X}_3$, etc.). When making pairwise comparisons, the potential to inflate alpha error is a major concern. This is because the number of possible comparisons increases rapidly as the number of groups in a study increases. There are many statistical procedures that can be used to control for the

BOX 4-7. Evaluating Statistical Significance

From the data presented in Boxes 4-4 and 4-5, we can calculate the F-statistic to determine if the difference between group means is statistically significant using the following formula.

$$F(df_{Numerator}, df_{Denominator}) = \frac{SS_{Between}/df}{SS_{Error}/df}$$

Because there are two groups in the study, the Numerator degrees of freedom (df) is 2 – 1 = 1. Because there are eight people in the study and two groups are being evaluated, the Denominator df is 8 – 2 = 6. Plugging the values from Boxes 4-4 and 4-5 into the formula gives us:

$$F(1,6) = \frac{3{,}200/1}{4{,}200/6} = \frac{3{,}200}{700} = 4.57$$

Finally, we must determine if $F(1,6) = 4.57$ is ≥ critical value (CV). As shown in the figure to the right, the F-distribution varies as a function of the number of groups involved in the analysis and the number of study participants. Each curve represents a different combination of these two factors. Each curve stops when it reaches the CV, assuming that alpha is set at 0.05.

In this example, we had 2 groups and 8 participants. Under these conditions, the critical value for the F-statistic is about 6.0. Thus, because the value we computed (i.e., 4.57) is less than the CV, we do **not** reject the null hypothesis. In so doing, we could be making a Type II (β) error (i.e., missing a true difference in the population mean weight for men compared to women). Note, that if the study had included 100 participants, the CV would have been considerably lower and we would have had more power to detect a true difference

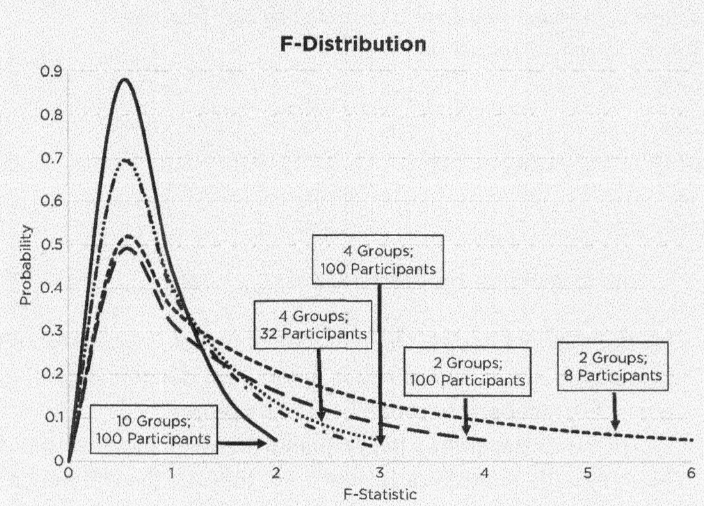

inflation of alpha error when multiple comparisons are necessary (e.g., Tukey's honestly significant difference, Bonferroni, Scheffe, Student-Newman-Keuls, Dunnett, Hochberg). Most of these procedures involve evaluating the difference between each pair of means for statistical significance with alpha set at a level below the conventional level of 0.05. When you are reading a paper where pairwise comparisons were used to follow up on a statistically significant F-test, check to see if the investigators used any statistical procedures to control for the potential inflation of alpha error. It they did not, beware of any statistically significant differences they report—they could be due to Type I (α) error.

Box 4-8 provides an example of a 1-way ANOVA from a fictitious study in which there were four groups of interest (see Box 4-9 for complete data). It includes a description of pairwise comparisons performed after a statistically significant F-test.

BOX 4-8. Example of 1-Way ANOVA With Four Groups

Imagine that a study is undertaken to assess the effect of three different medications on weight loss. A total of 32 people are enrolled in the study. Each participant is randomly assigned to one of four treatment groups: Placebo, Medication 1, Medication 2, or Medication 3. Participants are weighed before the initiation of therapy and again 6 months later. The outcome variable is "weight change over the 6-month duration of the study." The independent variable is "treatment group." Treatment group has four levels (i.e., Placebo, Medication 1, Medication 2, Medication 3). Findings from this fictitious study are summarized in the table below and complete data are provided in Box 4-9.

Mean Weight Change by Treatment Group

Treatment Group	N	Mean Weight Change
Placebo	8	+5 pounds
Medication 1	8	–15 pounds
Medication 2	8	–5 pounds
Medication 3	8	–45 pounds
Overall sample	32	–15 pounds

The null hypothesis being tested is $H_0{:}\mu_1 = \mu_2 = \mu_3 = \mu_4$. Thus, we will reject the null hypothesis if we find sufficient evidence to indicate a difference between any of the pairs of means of interest. (Note: There are a total of six pairs of means [i.e., μ_1 vs μ_2, μ_1 vs μ_3, μ_1 vs μ_4, μ_2 vs μ_3, μ_2 vs μ_4, μ_3 vs μ_4]).

Raw data from the study (see Box 4-9) were used to compute the **total sums of squares (SS)** as follows: $Total\ SS = (26-(-15))^2 + (16-(-15))^2 + (16-(-15))^2 + \ldots + (-35-(-15))^2 = 18{,}954$

Next, the between groups SS was calculated as follows:

$$\sum n_{Group}\left(\bar{X}_{Group} - \bar{X}_{Overall}\right)^2 = 8(-45-(-15))^2 + 8(-5-(15))^2 + 8(-15-(15))^2 + 8(5-(15))^2$$
$$= 11{,}200$$

Error SS can be computed as:

$$Error\ SS = Total\ SS - Between\ Groups\ SS = 18{,}954 - 11{,}200 = 7{,}754$$

R^2 can be computed as:

$$\frac{Between\ Groups\ SS}{Total\ SS} = \frac{11{,}200}{18{,}954} = 0.59$$

Thus, in this example, treatment group explains 59% of the variance in weight change over the 6-month follow-up period.

(continued)

BOX 4-8. Example of 1-Way ANOVA With Four Groups *(Continued)*

The F-statistic can be calculated as:

$$F(3,28) = \frac{SS_{Between}/df}{SS_{Error}/df} = \frac{11{,}200/3}{7{,}754/28} = 13.48$$

As can be seen in the figure to the right, when a study involves 4 groups and 32 participants, the critical value (CV) for the F-statistic (assuming alpha = 0.05) is about 3.0.

(In the figure, each curve stops at the CV. When alpha is set at 0.05, this is the point at which 95% of the distribution lies to the left of the point.)

Because the value we calculated (13.48) is greater than the CV, we would reject the null hypothesis and conclude that at least one of the group means differs from the others.

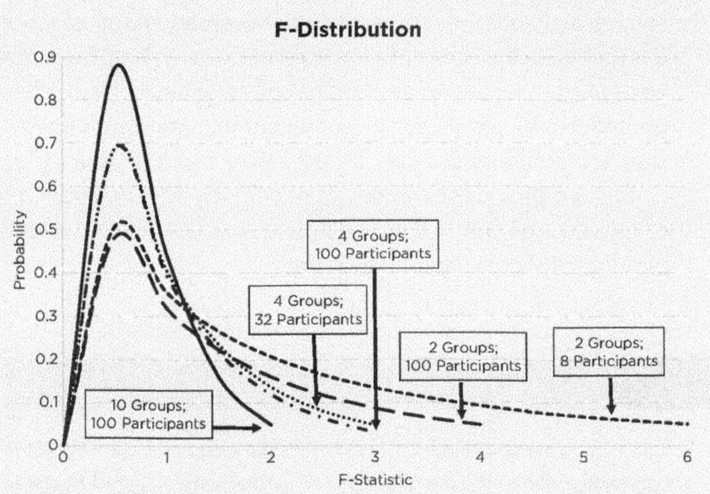

By comparing the F-statistic calculated to the CV, as we just did, one can only determine if the probability of observing a difference as large or larger than the one observed is less than 0.05 **if the null hypothesis is true**. However, the exact probability of observing a difference that large **if the null hypothesis is true** can be determined using an F-table.

In this example, the probability of observing a value of $F(3,28) = 13.48$, if **the null hypothesis is true**, is <0.0001. Because this large of a difference was observed, one concludes that it is **very unlikely** that the null hypothesis is true. Therefore, the null hypothesis is rejected.

Remember that the F-statistic is used to test the null hypothesis that **all** of the group means are equal to one another. If the F-test is statistically significant, investigators still need to determine which specific means differ from one another.

This example requires a total of 6 pairwise comparisons (i.e., Placebo vs Medication 1, Placebo vs Medication 2, Placebo vs Medication 3, Medication 1 vs Medication 2, Medication 1 vs Medication 3, Medication 2 vs Medication 3). The results of these comparisons are presented below. The rightmost column presents the *P* value associated with the overall F-test. The other cells in the table show the mean weight change in each group. The superscripts by the means are for reference. Whenever two means share the same superscript, it indicates that the difference between the means is **not** statistically significant. Thus, the differences between the Placebo, Medication 1, and Medication 2 groups are **not** statistically significant. However, the unique superscript by the mean weight change in the group taking Medication 3 indicates that participants in this group lost significantly more weight than participants in the other groups.

	Placebo	Med 1	Med 2	Med 3	p
Weight change (in pounds)	+5[a]	−15[a]	−5[a]	−45[b]	<0.0001

Factorial ANOVA

Factorial ANOVA is an extension of 1-way ANOVA that allows one to simultaneously examine the relationship between an outcome variable and **multiple** independent variables. (Remember that 1-way ANOVA is limited to situations where there is only one independent variable of interest.) Further, in addition to examining the relationship between each independent variable and the outcome variable in isolation, which are called main effects, one can also test for the presence of interactions among the independent variables. Interactions are present when the effect that one independent variable has on the outcome variable depends on the value of the other independent variable. Sometimes variables that are involved in

BOX 4-9. Raw Data and Group Means (SD) From Fictitious Weight Loss Study

Group	Sex	Before	After	Change
Placebo	M	340	366	26
Placebo	M	350	366	16
Placebo	M	350	366	16
Placebo	M	360	382	22
Placebo	F	290	286	–4
Placebo	F	300	289	–11
Placebo	F	300	290	–10
Placebo	F	310	295	–15
Placebo Mean (SD)		325 (27.77)	330 (43.15)	5 (16.62)
Med 1	M	340	331	–9
Med 1	M	350	350	0
Med 1	M	350	350	0
Med 1	M	360	365	5
Med 1	F	290	271	–19
Med 1	F	300	271	–29
Med 1	F	300	271	–29
Med 1	F	310	271	–39
Med 1 Mean (SD)		325 (27.77)	310 (42.68)	–15 (16.34)
Med 2	M	340	345	5
Med 2	M	350	360	10
Med 2	M	350	360	10
Med 2	M	360	375	15
Med 2	F	290	275	–15
Med 2	F	300	280	–20
Med 2	F	300	280	–20
Med 2	F	310	285	–25
Med 2 Mean (SD)		325 (27.77)	320 (43.59)	–5 (16.48)
Med 3	M	390	340	–50
Med 3	M	400	340	–60
Med 3	M	400	340	–60
Med 3	M	410	340	–70
Med 3	F	340	315	–25
Med 3	F	350	320	–30
Med 3	F	350	320	–30
Med 3	F	360	325	–35
Med 3 Mean (SD)		375 (27.77)	330 (11.02)	–45 (17.11)
Male Mean (SD)				–7.75 (32.52)
Female Mean (SD)				–22.25 (9.68)

interactions are called "effect modifiers." For that reason, interaction is sometimes referred to as "effect modification." These are good names because when two variables are involved in an interaction, one variable is modifying the effect of the other on the outcome variable.

Box 4-10 provides an example of a factorial ANOVA based on the fictitious weight loss study introduced previously. In the example, I add a second independent variable, sex, and test for the presence of an interaction between treatment group and sex. That is, I ask the following question: *Does the effectiveness of the various treatments (i.e., Placebo, Medication 1, Medication 2, Medication 3) depend on whether a patient is a man or a woman?*

As you look at the example provided in Box 4-10, notice that the error SS decreases when new independent variables that explain some of the variation in the outcome variable are included in the analysis. As a result, an independent variable that was not statistically significant before the introduction of the new independent variable can become statistically significant just because error variance has been reduced. To use an analogy, removing error variance is like removing the fuzziness from a picture. Once you remove the fuzziness, the images in the picture become clearer.

The information provided in Box 4-10 also reveals a statistically significant interaction between treatment group and sex. In the presence of a significant interaction, it is no longer possible to give simple answers to questions about main effects, such as, "*Which medication results in the greatest weight loss?*" In the presence of a statistically significant interaction, the answer to this question is "*It depends.*" In the example, it depends on the sex of the patient. For men, Medication 3 is most effective. For women, there is no evidence that any of the active medications (i.e., Medication 1, Medication 2, and Medication 3) is superior to the others.

Statistically significant interactions are often depicted graphically to help visualize the nature of the interaction. The data provided in Box 4-10 is shown graphically in Figure 4-1. The outcome variable (weight change) is plotted on the y-axis, and sex is indicated on the x-axis. Each line corresponds to a different treatment. For each treatment, the mean weight change for men is indicated at the beginning of the line and the mean weight change for women is indicated at the end of the line. For example, you can see that the mean weight loss for men taking Medication 3 was about 60 pounds, whereas women taking Medication 3 lost an average of about 30 pounds. Interactions can be identified in graphs when the lines associated with different groups are not all parallel to one another. Figure 4-1 is an example of a pattern of findings suggesting the presence of an interaction between treatment and sex. Clearly, the lines are not all parallel to one another.

The pattern of the lines in this type of figure conveys considerably more information than just whether or not an interaction is present. Figure 4-2 shows a main effect of both sex and treatment but with the absence of a sex-treatment interaction. (Note: The data portrayed in these figures do not correspond to the data provided in Box 4-9.) The slope of each line indexes the main effect of sex. The steeper the line is, the greater the effect of sex on weight change. The vertical distance between the lines indexes the main effect of treatment. The greater the vertical distance between the lines is, the greater the effect of treatment. Although the effect of sex is similar in both figures, the effect of treatment is quite distinct. In the left panel in Figure 4-2, Medication 3 results in the greatest weight loss, followed by Medication 1, followed by Medication 2. All three medications are superior to Placebo. In the panel on the right in Figure 4-2, although all three medications are still superior to Placebo, they are all similar to one another. That is, Medications 1, 2, and 3 all result in a loss of about 30 pounds among men and 50 pounds among women. The pattern of group means depicted in both panels in Figure 4-2 is consistent with a main effect of treatment, despite the lack of differences among the three active medications in the right panel. This is because the null hypothesis is that all of the means are equal to one another. Thus, differences between Placebo and the three active medications can lead to rejection of the null hypothesis, even when the active medications are equally effective.

The panels in Figure 4-3 depict other possible patterns of findings. The top left panel depicts a pattern consistent with a significant effect of sex (apparent from the slope of the lines) but no effect of treatment (because there is little distance between the lines). The top right panel depicts a pattern consistent with a

BOX 4-10. Example of Factorial ANOVA

Continuing with the fictitious weight loss example introduced in Box 4-8, we will add sex as a second independent variable. This will allow us to answer two questions:

1. Does weight loss differ between men and women? This question involves testing for the presence of a **main effect** of sex on weight loss.
2. Does the effectiveness of the specific treatments vary as a function of participant sex? This question involves testing for the presence of an **interaction** between treatment and sex.

The table below shows the mean weight loss observed in each treatment group stratified by sex and the mean weight loss for men and women. The values shown are based on the raw data provided in Box 4-9.

Mean Weight Change by Treatment Group and Sex

Sex	Placebo	Med 1	Med 2	Med 3	Mean
Male	+20	–1	+10	–60	–7.75
Female	–10	–29	–20	–30	–22.25
Overall	+5	–15	–5	–45	–15

Med, medication.

The data have not changed. Therefore,

Total SS = 18,954 and Between Groups SS for "Treatment" = 11,200, just as they did before.

Between Groups SS for "Sex" was calculated as follows:

$$\sum n_{Group}\left(\bar{X}_{Group} - \bar{X}_{Overall}\right)^2 = 16(-22.25-(-15))^2 + 16(-7.75-(-15))^2 = 1{,}682$$

Formulas for calculating the SS for the interaction between sex and treatment group are fairly complex. Therefore, I used a statistical analysis program called SAS to compute this value. The results of that analysis are shown to the right. They reveal that the SS for the interaction term is 5,286.

The SAS System

The ANOVA Procedure

Dependent Variable: Change

Source	DF	Sum of Squares	Mean Square	F Value	Pr > F
Model	7	18,168.00000	2,595.42857	79.25	<.0001
Error	24	786.00000	32.75000		
Corrected Total	31	18,954.00000			

R-Square	Coeff Var	Root MSE	Change Mean
0.958531	-38.15174	5.722762	-15.00000

Source	DF	ANOVA SS	Mean Square	F Value	Pr > F
Treatment_Group	3	11,200.00000	3,733.33333	113.99	<.0001
Sex	1	1,682.00000	1,682.00000	51.36	<.0001
Sex*Treatment_Group	3	5,286.00000	1,762.00000	53.80	<.0001

Coeff Var, coefficient of variation; DF, degrees of freedom; MSE, mean squared error; Pr, probability; SS, sum of squares.

(continued)

BOX 4-10. Example of Factorial ANOVA *(Continued)*

Because there are now two between groups SS terms and the SS term for the interaction, the formula for calculating the error SS becomes:

$$Error\ SS = Total\ SS - Between\ Groups\ SS_{Treatment} - Between\ Groups\ SS_{Gender} - Interaction\ SS$$

Thus, *Error SS* = 18,954 – 11,200 – 1,682 – 5,286 = 786.

The F-statistic for "Treatment" is calculated as $F(3,24) = \frac{SS_{Between}/df}{SS_{Error}/df} = \frac{11,200/3}{786/24} = 113.99$

The F-statistic for "Sex" is calculated as $F(1,24) = \frac{SS_{Between}/df}{SS_{Error}/df} = \frac{1,682/1}{786/24} = 51.36$

The F-statistic for the interaction term is calculated as

$$F(3,24) = \frac{SS_{Between}/df}{SS_{Error}/df} = \frac{5,286/3}{786/24} = 53.80$$

All of these F-statistics are very large, and all are statistically significant at $P < 0.0001$. However, because the interaction term is statistically significant, we cannot use information from this analysis to answer questions concerning the main effect of "Treatment" or "Sex." That is because, in this example, the significant interaction suggests that (a) the effectiveness of the four treatments depends on the sex of the patient and (b) the amount of weight lost by men and women depends on the type of treatment received.

When an analysis reveals a statistically significant interaction between two independent variables, the investigators usually stratify the sample on one of the independent variables and then rerun their analysis, looking at the main effect of the other independent variable within each stratum. Because we are most interested in the effect of treatment on weight loss, I stratified the sample by sex and reexamined the effect of treatment group on weight loss separately for men and women. The results for this analysis are shown below. Tukey's honestly significant difference test was used to perform post hoc comparisons.

Weight Loss (Pounds)

Sex	Placebo	Medication 1	Medication 2	Medication 3	p
Males	+20[a]	–1[b]	+10[a,b]	–60[c]	<0.0001
Females	–10[a]	–29[b]	–20[b]	–30[b]	<0.001

From the *P* values in the rightmost column, you can see that treatment had a statistically significant effect on weight loss among both men and women.

Within each row of the table, the difference in weight loss between groups that share a superscript is not statistically significant. You can see from the superscripts that, **among men**, Medication 3 produced significantly greater weight loss than any of the other treatments. In addition, Medication 2 was no more effective than placebo. In contrast, **among women**, all three treatments worked better than placebo, but the differences between the groups taking Medication 1, 2, and 3 were not statistically significant. That is, **among women**, there is not sufficient evidence to conclude that any of the medications are more effective than the others.

FIGURE 4-1. Significant Interaction Based on Data in Box 4-10

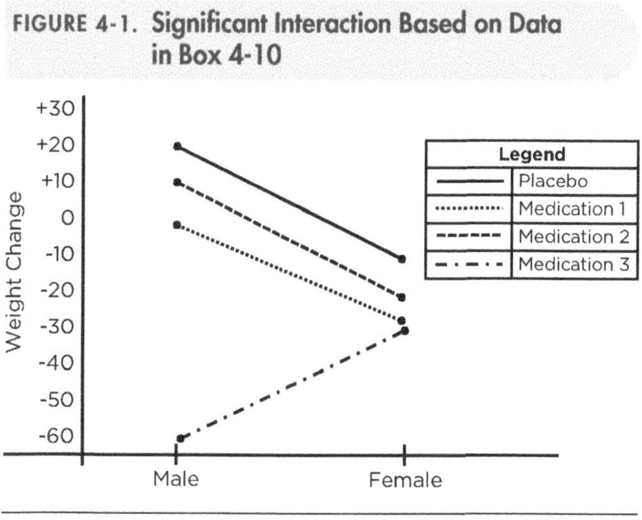

significant treatment effect (apparent from the distance between the lines) but no sex effect (because the lines are flat). Finally, the bottom panel depicts a pattern consistent with the absence of any main effects; the lines are flat with little distance between them.

Repeated Measures ANOVA

In 1-way ANOVA and factorial ANOVA, each study participant is assessed one time only. Repeated measures ANOVA is used when each participant is assessed multiple times. This situation most often arises within the context of crossover research designs. In these types of designs, each participant is exposed to each treatment being evaluated. For example, after enrolling in a study examining the effectiveness of several analgesics for chronic pain, participants might first take Medication A for 2 weeks. Then, they might undergo a "washout period" during which they take no medications. Then, they might take Medication B for 2 weeks, undergo another washout period, and so on until they have taken all of the medications being evaluated. Pain would be assessed while taking each medication.

FIGURE 4-2. Appearance of Main Effects of Both Sex and Treatment with No Interaction

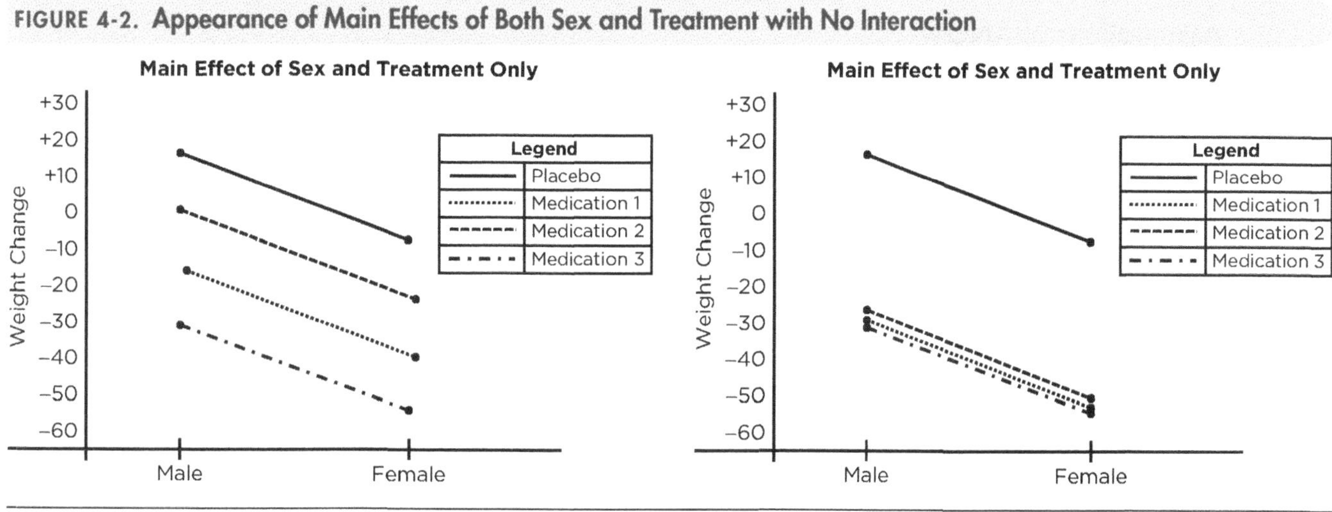

FIGURE 4-3. **Appearance of Other Alternative Findings**

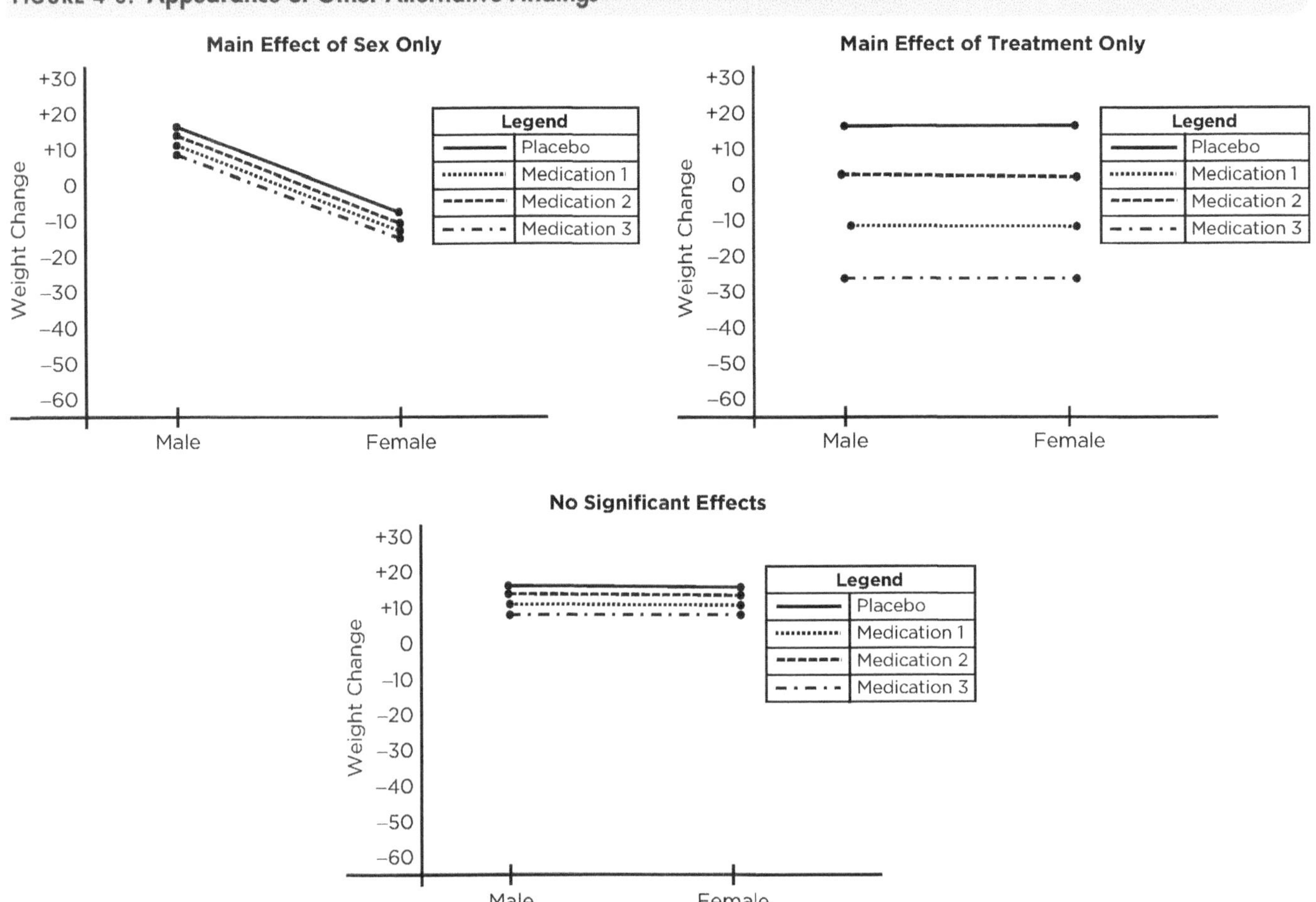

This type of design can be very powerful because it allows investigators to remove variance in the outcome variable that is due to individual variability in the same way that this is achieved when using paired t-tests. In these designs, "person" is treated as an independent variable. Thus, any variance that can be explained by individual differences is removed from the error SS, making it easier to detect relationships among the primary variables of interest.

Assumptions of ANOVA

The primary assumptions of ANOVA parallel those for t-tests:

1. The outcome variable is measured on a numerical scale.
2. The outcome variable is normally distributed in each group **or** N in each group ≥30.
3. The variance of the outcome variable is approximately the same in all groups. Small differences are not usually problematic. Further, if the number of people within each group is about the same, large differences in variance are not problematic. However, where there are large differences in variance (differences in the twofold range or greater) **and** large differences in group size (again, differences in the twofold range or greater), ANOVA should not be used. (Note: Regression procedures should be used in these instances.)
4. The observations in the sample are independent of one another. (Note: This assumption does **not** apply to repeated measures ANOVA, where clearly the observations in the sample are not independent of one another.)

Examples from the Literature

The main goal of this book is to help health care professionals develop the skills and confidence needed to read the medical literature. Therefore, this section focuses on a few examples of studies that have used the statistical procedures discussed in this chapter. In my discussion of these studies, I focus on issues pertaining to the interpretation of study findings.

The first study was conducted by Curington and colleagues.[1] This study examined the clinical outcomes of patients with type 2 diabetes who were switched from insulin glargine to NPH insulin. All patients received care at a charitable community pharmacy in Cincinnati. A total of 29 patients were enrolled in the study. Of these, 15 were using NPH insulin at baseline (referred to as the control group by study investigators), and 14 were switched from insulin glargine to NPH insulin as part of the study protocol (intervention group). (Note: It would have been more appropriate to label the group of patients taking NPH insulin at baseline as the "*comparison*" group. The term "control" group is best reserved for studies that involve randomization to treatment arm.) All patients were followed for 24 weeks. The primary outcome variables were HbA1c, 30-day average blood glucose, number of suspected and confirmed hypoglycemic episodes, total insulin dose, and medication adherence. Of the 29 patients enrolled in the study, only 17 completed the 24-week follow-up.

Table 1 in Box 4-11 shows the characteristics of study participants at baseline, stratified by group. Note that the far-right column provides *P* values. The footnote explains that data for continuous variables are presented as means ± SD and that between group differences for these variables were evaluated via t-tests. Although the authors do not say explicitly, the two groups are independent. Therefore, I am confident that they used independent groups t-tests.

I framed all of the continuous variables shown in Table 1 in rectangles. You can see that most of the between group differences are not statistically significant (i.e., $P > 0.05$). However, the total daily dose of insulin was significantly lower in the intervention group ($P = 0.02$), and people in the intervention group were a bit older ($P = 0.05$).

The primary study findings are presented in Table 2. At each time point, the investigators performed an independent groups t-test on each of the outcome variables—a total of 21 separate tests. This is an example of multiple comparisons, which creates a problem due to the potential to inflate Type I (α) error. Nonetheless, few differences were observed. The investigators in this study were limited in what they could do because of the small sample size. However, the findings in Table 2 are difficult to interpret because any differences at the follow-up assessments may have been due to differences at baseline. This is most evident from the significant difference in total daily dose of insulin at the 4-week follow-up. The lower daily dose of insulin taken by people in the intervention group at the 4-week follow-up is due to their lower dose at baseline. An alternative analytic strategy would have been to create change scores (like we did earlier in this chapter when discussing the fictitious weight loss study). This would have allowed the investigators to focus on **change** in the outcome variables following implementation of the intervention. (With a larger sample, a better approach is to use regression analysis to control for potential confounders such as baseline differences between groups. We will cover regression procedures in a later chapter.) Finally, whenever investigators report nonsignificant findings, readers should ask whether they had sufficient power to detect clinically meaningful effects. This study did not include a power analysis. The investigators acknowledge in the Discussion section that lack of power could have contributed to their findings. In addition, although not related to the primary study findings, lack of power is evident in Table 1. For example, individuals in the control group had been using insulin for an average of 9.2 years compared to 5.2 years in the intervention group. This seems like a large difference. Yet, it is not statistically significant due to the small sample size.

The second study examined the effect of a telephone call reminder program on medication adherence among older adults with hypertension.[2] The study used a quasi-experimental research design. All participants in the intervention group participated in at least one live interactive call with a pharmacist

BOX 4-11. NPH Insulin Study

Table 1
Baseline characteristics

Characteristic	Control: NPH insulin (n = 15)	Intervention: glargine to NPH (n = 14)	*P* value
Background			
Age (y)	53.0 ± 5.1	56.9 ± 4.9	0.05
Female, n (%)	11 (73.3)	9 (64.3)	0.70
Weight (kg)	115.8 ± 30.7	109.0 ± 18.2	0.48
BMI (kg/m^2)	40.0 ± 8.0	37.9 ± 3.9	0.39
Diabetes duration (y)	15.9 ± 8.2	12.1 ± 8.2	0.22
Insulin duration (y)	9.2 ± 7.5	5.2 ± 4.4	0.10
Ethnicity, n (%)			
Black	8 (53.3)	9 (64.3)	0.71
White	7 (46.7)	5 (35.7)	0.71
Education, n (%)			
High school graduate	14 (93.3)	13 (92.9)	1.00
College education	9 (60)	6 (42.9)	0.47
Oral antidiabetic agents, n (%)			
Metformin	9 (60)	7 (50)	0.72
Other	5 (33.3)	2 (14.3)	0.39
HbA_{1c}, % (mmol/mol)	9.0 ± 1.6 (75 ± 18)	8.8 ± 1.7 (73 ± 19)	0.79
30-day hypoglycemic events (baseline)			
Signs/symptoms (episodes)	2.1 ± 2.6	1.0 ± 1.5	0.20
Confirmed BG <70 mg/dL (episodes)	1.7 ± 3.9	0.6 ± 1.5	0.36
Insulin use			
TDD insulin (U)	108.4 ± 63.5	57.6 ± 38.3	0.02
Adherence (MMAS)	6.6 ± 1.9	6.2 ± 2.0	0.60

BMI, body mass index
Data presented as mean ± SD for continuous and n (%) for categoric parameters. *P* value determined by *t* test (continuous variables) or Fisher exact χ^2 test (categoric variables).
Abbreviations used: BG, blood glucose; MMAS, Morisky Medication Adherence Scale; TDD, total daily dose.

Table 2
Results

Characteristic	n	Control: NPH insulin	n	Intervention: glargine to NPH	*P* value
HbA_{1c}, % (mmol/mol)					
Baseline	15	9.0 ±1.6 (75 ±18)	14	8.8 ±1.7 (73 ±19)	0.79
Week 12	12	8.7 ±2.2 (72 ±24)	9	8.7 ±1.3 (71 ±14)	0.96
Week 24	10	8.0 ±1.9 (64 ±20)	7	7.8 ±1.6 (62 ±18)	0.79
Average BG (mg/dL)					
Week 4	15	173.9 ±48.0	14	172.8 ±34.2	0.95
Week 12	12	175.4 ±61.3	9	159.0 ±32.2	0.48
Week 24	10	179.0 ±73.9	7	141.6 ±46.6	0.26
Hypoglycemic symptoms (episodes)					
Baseline	15	2.1 ±2.6	14	1.0 ±1.5	0.20
Week 4	15	0.7 ±1.4	11	0.5 ±1.2	0.82
Week 12	12	1.6 ±1.6	9	0.6 ±1.0	0.09
Week 24	10	0.9 ±1.3	7	0.9 ±1.9	0.96
Hypoglycemia confirmed (BG <70 mg/dL, episodes)					
Baseline	15	1.7 ±3.9	14	0.6 ±1.5	0.36
Week 4	15	0.3 ±0.9	11	0.2 ±0.6	0.63
Week 12	12	0.7 ±1.1	9	0.3 ±1.0	0.48
Week 24	10	0.3 ±0.7	7	0.6 ±1.1	0.54
TDD (U)					
Baseline	15	108.4 ±63.5	14	57.6 ±38.3	0.02
Week 4	15	113.6 ±66.9	11	57.8 ±41.3	0.02
Week 12	12	103.9 ±71.2	9	62.8 ±32.7	0.13
Week 24	10	98.6 ±76.0	7	46.4 ±19.4	0.10
Adherence (MMAS)					
Baseline	15	6.6 ±1.9	14	6.2 ±2.0	0.60
Week 12	12	7.0 ±1.6	9	7.3 ±1.0	0.68
Week 24	10	6.7 ±1.6	7	6.5 ±2.0	0.83

Data presented as mean ±SD for continuous and n (%) for categoric parameters. *P* value determined by *t* test (continuous variables) or Fisher exact χ^2 test (categoric variables).
Abbreviations as in Table 1.

focused on the patient's medication use. Participants in the control group were drawn from patients who were served by the same call center and met study inclusion criteria but who did not participate in any calls. (As in the previous study, because participants were not randomly assigned to their treatment group, it would be most appropriate to refer to the group that did not receive the intervention as a "*comparison*" group.) Each patient in the intervention group was matched to a control on age, sex, county of residence, and medication adherence during the 6-month period prior to implementation of the intervention. Medication adherence was defined as the proportion of days covered (PDC), which reflects the number of days during the study period that patients were in possession of their antihypertensive medications based on their medication refill records. The PDC ranges from 0 to 100%, with higher scores reflecting greater adherence. Data analyses used a difference-in-differences approach. This approach involves comparing change over time in one group to change over time in the other group. There were a total of 563 pairs of patients (i.e., 563 intervention participants and 563 matched controls).

The primary findings from the study are shown in Table 2 in Box 4-12. The investigators used paired t-tests to determine that the increase in PDC from the preintervention period to the postintervention period was statistically significant in both the intervention and control groups (intervention: $\bar{X} = 17.33\%$, $SD = 33.56$; control: $\bar{X} = 13.83\%$, $SD = 32.34$). Using another paired t-test, they found that the difference in improvement between the two groups was also statistically significant ($X = 3.50\%$, $SD = 36.28$, $p = 0.022$). Thus,

BOX 4-12. Telephone Call Reminder Study

Table 2

Change in adherence 6-month postintervention period versus 6-month preintervention period for patients in the intervention and control groups

Proportion of days covered	Intervention group (n = 563)			Matched control group (n = 563)			Difference-in-differences	
	6-month postintervention	Change	*P* value	6-month postintervention	Change	*P* value	Difference-in-differences	*P* value[a]
Mean (SD)	80.5 (22.0)	17.33 (33.56)	<0.001[b]	76.1 (25.9)	13.83 (32.34)	<0.001[b]	3.50 (36.28)	0.022
No. patients ≥80%, n (%)	365 (64.8)	140 (24.9)	<0.001[c]	335 (59.5)	121 (21.5)	<0.001[c]	N/A	

SD, standard deviation

[a] *P* values compare the difference-in-differences (Changes in intervention group − Changes in matched control groups) using paired *t* test.

[b] *P* values compare changes between the 6-month preintervention and postintervention using paired *t* tests.

[c] *P* values compare changes between the 6-month preintervention and postintervention using McNemar test.

Appendix C

Subgroup analysis for adherence changes within intervention and control groups

PDC	Intervention group					Control group				
	N	6-month preintervention, PDC, mean (SD)	6-month postintervention, PDC, mean (SD)	Change in PDC, mean (SD)	*P* value[a]	N	6-month preintervention, PDC, mean (SD)	6-month postintervention PDC, mean (SD)	Change in PDC, mean (SD)	*P* value[a]
Medication treatment patterns										
Mono therapy	264	77.3 (25.9)	85.9 (18.8)	8.5 (29.4)	<0.001[b]	209	87.8 (19.2)	82.6 (23.4)	−5.3 (25.5)	<0.001
Dual therapy	214	53.1 (28.6)	78.4 (22.7)	25.3 (35.0)[c]	1	263	49.7 (23.7)	73.9 (26.6)	24.2 (30.4)[c]	1
Triple therapy	85	44.2 (23.9)	68.9 (24.1)	24.7 (35.5)[c]		91	39.8 (20.7)	67.5 (26.2)	27.6 (31.4)[c]	
Number of reminder calls										
1	374	66.4 (28.4)	80.1 (21.5)	13.7 (31.4)	<0.001	N/A				N/A
2	138	62.2 (29.4)	79.6 (23.3)	17.5 (34.2)	2					
≥3	51	41.8 (33.3)	85.2 (21.4)	43.4 (36.0)[d]						
Age (y)										
<70	128	59.2 (30.6)	80.7 (22.1)	21.5 (35.3)	0.136	119	60.9 (30.0)	77.2 (26.0)	16.4 (31.6)	0.237
70–80	228	62.3 (29.5)	79.6 (22.7)	17.3 (33.9)	3	232	60.9 (28.0)	76.1 (25.6)	15.2 (32.1)	3
>80	207	66.5 (30.0)	81.3 (21.1)	14.8 (31.9)		212	64.6 (30.8)	75.5 (26.3)	10.9 (33.0)	

Abbreviations used: PDC, Proportion of days covered; N/A, not available.

[a] *P* values compare changes in PDC between the 6-month preintervention and postintervention within group using analysis of variance test.

[b] Generalized estimating equation adjusted regression shows that the *P* value was statistically significant (*P* <0.05).

[c] Post hoc pairwise comparison using Bonferroni test indicates that change in PDC (dual and triple therapy) was statistically significantly higher compared to patients with monotherapy (*P* <0.05).

[d] Post hoc pairwise comparison using Bonferroni test indicates that change in PDC (≥3 reminder calls) was statistically significantly higher compared with patients receiving 1 or 2 reminder calls, respectively (*P* <0.05).

the investigators concluded that the telephone reminder intervention had a beneficial effect on medication adherence.

The table labeled Appendix C in Box 4-12 shows the results of subgroup analyses conducted to determine if certain subgroups of patients benefited from the intervention more than others. Data from the intervention and control groups were analyzed separately using 1-way ANOVA to test the null hypotheses that change over time was **not** related to (1) medication treatment patterns, (2) the number of reminder calls, and (3) patient age. Post hoc pairwise comparisons were used to examine the specific subgroups that differed from one another. In the first set of rows in Appendix C (designated by 1), you can see that there was a significant association between change in PDC and medication treatment pattern. In both the intervention and control groups, PDC increased less among people using monotherapy compared to those using either dual or triple therapy. However, there was no difference in PDC among those using dual versus triple therapy, as can be seen by the shared "c" superscripts. In the second set of rows (designated by 2), you can see that PDC increased more among people who received three or more calls than among those who received either one or two calls. Finally, in the last set of rows (designated by 3), you can see that change in PDC over time was not related to patient age. This conclusion can be reached on the basis of the *P* values of 0.136 and 0.237 provided for the intervention and control groups, respectively.

The third study examined factors associated with pharmacists' perceptions of the ease with which they could find a different position with specific characteristics.[3] This variable is called "perceived job alternatives" and includes four separate dimensions: environmental conditions (e.g., lower workload, less stress), professional opportunities (e.g., more intellectual challenge, more patient contact), compensation (e.g., better pay, better benefits), and coworkers (e.g., better pharmacist and technician coworkers). The independent variables used to predict scores on the different dimensions of perceived job alternatives include demographics (e.g., age, gender), practice characteristics (e.g., primary work setting), and work life attitudes (e.g., job satisfaction, professional commitment).

Data were collected via a cross-sectional survey completed by a nationally representative sample of 1,574 practicing pharmacists. Although no power analysis was reported in this paper, lack of power is unlikely to be a problem given the fairly large sample size. However, in large samples, readers must remember that small differences that are not clinically meaningful may be statistically significant. Therefore, readers should always ask whether any statistically significant differences reported are clinically meaningful.

The table in Box 4-13 shows the results of analyses examining differences in pharmacist ratings on the four dimensions of perceived job alternatives (i.e., environmental conditions, professional opportunities, compensation, coworkers) as a function of demographic and practice characteristics. Note that whenever the independent variable involved two groups (e.g., gender, race, job position), t-tests were used to assess between group differences. When the independent variable involved more than two groups (e.g., age classification, primary work setting), 1-way ANOVA was used. You can see from the table that younger pharmacists (≤ 30 years old) perceived that it would be easier to find a different position with better environmental conditions, professional opportunities, and compensation compared to older pharmacists (> 60 years old). You can also see from the table that pharmacists licensed since the year 2000 perceived that it would be easier to find a different position with better environmental conditions, professional opportunities, compensation, and coworkers compared to pharmacists licensed earlier. Note that these two sets of findings are unlikely to be independent because age and year of licensure are probably highly correlated. The data reported in Box 4-13 do not take any correlations among the independent variables into consideration. However, in other analyses reported in the paper, the investigators used regression analyses to control for intercorrelations among the independent variables. We will return to this study to look at those findings in Chapter 7, which covers linear regression. Finally, beware of the potential inflation of Type I (α) error by all of the comparisons made in Box 4-13. It is likely that some of the significant findings reported are due to Type I (α) error. For this reason, the analyses reported in Box 4-13 are best thought of as exploratory.

BOX 4-13. Perceived Job Alternatives Study

Table 4

Means and standard deviations of perceived job alternatives dimensions according to independent variables

Characteristic	Environmental conditions	Professional opportunities	Compensation	Coworkers
Demographic variables				
Gender[a]				
Male	11.72 ± 3.91	12.91 ± 3.56	7.20 ± 2.46[*]	4.59 ± 1.60
Female	11.98 ± 3.72	13.14 ± 3.50	7.66 ± 2.42	4.52 ± 1.64
Age (y)[b]				
≤30	13.09 ± 3.62[c]	13.85 ± 3.53[c]	7.98 ± 2.45[c]	4.68 ± 1.52
31-40	12.17 ± 3.93[c,d]	13.35 ± 3.55[c]	7.67 ± 2.34[c,d]	4.73 ± 1.64
41-50	11.64 ± 3.80[d]	12.88 ± 3.49[c,d]	7.43 ± 2.50[c,d]	4.45 ± 1.60
51-60	11.67 ± 3.69[d]	3.07 ± 3.37[c,d]	7.35 ± 2.36[c,d]	4.54 ± 1.62
>60	11.17 ± 3.68[d]	12.09 ± 3.63[d]	7.01 ± 2.65[d]	4.29 ± 1.69
Race[a]				
White	11.94 ± 3.79	13.02 ± 3.53	7.54 ± 2.47[*]	4.48 ± 1.62[*]
Nonwhite	11.56 ± 3.91	13.19 ± 3.55	7.08 ± 2.28	4.84 ± 1.63
Marital status[b]				
Single	12.24 ± 3.77	13.38 ± 3.54	7.64 ± 2.53	4.63 ± 1.62
Married or partnered	11.82 ± 3.66	12.98 ± 3.92	7.46 ± 2.46	4.51 ± 1.55
Divorced or widowed	11.70 ± 3.83	13.05 ± 3.49	7.44 ± 2.44	4.75 ± 1.64
Degree held[a]				
PharmD	12.19 ± 3.88[*]	13.23 ± 3.59	7.63 ± 2.49	4.61 ± 1.59
No PharmD	11.57 ± 3.69	12.82 ± 3.51	7.35 ± 2.34	4.48 ± 1.67
Year of licensure[a]				
Before 2000	11.60 ± 3.70[*]	12.82 ± 3.43[*]	7.34 ± 2.46[*]	4.47 ± 1.65[*]
Since 2000	12.34 ± 3.91	13.45 ± 3.63	7.69 ± 2.42	4.69 ± 1.56
Practice variables				
Primary work setting[b]				
Community	11.85 ± 4.01[†]	13.07 ± 3.48	7.39 ± 2.45	4.61 ± 1.57
Other patient care	11.23 ± 3.77	13.08 ± 3.77	7.61 ± 2.70	4.47 ± 1.65
Health-system pharmacy	12.15 ± 3.56	12.95 ± 3.50	7.47 ± 2.33	4.49 ± 1.67
Other nonpatient care	12.32 ± 3.15	13.36 ± 3.46	7.76 ± 2.26	4.64 ± 1.72
Work status[a]				
Full-time	11.90 ± 3.86	13.04 ± 3.52	7.41 ± 2.44[*]	4.54 ± 1.62
Part-time	11.60 ± 3.36	13.15 ± 3.56	8.05 ± 2.40	4.53 ± 1.75
Job position[a]				
Manager	11.77 ± 3.98	12.46 ± 3.60[*]	7.10 ± 2.58[*]	4.47 ± 1.65
Staff	11.92 ± 3.71	13.34 ± 3.45	7.65 ± 2.35	4.59 ± 1.61
Years with current employer[b]				
≤5	11.71 ± 3.77	13.39 ± 3.56	7.89 ± 2.51[c]	4.67 ± 1.58[c]
6-10	12.19 ± 3.89	12.98 ± 3.70	7.31 ± 2.53[d]	4.53 ± 1.63[c,d]
11-15	11.82 ± 3.60	12.96 ± 3.34	7.32 ± 2.20[c,d]	4.64 ± 1.67[c,d]
>15	11.82 ± 3.89	12.72 ± 3.40	7.12 ± 2.36[d]	4.32 ± 1.59[d]

Pharmacists with higher responses perceived that it would be easier to find a job with these aspects.

[a] *t* tests were used to test differences in mean scores across levels of the independent variables.

[b] One-way analysis of variance (ANOVA) was used to test differences in mean scores across levels of the independent variables.

[c,d] Within the same perceived job alternatives dimension, means followed by the same letter are not significantly different at the 0.05 level with the use of Scheffé post hoc tests.

[*] Statistically significant association via *t* test at $P < 0.05$.

[†] The overall F test via one-way ANOVA at $P < 0.05$ was statistically significant. However, Scheffé post hoc pairwise comparisons revealed no statistically significant differences.

Self-Study Questions

1. In ANOVA, as the difference in observed means increases, what happens to the between groups sums of squares (SS)?

   A. The between groups SS increases.
   B. The between groups SS stays the same.
   C. The between groups SS decreases.

2. Is the following statement true or false? Addition of predictor variables to an ANOVA has no effect on the F-test associated with predictor variables that have been added previously. (True/False)

3. Is the following statement true or false? A variable involved in an interaction is sometimes called an effect modifier. (True/False)

4. As predictor variables are added to an ANOVA, which of the following tend to decrease?

   A. Error SS
   B. Between-groups SS
   C. Total SS
   D. Error SS **and** total SS

5. In a journal article, the authors perform an ANOVA and report that $F(2,298) = 0.84$, ns. (The abbreviation "ns" means Not Significant.) The next step in the analysis is to:

   A. Perform a Tukey's honestly significant difference test
   B. Perform a Student-Newman-Keuls test
   C. Perform a Bonferroni correction
   D. Stop; no further analyses should be performed since the overall F-test was not significant

6. Imagine that you are given the data from a trial that randomly assigned 400 participants to one of four treatments for hypertension. The outcome that was being studied in this trial was blood pressure, measured in mmHg. Given just this information, what type of statistical analysis would be most appropriate to assess treatment effect?

   A. A 1-sample t-test
   B. A 1-way ANOVA
   C. A paired t-test
   D. Factorial ANOVA

7. In an ANOVA, the between groups SS reflects:

   A. The portion of variance in the independent variable that is explained by the dependent variable
   B. The portion of variance in the dependent variable that is explained by the independent variable
   C. The portion of variance in the independent variable that is **not** explained by the dependent variable
   D. The portion of variance in the dependent variable that is **not** explained by the independent variable

8. Assume that a team of investigators is studying the impact of lifestyle modifications on weight loss. They assign 300 subjects to one of the following three options: exercise only, low-carbohydrate diet only, and low-fat diet only. During the course of the study, each participant is assigned to one of the treatment arms for one month and then their weights are assessed. After this month, they are switched to one of the other two treatment arms for an additional month and have their weight assessed again. Finally, they enter the third treatment arm and have their weight assessed at the end of that month. At the end of the trial, each of the 300 participants has tested each of the lifestyle modifications for 1 month. To analyze these data, the investigators would probably use:

   A. 1-Way ANOVA
   B. Factorial ANOVA
   C. Repeated measures ANOVA
   D. Kruskal-Wallis ANOVA

9. If all other things are held constant, as alpha error increases:

   A. Power decreases
   B. The chance of missing a true effect increases
   C. The chance of incorrectly rejecting the null hypothesis increases
   D. Beta error decreases
   E. Both C and D

10. Which of the following would usually be considered an acceptable level of power in a study?

    A. 0.05
    B. 0.60
    C. 0.80
    D. 0.90
    E. Both C and D

11. All other things held constant, as sample size increases:

A. Alpha error usually decreases
B. Power usually decreases
C. Power usually increases
D. The magnitude of the true difference usually increases

12. Imagine that a study is conducted examining the effect of a new medication on bone density. Individuals in the study are randomly assigned to receive either the new medication or placebo. Individuals then are followed for 1 year, and bone density is assessed at the end of the year. In the results of the paper reporting study findings, the authors write that the bone density of people taking the new medication was greater than those taking placebo and that the mean difference was 0.04 g/cm^2 (95% CI: –0.02 to 0.10 g/cm^2). Based just on these findings, what would you conclude?

A. The difference between people taking placebo versus the new medication was statistically significant.
B. The difference between people taking placebo versus the new medication was **not** statistically significant.
C. The difference between people taking placebo versus the new medication was clinically meaningful.
D. There is insufficient information presented to draw any conclusions.

13. Another study assessed the effect of the same medication discussed in the last question. This time a before-after study design was used. All 100 people in the study took the new medication. Bone density was assessed at two points in time: before the initiation of therapy and again 6 months later. The mean difference in bone density between these two time periods was 0.15 g/cm^2 (SD=0.2 g/cm^2). What is the 95% CI for the difference score?

A. 0.13 to 0.17 g/cm^2
B. –0.05 to 0.35 g/cm^2
C. 0.11 to 0.19 g/cm^2
D. –0.25 to 0.55 g/cm^2
E. The 95% CI cannot be determined from the information provided.

14. Which of the following statistical tests would be most appropriate to use to analyze the data in the study described in Question 13?

A. 1-sample t-test
B. Paired t-test
C. Independent groups t-test
D. ANOVA

15. Imagine that the same set of data is analyzed using both CIs and an appropriate t-test. How will the conclusions drawn using these different approaches compare?

A. They will **always** lead to the same conclusion with respect to whether the null hypothesis should be accepted or rejected.
B. They will **usually** (but **not** always) lead to the same conclusion with respect to whether the null hypothesis should be accepted or rejected.
C. As a general rule, they will lead to different conclusions with respect to whether the null hypothesis should be accepted or rejected.

16. Is the following statement true or false? A difference observed in a study can be statistically significant without being clinically meaningful. (True/False)

17. T-tests assume that the dependent variable is measured on what type of scale?

A. Nominal
B. Dichotomous
C. Ordinal
D. Numerical
E. Either C or D

18. When one looks at a figure presenting results of a factorial ANOVA, interactions are usually detected by:

A. The point at which different lines intersect the y-axis
B. The point at which different lines intersect the x-axis
C. A lack of parallelism among the lines corresponding to the different groups
D. Either A or B

19. Imagine that you are reading a paper. It states that the sample size was determined so that the study would have 80% power to detect a change in blood pressure of 10 mmHg. Which of the following is a correct interpretation of this statement?

A. If the drug alters blood pressure by less than 10 mmHg, the investigators have an 80% chance of correctly identifying this effect.
B. If the drug alters blood pressure by 10 mmHg or more, the investigators have an 80% chance of correctly identifying this effect.
C. If the drug alters blood pressure by 10 mmHg or more, the investigators have a 20% chance of failing to detect this effect.
D. Both B and C
E. Both A and C

20. Imagine that you are reading a paper. It states that the study has 50% power to detect a change in blood pressure of 10 mmHg. Which of the following is a correct interpretation of this statement?

A. If the drug alters blood pressure by less than 10 mmHg, the investigators had a 50% chance of correctly identifying this effect.
B. If the drug alters blood pressure by 10 mmHg or more, the investigators had a 50% chance of correctly identifying this effect.
C. If a change in blood pressure of 10 mmHg is clinically meaningful, the study was **not** sufficiently powered.
D. Both B and C

21. When performing a t-test, the null hypothesis is rejected when:

A. The t-statistic is greater than the critical value
B. The investigators conclude that the medication under investigation is effective
C. The difference between the means being compared is unlikely to be "0"
D. All of the above

22. A study states: "Postintervention cases had shorter hospital stays compared with preintervention cases (median 6 vs 7 days, respectively; $P = 0.026$)." If alpha was set at 0.05, would the investigators conclude that this difference was statistically significant?

A. **Yes**, they would conclude that the difference is statistically significant.
B. **No**, they would **not** conclude that the difference is statistically significant.
C. Statistical significance cannot be determined from the information provided.

23. If alpha is set at 0.05 in a study, how likely is it that the investigators will conclude that a medication is effective when it is not?

A. They have a 5% chance of concluding that it is effective if it is not.
B. They have a 95% chance of concluding that it is effective if it is not.
C. They have an 80% chance of concluding that it is effective if it is not.
D. This is a trick question; they would never conclude that it is effective if it is not.
E. The likelihood cannot be determined from the information provided.

24. Clinicians often prefer CIs over hypothesis testing because:

A. CIs are more likely to lead to the correct conclusion
B. CIs are easier to compute
C. CIs provide more useful information
D. A and B
E. All of the above

25. Imagine that you are reading a journal article. It states that t=4.25, $P<0.04$. On the basis of this test, the authors conclude that there is a statistically significant difference between the treatments being evaluated. The value "$P<0.04$" means that:

A. The investigators were willing to accept a 5% chance of incorrectly rejecting the null hypothesis
B. The probability is less than 4% that a difference as large as the one observed would have occurred if, in reality, the treatments did not differ (i.e., in reality, the null hypothesis is true)
C. The study is adequately powered to identify the smallest clinically meaningful difference
D. The difference between the treatments is clinically meaningful

26. Performing multiple t-tests is a problem because:

A. It increases error variance
B. It inflates alpha error
C. It takes more time
D. It leads to computational errors
E. This is a trick question; performing multiple t-tests is not a problem

27. In the formulas for t-tests, the denominator term indexes:

A. The observed difference in means
B. Alpha error
C. Beta error
D. Sampling error
E. Power

28. What is the probability of making at least one alpha error if you perform five separate independent groups t-tests with alpha set at 0.01 for each test?

A. 1%
B. 5%
C. 10%
D. 15%
E. 20%

29. Which of the following is **not** an assumption of ANOVA?

A. The variance in the all groups is approximately equal.
B. The dependent variable is assessed on a numerical scale.
C. All predictor variables have no more than two groups.
D. Observations are independent of one another.

30. Which of the following is **not** an assumption of t-tests?

A. The outcome variable is measured on an ordinal scale.
B. The outcome variable is normally distributed, or the sample size is large enough to assume that the sampling distribution is normally distributed.
C. There cannot be more than two groups.

References

1. Curington R, Espel M, Heaton PC, et al. Clinical outcomes of switching from insulin glargine to NPH insulin in indigent patients at a charitable pharmacy: The Charitable Insulin NPH: Care for the Indigent study. *J Am Pharm Assoc.* 2017;57:S229–S35.
2. Park H, Adeyemi A, Want W, Roane TE. Impact of a telephonic outreach program on medication adherence in Medicare Advantage Prescription Drug (MAPD) plan beneficiaries. *J Am Pharm Assoc.* 2017;57:62–6.
3. Rojanasarot S, Gaither CA, Schommer JC, et al. Exploring pharmacists' perceived job alternatives: results from the 2014 National Pharmacist Workforce Survey. *J Am Pharm Assoc.* 2017;57:47–55.

Ordinal Outcome Variables

5

After reading this chapter, you should be able to do the following:

1. Describe the distinction between parametric and nonparametric statistics.
2. Explain the logic underlying the use of nonparametric statistics to analyze (1) ordinal outcome measures and (2) numerical outcome measures when the assumptions of parametric procedures are not met.
3. Describe the situations in which the following statistical tests would be used: (1) sign test, (2) Wilcoxon signed rank test, (3) Wilcoxon rank sum test, (4) Kruskal–Wallis analysis of variance (ANOVA), and (5) Friedman 2-Way ANOVA by ranks.
4. Interpret findings from studies that assess between group differences using the statistical tests listed above.

When an outcome variable is assessed on a numerical scale (i.e., interval or ratio) and observations are normally distributed, investigators use parametric procedures (e.g., t-tests, analysis of variance [ANOVA]) to examine differences involving means. Parametric procedures can be used for this purpose even if the outcome variable is not normally distributed as long as each mean estimate is based on a sample size of 30 or more. In studies of this size, the sampling distribution of the means can be assumed to be normal even if the observations in the sample are not.

This chapter covers nonparametric statistical tests that are used to analyze (1) ordinal outcome measures and (2) numerical outcome variables if the assumptions that underlie parametric procedures are not met. Unlike parametric procedures, nonparametric procedures do not make any assumptions about the probability distribution of the outcome measure. Nonparametric statistical tests usually involve converting raw scores on the outcome variable into ranks and then analyzing the ranks. The ranks maintain the fact that people who score higher on the variable have more of the characteristic of interest but ignore the precise differences between observations. For example, imagine that in a study of chronic pain, an investigator asks five people to rate their pain on a 10-point scale ranging from "1 = none at all" to "10 = worst pain imaginable." The ratings in the top row of Table 5-1 are obtained. The second row shows how the raw scores are converted to ranks. The ranks retain the order of the pain ratings. That is, the person with the least pain has the lowest rank and the person with the most pain has the highest rank. However, the ranks ignore how far the raw scores are apart. This is because the distance that separates adjacent numbers on an ordinal scale cannot be assumed to be equal across the range of the scale. Therefore, this information is ignored in statistical analyses involving ordinal outcome variables.

In this chapter, we will cover nonparametric statistical tests that are used in the four analytic situations shown in Table 5-2. These are the same situations discussed in Chapter 4 of this book in relation to t-tests and ANOVA. It may help to think of the nonparametric tests as alternatives to the parametric tests when the assumptions of the parametric tests are not met. Therefore, I have included both types of tests in the table.

TABLE 5-1. Fictitious Pain Rating Study

Characteristic	Person 1	Person 2	Person 3	Person 4	Person 5
Pain rating (raw score)	7	10	4	8	1
Rank	3	5	2	4	1

TABLE 5-2. Four Analytic Situations for Parametric and Nonparametric Tests

Analytic Context	Parametric–Numerical	Nonparametric–Ordinal
1 Sample; 1 data collection point	1-Sample t-test	Sign test
1 Sample; 2 data collection points	Paired t-test	Wilcoxon signed rank test
2 Samples; 1 data collection point	Independent groups t-test	Wilcoxon rank sum
More complex designs	ANOVA	Kruskal–Wallis ANOVA
	Factorial ANOVA	Friedman 2-way ANOVA by ranks
	Repeated measures ANOVA	

One Sample Assessed One Time: Sign Test

In this situation, investigators collect data from only one sample and compare the data they obtain to a reference population. The sign test is based on the notion that, if the distribution of a variable in a sample is the same as its distribution in a reference population, half of the values in the sample will be below the median of the reference population and half of the values in the sample will be above the median of the reference population. The binomial test can be used to calculate the probability that the pattern of data observed in the sample would have been observed **if the null hypothesis was true**. Box 5-1 provides an example of using the sign test to test a hypothesis involving an ordinal outcome variable.

One Sample Assessed Two Times: Wilcoxon Signed Rank Test

In this situation, investigators want to determine if the outcome changes over time. The Wilcoxon signed rank test is used for this purpose. This test is based on the notion that, **if the null hypothesis is true**, change should be equally likely in both directions. That is, people should be as likely to get worse as they are to get better. Moreover, the magnitude of change should be similar in both directions. That is, if some people get a lot better, one would expect some people to get a lot worse—**if the null hypothesis is true**. This is the same logic that underlies paired t-tests. When using paired t-tests, we expect the mean change over time to be "0" if the null hypothesis is true. However, when using Wilcoxon signed rank tests, raw scores are converted to ranks and the null hypothesis tested is that the mean of the signed ranks is "0." The signed ranks capture both the direction and the magnitude of change over time relative to others in the sample but do not rely on the precise change scores that are used for paired t-tests. Boxes 5-2 and 5-3 provide an example of using the Wilcoxon signed rank test to test a hypothesis involving an ordinal outcome variable.

BOX 5-1. Example of Sign Test

Imagine that 10 children take part in a study to determine if a recently marketed medication for allergic rhinitis is less effective in children than in adults. Data suggest that the median symptom relief reported among adults who take the medication is 7.5 on a 10-point scale, where "1 = No relief at all" and "10 = Complete relief of symptoms." The amount of symptom relief reported by the 10 children in the study is shown below.

Child	1	2	3	4	5	6	7	8	9	10
Symptom relief	1	10	2	6	8	3	4	5	4	2
Sign	–	+	–	–	+	–	–	–	–	–

In this example, if the medication were equally effective in children as in adults, 5 children should have scored above 7.5. However, only 2 children actually did so.

We can use the binomial formula to calculate the probability of observing this outcome if the medication was equally effective in children and adults.

In this example, n = 10, x = 2, and $\pi = 0.50$. Note that $\pi = 0.50$ because half of the participants are expected to score above the median **if the null hypothesis is true**.

Plugging these values into the binomial formula gives us $\frac{10!}{2!(8!)}\left[.5^2(.5)^8\right] = 0.044$.

Because the *P* value is less than 0.05, we reject the null hypothesis and conclude that the medication is not as effective in children as it is in adults.

BOX 5-2. Example of Wilcoxon Signed Rank Test

Imagine that 10 patients with allergic rhinitis take part in a study. All patients rate their symptom severity on a scale that ranges from "0 = Not at all severe" to "100 = Extremely severe." All patients then receive an experimental medication. After 36 hours of treatment, patients again rate their symptom severity. Data from this fictitious study are shown below.

Patient	1	2	3	4	5	6	7	8	9	10
After	50	63	40	30	15	69	70	45	5	22
Before	35	45	60	62	65	70	75	80	85	90

The first step in computing the Wilcoxon signed rank test involves subtracting each patient's "Before" rating from their "After" rating. The results of these calculations are shown below. Note that negative values reflect symptom improvement.

Change	+15	+18	−20	−32	−50	−1	−5	−35	−80	−68

Next, the symptom change scores are converted to ranks without regard to sign (i.e., whether the change score is "+" or "−").

Rank	3	4	5	6	8	1	2	7	10	9

Next, the sign from the change score is carried forward to the rank as shown below.

Signed rank	+3	+4	−5	−6	−8	−1	−2	−7	−10	−9

Next, the sum of the positive and negative ranks is computed separately. Thus,

$$R_{Positive} = 3 + 4 = 7;\ R_{Negative} = 5 + 6 + 8 + 1 + 2 + 7 + 10 + 9 = 48$$

(continued)

BOX 5-2. Example of Wilcoxon Signed Rank Test *(Continued)*

Note that if the sum of the positive and negative ranks were the same, both of these values would equal: $\frac{7+48}{2} = 27.5$, which is the expected value under the null hypothesis.

The Wilcoxon signed rank statistic is derived by subtracting this expected value from the sum of the positive ranks. Thus,

$$S = 7 - 27.5 = -20.5$$

Box 5-3 shows the printout obtained when performing this analysis using Proc Univariate in SAS. Tables can be used to determine the exact probability of observing an S value as large or larger than the observed **if the null hypothesis is true**. In addition, if one assumes that n is 10 or greater, statistical significance can be estimated using a paired t-test to test the null hypothesis that the mean of the signed ranks is "0." Both types of tests are performed automatically by SAS. As shown in Box 5-3, they yielded very similar probabilities for this example, $P = 0.0376$ and $P = 0.0371$, for the t-test and exact signed rank test, respectively. Because $P < 0.05$, we reject the null hypothesis and conclude that the medication reduces symptom severity.

BOX 5-3. SAS Printout for Wilcoxon Signed Rank Test Example

The UNIVARIATE Procedure
Variable: Symptom_Severity_Change

Moments

N	10	**Sum Weights**	10
Mean	–25.8	**Sum Observations**	–258
Std Deviation	33.485652	**Variance**	1121.28889
Skewness	–0.2706566	**Kurtosis**	–1.0114155
Uncorrected SS	16748	**Corrected SS**	10091.6
Coeff Variation	–129.78935	**Std Error Mean**	10.5890929

Basic Statistical Measures

Location		Variability	
Mean	–25.8000	**Std Deviation**	33.48565
Median	–26.0000	**Variance**	1121
Mode		**Range**	98.00000
		Interquartile Range	49.00000

Tests for Location: Mu0=0

Test		Statistic	P Value	
Student's t	**t**	–2.43647	**Pr > |t|**	0.0376
Sign	**M**	–3	**Pr ≥ |M|**	0.1094
Signed Rank	**S**	–20.5	**Pr ≥ |S|**	0.0371

SS, sum of squares; coeff, coefficient; Std, standard.

Two Samples Assessed One Time: Wilcoxon Rank Sum Test (AKA Mann–Whitney U Test)

This test is comparable to an independent groups t-test. However, analyses are performed on ranked data rather than the original raw scores. When using independent groups t-tests, **if the null hypothesis is true**, we expect the means in the two groups to be the same (i.e., the expected difference between group means is "0"). However, when using the Wilcoxon rank sum test (also known as the Mann–Whitney U test), raw scores are converted to ranks, and the null hypothesis tested is that the mean of the summed ranks is the same in the two groups (i.e., the expected difference between the means of the summed ranks is "0"). The ranked data retain information about each participant's location in the distribution of the outcome variable but discard information concerning the precise distance between observations. Boxes 5-4 and 5-5 provide an example of using the Wilcoxon rank sum test to test a hypothesis involving an ordinal outcome variable.

BOX 5-4. Example of Wilcoxon Rank Sum Test

Imagine that 20 people with allergic rhinitis take part in a study. Half receive an experimental medication, and half receive a placebo. After 36 hours of treatment, participants rate their symptom relief on a scale of 0 to 100. Data from the study are shown in the table below.

In the table, participants in the experimental (E) and placebo (P) groups have been combined. Their ratings on the symptom relief scale were then used to rank them from the patient who experienced the least symptom relief (Patient 9) to the patient who experienced the greatest symptom relief (Patient 6).

Patient	9	3	16	7	1	18	13	4	19	10
Rating	4	8	12	16	20	24	28	32	36	40
Rank	1	2	3	4	5	6	7	8	9	10
Group	P	P	P	P	P	P	P	E	E	E

Patient	5	15	12	8	17	2	11	20	14	6
Rating	44	48	52	56	60	64	68	72	76	80
Rank	11	12	13	14	15	16	17	18	19	20
Group	P	P	P	E	E	E	E	E	E	E

Next, the ranks were summed for each group separately. Thus,

$$RankSum_{Placebo} = 1+2+3+4+5+6+7+11+12+13 = 64$$

$$RankSum_{Exp} = 8+9+10+14+15+16+17+18+19+20 = 146$$

Note that (1) the expected value for the RankSum in both groups under the null hypothesis is $\frac{64+146}{2} = 105$ and (2) the absolute difference between the RankSums and the expected value under the null hypothesis is 41 for each group (i.e., $|146-105| = 41; |64-105| = 41$).

Box 5-5 shows the printout obtained when performing this analysis using Proc NPar1Way in SAS. Tables can be used to determine the exact probability of observing a test statistic as large or larger than the one observed **if the null hypothesis is true**. In addition, if one assumes that n in both groups is 10 or greater, statistical significance can be estimated using a z- or t-test to test the null hypothesis that the mean of the summed ranks is the same in both groups. Both types of tests are performed automatically by SAS. As shown in Box 5-5, they yielded similar probabilities for this example, $P = 0.0022$ and $P = 0.0064$, for the z and t-test, respectively. Because $P < 0.05$, we reject the null hypothesis and conclude that the experimental medication provided more symptom relief than the placebo.

BOX 5-5. SAS Printout for Wilcoxon Rank Sum Test Example

The NPAR1WAY Procedure

Wilcoxon Scores (Rank Sums) for Variable Rank
Classified by Variable Group

Group	N	Sum of Scores	Expected Under H_0	Std Dev Under H_0	Mean Score
Experimental	10	146.0	105.0	13.228757	14.60
Placebo	10	64.0	105.0	13.228757	6.40

Wilcoxon Two-Sample Test

Statistic	146.0000
Normal Approximation	
Z	3.0615
One-Sided Pr > Z	0.0011
Two-Sided Pr > |Z|	0.0022
t Approximation	
One-Sided Pr > Z	0.0032
Two-Sided Pr > |Z|	0.0064

Z includes a continuity correction of 0.5.

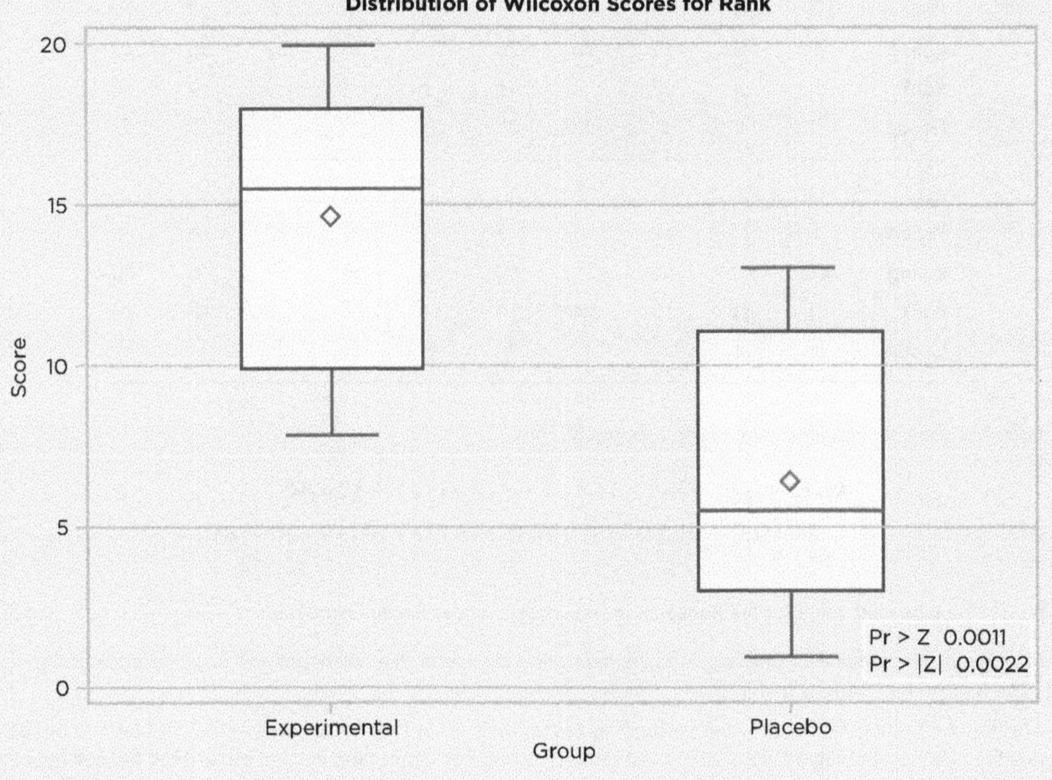

Std, standard; dev, deviation.

More Complex Designs

In this chapter, I have focused on the simplest research designs so that you can develop a basic understanding of the logic that underlies the use of nonparametric statistics to analyze ordinal outcome measures and numerical outcome measures when the assumptions required for parametric statistics are not met. The other types of nonparametric analyses for ordinal variables that you may encounter in the literature are (1) Kruskal–Wallis ANOVA, which is the nonparametric alternative to 1-way ANOVA, and (2) Friedman 2-way ANOVA by ranks, which is the nonparametric alternative to repeated measures ANOVA. The logic underlying these more complex procedures is similar to that described previously. That is, raw scores are converted to ranks and it is the ranks that are analyzed.

Examples from the Literature

We will now review selected findings from three recent studies that have used some of the tests described in this chapter to analyze study data. The first study examined the effect of a telephone call reminder program on medication adherence among older adults with hypertension.[1] We discussed some of the findings from this study in Chapter 4 of this book. You may remember that the study used a quasi-experimental research design. All participants in the intervention group (n = 563) participated in at least one live interactive call with a pharmacist focused on the patient's medication use. The study included both an **unmatched** and a **matched** control group. (In Chapter 4, we focused only on analyses involving the matched control group.) The unmatched control group included 9,188 patients who were served by the same call center as intervention patients and met study inclusion criteria but who did not participate in any calls. To form the matched control group, each patient in the intervention group was matched to a patient in the pool of 9,188 patients on age, gender, county of residence, and medication adherence during the 6-month period prior to implementation of the intervention. This resulted in 563 pairs of patients (i.e., 563 intervention patients and 563 matched controls).

Box 5-6 shows the results of analyses comparing intervention patients to both the matched and the unmatched control patients **at baseline**. The footnotes attached to the *P* values (circled for ease of reference) describe the types of tests that were performed to derive the *P* values. In the **unmatched analyses**, footnote "b" states that χ^2 tests were used to test differences involving categorical variables (we will cover this test in a later chapter) and that independent t-tests or Mann–Whitney U tests (equivalent to a Wilcoxon rank sum test) were also used to assess differences between the intervention and control groups. This footnote would have been clearer if the investigators had stated that these last two tests were used to assess differences involving numerical variables. However, I am confident that this is what they did. Nonetheless, it is not clear when t-tests versus Mann–Whitney U tests were used for the five numerical variables included in Box 5-6. (Note: I have framed these variables in rectangles.)

In the **matched analyses**, footnote "c" states that the McNemar test was used to test differences involving categorical variables (we will cover this test in a later chapter) and that paired t-tests or Wilcoxon signed rank tests were used to compare continuous variables between the intervention and the matched control group. Note the shift to paired tests given the paired design of this portion of the study. That is, although there were a total of 1,126 participants (i.e., 563 $*$ 2) in this portion of the study, data analyses focused on differences between the 563 matched pairs.

It is not clear why the investigators used both nonparametric and parametric tests to evaluate between group differences involving the numeric variables in Box 5-6. My hunch is that some of the numerical variables were not normally distributed and the investigators wanted to be certain that this did not bias their findings.

Because the main analyses in this study involved comparisons between the intervention group and the **matched** control group, the primary thing to look at in Box 5-6 is whether the intervention group and

BOX 5-6. Telephone Call Reminder Study

Table 1
Baseline comparisons of MTM intervention and control groups

Baseline characteristic	Unmatched			Propensity score matched[a]		
	Intervention group (n = 563)	Control group (n = 9188)	*P* value[b]	Intervention group (n = 563)	Matched control group (n = 563)	*P* value[c]
Age (y), mean (SD)	76.1 (8.3)	75.0 (9.0)	0.146	76.1 (8.3)	76.3 (8.0)	0.486
Sex, n (%), male	220 (39.1)	3701 (40.3)	0.595	220 (39.1)	201 (35.7)	0.195
County, n (%)						
Broward County	345 (61.3)	4766 (51.9)	<0.001	345 (61.3)	327 (58.1)	0.105
Miami-Dade County	218 (38.7)	4422 (48.1)		218 (38.7)	236 (41.9)	
Rx Treatment						
No. antihypertensive prescriptions, mean (SD)	7.0 (4.4)	7.6 (4.2)	0.001	7.0 (4.4)	6.9 (3.9)	0.804
No. non-antihypertensive prescriptions, mean (SD)	5.7 (3.6)	5.8 (3.7)	0.633	5.7 (3.6)	5.9 (3.7)	0.286
Days of supply, mean (SD)	43 (20.6)	45 (20.1)	0.037	43 (20.6)	44 (19.7)	0.568
Proportion of days covered						
Mean (SD)	63.1 (29.9)	70.6 (27.59)	<0.001	63.1 (29.9)	62.3 (29.4)	0.285
No. patients <80%, n (%)	338 (60.0)	4700 (51.2)	<0.001	338 (60.0)	349 (62.0)	0.266

MTM, medication therapy management; SD, standard deviation.
[a] Intervention and control groups matched on age, sex, county, and baseline proportion of days covered.
[b] χ^2 tests to compare distributions of categorical variables and independent *t* test or Mann-Whitney *U* test between intervention and control groups.
[c] McNemar test to compare distributions of categorical variables and paired *t* test or Wilcoxon signed rank test compare continuous variables between intervention and matched control groups.

the matched control group were similar at baseline. You can see from the analyses involving the **unmatched** control group that several statistically significant between-group differences are apparent. For example, unmatched control patients were taking more antihypertensive medications at baseline than those in the intervention group: $\bar{X}'s = 7.6(SD = 4.2)$ versus $7.0(SD = 4.4)$, $P = 0.001$, respectively. Unmatched control patients also were more adherent (as assessed by the proportion of days covered) than those in the intervention group: $\bar{X}'s = 70.6(SD = 27.59)$ versus $63.1(SD = 29.9)$, $P = 0.001$, respectively. These types of between group differences can introduce a serious bias in intervention studies, especially studies in which participants are not randomized to treatment condition. The investigators attempted to remove this bias by utilizing the matched control group in their main analyses. You can see from the second set of columns in Box 5-6 that the matching appears to have been successful. That is, none of the differences observed between intervention and unmatched control participants are evident in the analyses comparing intervention and matched control participants.

The second study examined the impact of California Senate Bill 41, which authorized pharmacists to sell syringes without a prescription.[2] The bill was part of prevention measures designed to reduce the spread of human immunodeficiency/hepatitis C virus by improving injection drug users' (IDUs) access to syringes. The study used a cross-sectional research design. Data were collected via an interviewer-administered survey. A total of 404 pharmacists and other pharmacy staff recruited from 212 pharmacies were interviewed. The primary outcome variable was whether or not the respondent stated that he/she would sell syringes to a person who is a known or suspected injector of illicit drugs. Under "Data Analysis," the authors state: "We then conducted a univariate analysis of factors associated with self-reported sales to IDUs by means of Wilcoxon rank sum tests for continuous variables and the Pearson chi-square test for categoric variables. Likert-type scale responses to knowledge, attitudes, and beliefs questions were collapsed to create binary variables (i.e., agree and strongly agree versus disagree and strongly disagree)" (p. 680). By "univariate analysis," the authors mean that they looked at the association of each independent variable with the outcome variable without controlling for any other predictor variables. This is the same analytic strategy that we have used thus far in this book. The term "Likert-type scale" is often used to refer to scales that assess beliefs and attitudes using a limited number of response options (e.g., strongly agree, agree, disagree, strongly disagree). In this study, the investigator used a 4-point Likert scale to assess knowledge, attitudes, and beliefs. This type of scale has ordinal properties. However, in the description of the analyses performed, the investigator indicates that these variables were dichotomized as either

(1) agree or strongly agree versus (2) disagree or strongly disagree. The results of these analyses are shown in Box 5-7. In the top row of the table, you can see that a total of 386 respondents were included in the analyses. (Eighteen respondents were excluded from these analyses, primarily because their pharmacy did not sell syringes at all.) Of the 386 respondents included in the analysis, 113 reported that they would sell syringes to IDUs and 273 indicated that they would not do so. The Wilcoxon rank sum test was used to determine whether age or number of pharmacists at the pharmacy differed between respondents who said that they would sell syringes to IDUs compared to those who said they would not do so. I determined this because age and the number of pharmacists at the pharmacy were measured on an ordinal scale, as can be seen from the reporting of the median and interquartile range for these variables. All of the other predictor variables are categorical (i.e., nominal). (We will discuss the types of analyses used to assess between group differences involving these types of variables in a later chapter.) You can see from the table that neither age nor number of pharmacists at the pharmacy differs between respondents who said that they would sell syringes to IDUs and those who said they would not do so. The *P* values associated with both of these variables are greater than 0.90. Finally, there is an issue with the analyses reported in Box 5-7 that warrants mention. The types of analyses performed assume that the observations in the data set (i.e., the 404 respondents) are independent of one another. However, one might question whether it is appropriate to consider pharmacists and pharmacy staff who work in the same pharmacy as independent

BOX 5-7. Nonprescription Syringe Sale Study

Table 2
Factors associated with self-reported nonprescription syringes to IDUs, Fresno and Kern Counties, n (%)

Factor	Total (n = 386)	Sell to IDUs (n = 113)	Do not sell to IDUs (n = 273)	*P* value
Median age, y (IQR)	34 (28–47)	35 (30–43)	34 (28–51)	0.968
Gender				0.283
Male	164 (42.7)	53 (46.9)	111 (40.7)	
Female	220 (57.3)	60 (53.1)	160 (58.6)	
Pharmacist				0.049
Yes	192 (49.7)	65 (57.5)	127 (46.5)	
No	194 (50.3)	48 (42.5)	146 (53.5)	
Pharmacy type				< 0.001
Chain	281 (89.4)	101 (89.4)	180 (65.9)	
Independent and other	105 (27.2)	12 (10.6)	93 (34.1)	
Number of pharmacists at location (IQR)	2 (2–3)	2 (2–3)	2 (2–4)	0.936
Sales policies based on:				< 0.001
Store policy only	172 (45.6)	34 (31.2)	138 (51.5)	
Discretion only	46 (12.2)	12 (11.0)	34 (12.7)	
Both	159 (42.2)	63 (57.8)	96 (35.8)	
Agree or strongly agree that:				
It is legal for IDUs 18 years of age or older to purchase a syringe in a pharmacy without a prescription.	236 (61.1)	94 (83.2)	142 (52.0)	< 0.001
Selling syringes to IDUs prevents infections such as HIV and HCV.	325 (84.2)	101 (89.4)	224 (82.1)	0.072
Only people who have a medical condition such as diabetes should be able to buy syringes.	207 (53.6)	34 (30.1)	173 (63.4)	< 0.001
I am concerned that providing syringes to IDUs encourages drug use.	233 (60.4)	47 (41.6)	186 (68.1)	< 0.001
IDUs are a disruption to my pharmacy.	155 (40.2)	34 (30.1)	121 (44.3)	0.009
Selling syringes to IDUs is not good business for pharmacies like mine.	201 (52.1)	31 (27.4)	170 (62.3)	< 0.001
Pharmacies that sell syringes to IDUs should provide information on how to get drug treatment.	316 (81.9)	91 (80.5)	225 (82.4)	0.662
Pharmacies that sell syringes to IDUs should provide information on how to prevent infection with HIV/HCV.	338 (87.6)	96 (85.0)	242 (88.6)	0.318
Pharmacies can be an important resource for IDUs who may not access health care in the community.	317 (82.1)	100 (88.5)	217 (79.5)	0.036
I am willing to provide information and resources to IDUs who purchase syringes at my pharmacy.	324 (83.9)	104 (92.0)	220 (80.6)	0.005
I am concerned that some people purchasing syringes without a prescription would feel uncomfortable if given HIV-related information and resources.	264 (68.4)	68 (60.2)	196 (71.8)	0.025
I am concerned that some people purchasing syringes without a prescription would feel uncomfortable if given information on how to access drug treatment.	268 (69.4)	68 (60.2)	200 (73.3)	0.011

IDU, injection drug user; HIV, human immunodeficiency virus.
Abbreviations used: IQR, interquartile range; HCV, hepatitis C virus; others as in Table 1.

observations. This is most apparent in predicator variables such as pharmacy type, number of pharmacists at location, and sales policies. One would expect all pharmacists and pharmacy staff at a single pharmacy to give the same answer to these questions; thus, their responses would not be independent of one another. In this study, it would have been preferable to have only included one respondent per pharmacy or to have performed a more sophisticated analysis that incorporated a "cluster effect." This type of analysis would have adjusted estimates and *P* values to reflect that the 404 respondents were clustered within 212 pharmacies.

The third study evaluated the effectiveness of a refill synchronization program implemented in two community pharmacies.[3] This study involved a retrospective analysis of the prescription refill records of 68 patients taking at least two medications who volunteered to participate in a medication synchronization program. One outcome variable was "refill consolidation." The authors state that "Refill consolidation reflects the extent to which patients collect all of their prescription medications during a single visit to a pharmacy (i.e., high consolidation) versus returning to the pharmacy to obtain individual refills on multiple occasions (i.e., low consolidation). A refill consolidation score can be calculated by subtracting from 1 the quotient of the number of distinct dates the pharmacy was visited divided by the total number of medications filled during the observation period. For example, a patient taking four chronic medications may visit their pharmacy twice over 200 days, each time receiving 100-day supplies of all four medications $\left(\textit{refill consolidation score} = \left(1-\left(\frac{2}{8}\right)\right) = 0.75\right)$. A low consolidation score would result if the same patient visited the pharmacy 8 times over 200 days, obtaining only 1 of their medications at each visit $\left(\textit{refill consolidation score} = \left(1-\left(\frac{8}{8}\right)\right) = 0\right)$. The values of refill consolidation range between 0 and 1, with higher values representing higher consolidation" (p. 656). The investigators used the Wilcoxon signed rank test to assess change in refill consolidation scores before and after participation in the medication synchronization program. They found that the median refill consolidation score increased from 0.44 during the preenrollment period to 0.67 during the postenrollment period. This difference was statistically significant ($P < 0.01$). Thus, the synchronization program was successful in improving refill consolidation.

Self-Study Questions

1. Imagine that you are reading a paper. Fifty people with arthritis are given a medication. Patients rate their pain on a 5-point scale before the initiation of therapy and again 2 months later. There is no control group. Pain is rated on a 4-point scale (i.e., 1 = no pain, 2 = mild pain, 3 = moderate pain, 4 = severe pain). Assume that this pain scale had ordinal (but not interval) properties. What is the most appropriate statistical test to use to analyze these data?

   A. 1-Sample t-test
   B. Paired t-test
   C. 1-Way ANOVA
   D. Wilcoxon signed rank test

2. Is the following statement true or false? Parametric procedures are appropriate to use in small samples when the dependent variable is not normally distributed. (True/False)

3. Imagine that you are an investigator who is testing a new relaxation technique on older adults (>65 years). Your technique has already been tested on people in other age groups, and you know that the average score on a 10-point scale is 7 points. On this scale, 1 = feel totally relaxed and 10 = feel totally wired. You want to determine if older adults rate your relaxation techniques differently than people in other age groups. You give the rating scale to 15 older adults. What type of test would you use to analyze these data?

   A. 1-Sample t-test
   B. Sign test
   C. Wilcoxon rank sum test

4. What is the null hypothesis for the relaxation study described in Question 3?

   A. There is no difference in ratings between older adults and other age groups.
   B. There is a difference in ratings between older adults and other age groups.
   C. Older adults score higher than other age groups.
   D. Older adults score lower than other age groups.

5. Imagine that an investigator wants to compare the effectiveness of Tylenol and Ecotrin. Sixty patients with chronic pain are recruited into the study. Half receive Tylenol, and half receive Ecotrin. Following 2 weeks of therapy, subjects rate their pain on a 5-point scale where 1 = no pain, 2 = mild pain, 3 = moderate pain, 4 = severe pain, and 5 = excruciating pain. Assume that this pain scale had ordinal (but not interval) properties. Which of the following is the most appropriate test to use in comparing the effectiveness of the two medications?

   A. Binomial test
   B. 1-Way ANOVA
   C. Independent groups t-test
   D. Wilcoxon rank sum test

6. Imagine that a crossover study is conducted evaluating the effect of a new analgesic on chronic pain. People are randomly assigned to receive either the medication or a placebo for 7 days. At the end of the 7-day period, all individuals undergo a 14-day washout period. At the end of the washout period, individuals who took the medication during the first period receive the placebo for a second 7-day period, and individuals who took the placebo during the first period receive the medication for the second 7-day period. Pain is assessed on a 5-point scale where 1 = no pain, 2 = just a little pain, 3 = a moderate amount of pain, 4 = a lot of pain, and 5 = excruciating pain. Which of the following statistics would be most appropriate to use to analyze the data from this study?

   A. Binomial test
   B. Independent groups t-test
   C. Wilcoxon signed rank test
   D. 1-Sample t-test

7. If the dependent variables in a study are measured on ordinal scales, they should be analyzed using what type of statistical procedures?

   A. Parametric procedures
   B. Nonparametric procedures
   C. Either type (It really does not matter.)

References

1. Park H, Adeyemi A, Want W, Roane TE. Impact of a telephonic outreach program on medication adherence in Medicare Advantage Prescription Drug (MAPD) plan beneficiaries. *J Am Pharm Assoc.* 2017;57(1):62–6.
2. Pollini RA. Self-reported participation in voluntary nonprescription syringe sales in California's Central Valley. *J Am Pharm Assoc.* 2017;57(6):677–85.
3. Blackburn DF, Tran D, Quiring C. Evaluation of a refill synchronization program in two community pharmacies. *J Am Pharm Assoc.* 2016;56(6):656–9.

Nominal Outcome Variables

6

After reading this chapter, you should be able to do the following:

1. Describe the logic underlying the use of nonparametric statistics to analyze nominal outcome variables.
2. Describe situations in which the following statistical tests would be used: binomial, z approximation, chi-square, Fisher's exact, and McNemar.
3. Interpret findings from studies that assess between group differences using the statistical tests listed above.
4. Explain how confidence intervals can be used to assess between group differences involving proportions.

In this chapter, we will cover nonparametric tests used to assess between group differences when the outcome variable is measured on a nominal scale (i.e., categorical variables). Nonparametric procedures involving nominal outcome variables usually assess whether observed differences in proportions are so large that they are unlikely to have occurred if the null hypothesis is true. Many of these procedures are based on the multiplication rule for independent events discussed in this book in Chapter 3, "Probability and Statistical Inference." This rule allows one to calculate the probability that two events will occur together if the events are independent. The assumption of independence is a form of the null hypothesis.

In this chapter, we will cover nonparametric tests that are used in the three analytic situations shown in Table 6-1 to evaluate between group differences involving **nominal** outcome variables. It may help to think of the tests covered in this chapter as alternatives to t-tests when the outcome variable is assessed on a nominal scale. Therefore, I have included the three types of t-tests discussed previously in the table as well. Within each of the three analytic situations, confidence intervals (CIs) can also be computed to examine between group differences. Therefore, in addition to the statistical tests shown in the table, we will discuss the appropriate CIs that should be computed for each analytic situation and how to interpret the results of these computations.

One Sample Assessed One Time: Binomial Test or Z Approximation

Sometimes investigators want to know if the outcomes experienced by people within a specific population subgroup (e.g., women taking prednisone) are similar to those experienced by people in the general population. If the outcome variable were numerical, the investigators could use a 1-sample t-test to compare the mean from a sample drawn from the population subgroup to an established population norm. So, this is a parallel situation where the outcome variable is assessed on a nominal

TABLE 6-1. Research Designs

Analytic Situation	Parametric–Numerical	Nonparametric–Nominal
1 Sample; 1 data collection point	1-Sample t-test	Binomial test Z approximation
1 Sample; 2 data collection points	Paired t-test	McNemar test
2 Samples; 1 data collection point	Independent groups t-test	Chi-square test Fisher's exact test Z approximation

scale and data are summarized using proportions. If the sample size is small, the investigators could use the binomial test to compute the probability of observing a particular outcome if the null hypothesis is true. Here, the null hypothesis is $\rho_{PopulationOfInterest} = \rho_{GeneralPopulation}$, where ρ represents the population proportions. Box 6-1 provides an example of how the binomial formula might be used in a small study to evaluate the effectiveness of an experimental medication.

In larger samples, a z approximation test can be used to test the null hypothesis that $\rho_{PopulationOfInterest} = \rho_{GeneralPopulation}$. This test assumes that both $\rho(n)$ **and** $(1 - \rho)n$ are no less than 5, where ρ is the proportion observed in the general population and *n* is the sample size. If these sample size assumptions are met, a CI can also be computed for the proportion observed in the sample. If the CI for the sample proportion does not include the proportion observed in the general population, one rejects the null hypothesis and concludes that the proportions differ. Conversely, if the CI for the sample proportion includes the proportion observed in the general public, one does **not** reject the null hypothesis. In this case, there would be insufficient evidence to conclude that the proportions differ. Box 6-2 provides an example of using a z approximation test and the CI approach to evaluate the effectiveness of an experimental medication in a study where the sample size requirements (i.e., $\rho(n) > 5$ **and** $(1 - \rho)n > 5$) are met.

BOX 6-1. Example of Binomial Test

Imagine that the 1-year survival rate from Disease A is 30% with the best therapy currently available. A study is conducted in which 10 patients with Disease A are treated with a new experimental drug. At the conclusion of a 1-year follow-up period, 80% of the patients in the study are still alive.

If the drug had no effect on survival, how likely is it that this outcome would have been obtained? (Note: The phrase "If the drug had no effect on survival" is equivalent to saying "If the null hypothesis is true." Thus, we are asking how likely it is that 8 people in the study would have survived if the experimental medication had no effect on the likelihood of surviving.)

This question can be answered using the binominal formula shown to the right where ρ is the probability of 1-year survival with the best therapy currently available, *n* is the number of people in the study, and *x* is the number of people in the study who were alive after 1-year of follow-up.

$$\frac{n!}{x!(n-x)!}\left[\rho^{x}(1-\rho)^{n-x}\right]$$

Plugging the values from the example into the formula, we find that the probability of 8 patients in this study being alive at the end of the 1-year follow-up period is 0.0014 if the experimental medication had no effect on survival.

$$\frac{10!}{8!2!}\left[0.3^{8}(0.7)^{2}\right] = 0.0014$$

Because this *P* value is small, it is **pretty unlikely that the medication has no effect** on the probability of survival. Thus, we reject the null hypothesis and conclude that the medication does improve the 1-year survival rate for Disease A.

BOX 6-2. Z Approximation and Confidence Interval Approach

Continuing with the example from Box 6-1, imagine that the 1-year survival rate from Disease A is 30% with the best therapy currently available. Given the results of the study reported in Box 6-1, imagine that a second study is conducted, this one involving 100 patients with Disease A, all of whom are treated with the experimental drug used in the smaller study. At the end of a 1-year follow-up period, 80% of the patients in the study are still alive. The question we want to answer is the same as in Box 6-1: if the drug had no effect on survival, how likely is it that this outcome would have been obtained?

We could use the binomial formula to calculate the probability directly as shown to the right.

$$\frac{100!}{80!20!}\left[0.3^{80}(0.7)^{20}\right] < 0.0001$$

However, using the binomial formula to compute probabilities becomes challenging as sample size increases. Therefore, we could instead use a z approximation test and compute a confidence for the proportion if sample size requirements are met. We can see from the following that these requirements are met: $\rho(n) = 0.3(100) = 30$, $(1 - \rho)n = (0.7)100 = 70$

The formula for the z approximation test is shown to the right. Although the denominator looks complex, it is simply the formula for the standard error (SE) of the proportion. Thus, this formula converts the raw difference between the proportions into SE units.

$$z = \frac{p_{Sample} - p_{GeneralPopulation}}{\sqrt{\frac{p_{GeneralPopulation}(1 - p_{GeneralPopulation})}{n}}}$$

Plugging the values from the example into this formula yields: $z = \frac{0.8 - 0.3}{\sqrt{\frac{0.3(0.7)}{100}}} = 10.9$

The *P* value associated with $z = 10.9$ is <0.0001. This is much smaller than the *P* value calculated in the small study with 10 subjects (Box 6-1) because the SE decreases as sample size increases. Still, the conclusion is the same. We reject the null hypothesis and conclude that the medication does improve the 1-year survival rate for Disease A.

We could also compute a 95% confidence interval (CI) for the sample proportion using the following formula, $p \pm 2\sqrt{\frac{p(1-p)}{n}}$. Note that the portion to the right of the critical value (i.e., 2) is the SE for the proportion observed in the sample. Plugging values from the example into this formula yields:

$$0.8 \pm 2\sqrt{\frac{0.8(1-0.8)}{100}} = 0.8 \pm 0.08 = 0.72 \textit{ to } 0.88$$

This CI does not include the survival rate observed with the best therapy currently available (i.e., 0.30). Thus, we would again conclude that the medication improves the 1-year survival rate for Disease A.

Assessing Change Over Time: McNemar Test

When investigators are interested in assessing change over time and the outcome variable is assessed on a **nominal scale**, the McNemar test can be used to determine whether the pattern of change observed is different than one would expect if the null hypothesis is true. The formula for the McNemar test is based on the 2 × 2 contingency table shown in Table 6-2. The rows indicate whether a person had a particular characteristic (i.e., their status on the outcome variable) at Time 1. The columns indicate whether the **same person** had the characteristic at Time 2. Each person in a study is counted in one cell of the table. For example, everyone who had the characteristic at both Time 1 and Time 2 would be counted in Cell A, whereas everyone who did not have the characteristic at either Time 1 or Time 2 would be counted in Cell D. The formula for computing the McNemar test ignores people in these cells because they experienced no change over time. Instead, the test focuses on people in Cells B and C. Everyone counted

TABLE 6-2. **Design for McNemar Test**

	Time 2	
Time 1	**Has Characteristic**	**Does Not Have Characteristic**
Has characteristic	A	B
Does not have characteristic	C	D

in Cell B had the characteristic at Time 1 but not at Time 2, whereas everyone counted in Cell C did not have the characteristic at Time 1 but did have it at Time 2. If the only change that occurred over time was random variation (i.e., some people get better, and some people get worse just by chance), we would expect an approximately equal number of people in Cells B and C. However, if something occurs between Time 1 and Time 2 that causes a shift in one direction, an imbalance will occur. In essence, the McNemar test assesses the likelihood that any imbalance between Cells B and C is due to random variation.

The formula for the McNemar test is $McNemar\ \chi^2 = \frac{(|b-c|)^2}{b+c}$. The McNemar test is a type of χ^2 test. The most important thing to notice in the formula for this test is that as the difference between Cells B and C increases, the McNemar χ^2 statistic increases. Box 6-3 provides an example of how the McNemar χ^2 test might be used in a study evaluating the effectiveness of a medication therapy management intervention.

Two Samples Assessed One Time: Chi-Square, Fisher's Exact, and Z Approximation Tests

When investigators are interested in assessing differences between two or more independent groups and the outcome variable is assessed on a **nominal scale**, the Pearson chi-square test may be used if sample size requirements are met. Often, the Pearson chi-square test is referred to simply as the chi-square test. For ease of reference, I will refer to this test simply as the chi-square test in this chapter. Chi-square tests involve analyzing contingency tables, such as the one shown in Table 6-3, to determine how likely it is that the observed cell frequencies would have occurred if the variables included in the table are independent (i.e., if the null hypothesis is true). The larger the difference between observed and expected frequencies, the less likely it is that the null hypothesis of independence is true.

Chi-square tests are used when both the independent variable and the outcome variable are measured on a nominal scale. However, the results of chi-square tests are only valid if the following sample size requirements are met: (1) the expected value in each cell must be at least 2, and (2) at least 80% of the cells must have an expected value of at least 5. Box 6-4 provides an example of using the chi-square test to assess the effectiveness of an experimental medication in reducing mortality rates from a specific type of cancer. The example explains how the expected values for each cell in the contingency table are calculated.

If the sample size requirements for the chi-square test are not met, Fisher's exact test can sometimes be used as an alternative. Fisher's exact test calculates the exact probability of observing a specific distribution of cell frequencies given the table marginals if the null hypothesis is true. The null hypothesis is that the cell frequencies are the same across the groups being compared after any differences in group size are taken into consideration. To determine the probability that the null hypothesis is true, one must calculate not only the probability of observing the specific distribution of cell frequencies that was observed, but also the probability of observing even more extreme imbalances across the cells. Box 6-5 provides an example of how Fisher's exact test might be used in a small study evaluating the effectiveness of an experimental cancer medication.

BOX 6-3. Example of McNemar Test

Imagine that a team of investigators wants to know if a medication therapy management (MTM) intervention targeting people with hypertension improves blood pressure control. A sample of 100 patients with hypertension have their blood pressure taken prior to participating in the intervention and again 3 months later.

The research question being addressed is as follows: Does the MTM intervention improve blood pressure control? Data from the study are presented in the table below.

Before	After	
	Controlled	Not Controlled
Controlled	40	10
Not controlled	36	14

In this example, 36 patients did not have their blood pressure under control before the intervention but did have it under control after the intervention, whereas10 individuals had their blood pressure under control before the intervention but did not have it under control after.

Plugging these values into the McNemar formula gives us $\frac{(|10-36|)^2}{10+36} = 14.7$.

The chi-square distribution with 1 degree of freedom is shown in the figure below. If alpha is set at 0.05, the critical value (CV) for this test is 3.84. Therefore, since the value computed (i.e., 14.7) exceeds the CV, we reject the null hypothesis and conclude that the MTM intervention improves blood pressure control.

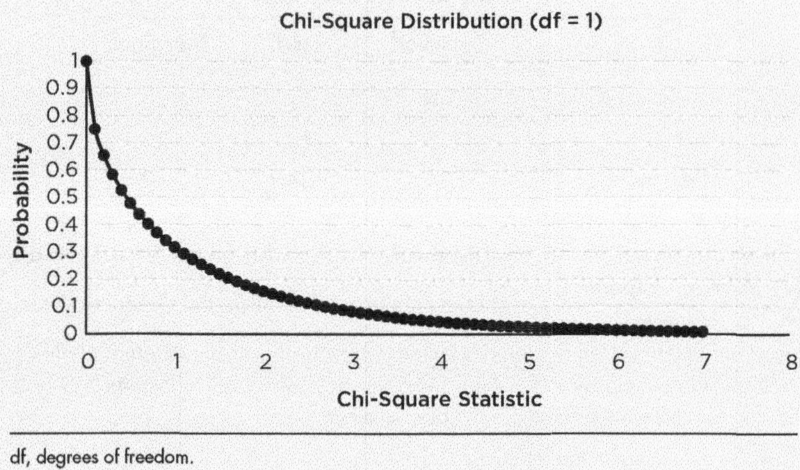

df, degrees of freedom.

If you play with the numbers in this example, you will see that if the values in Cells A and D remained unchanged but the values in Cells B and C were both 23 (i.e., (36+10)/2), the McNemar χ^2 would equal 0. This is the pattern that would be expected if the null hypothesis were true and any variation over time was due to chance.

TABLE 6-3. 2 × 2 Contingency Table Structure

Group	Outcome Experienced		Marginals
	Yes	No	
Group 1	A	B	A+B
Group 2	C	D	C+D
Marginals	A+C	B+D	A+B+C+D

BOX 6-4. Example of Chi-Square Test

Imagine that an investigator wants to know if an experimental medication reduces the mortality rate among patients with a specific type of cancer. The investigator enrolls 40 people with the type of cancer under investigation into a study and gives 20 the experimental drug and 20 a placebo. The results of the study are tabulated below. What do you conclude from these findings?

Observed			
Group	**Survived**	**Died**	**Marginals**
Experimental drug	12	8	20
Placebo	4	16	20
Marginals	16	24	40

First, we must calculate the **expected value** for each cell in the table. The "expected values" are the cell frequencies that are expected **if the null hypothesis is true.**

The expected value for each cell is computed by multiplying the marginals for the cell and dividing the product by the sample size. Thus, the expected number of survivors among people taking the experimental drug is computed as [[(16) * (20)]/40 = 8.] The expected values for each cell are shown below.

Expected Values			
Group	**Survived**	**Died**	**Marginals**
Experimental drug	8	12	20
Placebo	8	12	20
Marginals	16	24	40

The expected values shown demonstrate that we meet the sample size requirements to use the chi-square test. The formula for this test is $\chi^2 = \sum \frac{(Observed - Expected)^2}{Expected}$. As you can see from this formula, the chi-square statistic increases as the difference between observed and expected frequencies increases. For each cell, the difference between observed and expected frequencies is considered relative to the expected frequency (which reflects sampling variability). The larger the chi-square statistic, the less likely it is that the null hypothesis is true.

Plugging the values from the example into the formula yields:

$$\sum \frac{(12-8)^2}{8} + \frac{(8-12)^2}{12} + \frac{(4-8)^2}{8} + \frac{(16-12)^2}{12} = 6.67$$

For this example, we will set alpha at 0.05. This determines the critical value (CV) for the test, which is 3.84 for a chi-square statistic with 1 degree of freedom (df). Because the value we calculated in this case is larger than the CV, we reject the null hypothesis and conclude that the experimental drug improves the chances of survival for patients with the type of cancer under investigation.

A note about df. Within the context of a chi-square statistic, df varies as a function of the number of rows and columns in the table being analyzed. In a 2 × 2 table such as the one analyzed in this example: $df = (2 - 1) * (2 - 1) = 1$.

BOX 6-4. Example of Chi-Square Test *(Continued)*

If we had instead analyzed a 4 × 2 table as shown below, df would have been: $df = (4 - 1) * (2 - 1) = 3$. The CV for the chi-square statistic depends on the df associated with the test. For example, the CV for the chi-square statistic with 3 df is 7.81.

	Outcome Experienced		
Group	**Yes**	**No**	**Marginals**
Medication 1	A	B	A+B
Medication 2	C	D	C+D
Medication 3	E	F	E+F
Medication 4	G	H	G+H
Marginals	A+C+E+G	B+D+F+H	A+B+C+D+E+F+G+H

In published papers, you might see the results of a chi-square test reported in the following format: $\chi^2\,(1) = 6.67$. The df associated with the test is shown in parentheses.

BOX 6-5. Example of Fisher's Exact Test

Imagine that an investigator wants to know if an experimental medication reduces the mortality rate among patients with a specific type of cancer. The investigator enrolls 10 people with the type of cancer under investigation into a study and gives 5 the experimental drug and 5 a placebo. All patients are followed for 1 year. At the end of the year, the investigators record whether or not each patient is still alive. The results of the study are tabulated below. What do you conclude from these findings?

	Observed		
Group	**Survived**	**Died**	**Marginals**
Experimental drug	3	2	5
Placebo	1	4	5
Marginals	4	6	10

First, we will confirm that the sample size is too small to meet the requirements for the chi-square test. The expected value in the cell for those who took the experimental drug and survived is $\frac{(4*5)}{10} = 2$. Because there are only four cells in the table, this cell represents 25% of the cells in the table. Therefore, we do not meet the requirement for the chi-square test that at least 80% of the cells must have an expected value of 5 or more. In fact, the expected values in all of the cells range from 2 to 3. Because we do not meet the requirements for the chi-square test, we will use the Fisher's exact test.

The formula for Fisher's exact test is $\frac{(A+B)!*(C+D)!*(A+C)!*(B+D)!}{(A!)(B!)(C!)(D!)n!}$, where the terms A through D correspond to the four cells in the 2 x 2 table, as in the McNemar test, and N is the total sample size.

Plugging the values from the example into this formula yields: $\frac{5!*5!*4!*6!}{(3!)(2!)(1!)(4!)10!} = 0.238$

We also have to calculate the probability of observing more extreme imbalances across the cells. In this example, there is only one scenario that would result in a more extreme imbalance (without changing the marginals): 4 people who received the experimental drug might have survived, and all 5 people who received the placebo might have died. Plugging these values into the equation yields: $\frac{5!*5!*4!*6!}{(4!)(1!)(0!)(5!)10!} = 0.024$

Finally, we must add these two probabilities together and multiply by 2 to convert from a 1-tailed hypothesis test to a 2-tailed test. This yields: $(0.238 + 0.024) * 2 = 0.52$.

Thus, even though 60% of the people who received the experimental drug survived and only 20% of the people who received the placebo survived, we still cannot reject the null hypothesis that the experimental drug has no effect on the chances of surviving. This example highlights the limited power that small studies have to detect even fairly large effects.

If the sample size in a study is sufficiently large, differences in proportions can be analyzed using a z approximation test. This test is based on the same z distribution that we have discussed previously. When used to assess differences between proportions, the z test is an "approximate" test because nominal variables are not continuous and the z distribution describes the distribution of continuous variables. However, as sample size increases, distributions based on proportions begin to look continuous. For example, imagine that you have only two people in a study. The proportion of people who could experience an outcome of interest could take one of only three possible values: 0, 0.5, or 1.0. That is, neither person could experience the outcome, one person could experience the outcome, or both people could experience the outcome. If five people were in the study, the proportion of people who could experience the outcome of interest could take one of six possible values: 0, 0.2, 0.4, 0.6, 0.8, or 1.0. So, the possible distribution of proportions is a bit closer to continuous. If 100 people took part in the study, the proportion of people who could experience the outcome could take one of 101 values: 0, 0.01, 0.02, 0.03 ··· 0.97, 0.98, 0.99, 1.0. Thus, as sample size increases, the number of possible proportions increases and begins to approximate a continuous distribution.

The specific sample size requirements are (1) p_1n_1 **and** p_2n_2 must be >5 **and** $(1 - p_1)n_1$ **and** $(1 - p_2)n_2$ must be >5, where p_1 and n_1 are the proportion observed in one group and the sample size in that group and p_2 and n_2 are the proportion observed in the other group and the sample size in that group. If these sample size requirements are met, investigators can also compute a CI for the difference between proportions. If the null hypothesis is true, one would expect the difference between the proportions in the two groups to be 0. Box 6-6 provides an example of using the z approximation test to evaluate the effectiveness of an experimental cancer medication in a study involving 150 patients. Box 6-6 also includes the computations required to compute a CI for the difference in proportions between the two groups and interpret the results of these computations.

Examples from the Literature

We will now review selected findings from three recent studies that have used some of the tests described in this chapter to analyze study data. The first study examined the effect of a telephone call reminder program on medication adherence among older adults with hypertension.[1] We have discussed some of the findings from this study in previous chapters. Remember that the study used a quasi-experimental research design. All patients in the intervention group (n = 563) participated in at least one interactive call with a pharmacist focused on the patient's medication use. The study included both an **unmatched** and a **matched** control group. The unmatched control group included 9,188 patients who were served by the same call center as intervention patients and met study inclusion criteria but who did not participate in any calls. To form the matched control group, each patient in the intervention group was matched to a patient in the pool of 9,188 patients on age, sex, county of residence, and medication adherence during the 6-month period prior to implementation of the intervention, resulting in 563 matched pairs (i.e., 563 intervention patients and 563 matched controls).

The first table in Box 6-7 shows the results of analyses comparing intervention patients to both the matched and the unmatched control patients **at baseline**. The footnotes attached to the *P* values (circled for ease of reference) describe the types of tests that were performed to derive the *P* values. In the **unmatched analyses**, footnote "b" states that χ^2 tests were used to test differences involving categorical variables and that independent t-tests or Mann–Whitney U test were also used to assess differences between the intervention and control groups. (We discussed results of the t-tests and Mann–Whitney U tests in Chapter 5 of this book.) Three categorical (i.e., nominal) variables are shown in the table: sex, county, and number of patients who had proportion of days covered (PDC) values less than 80%. (Note: I have framed these variables in rectangles in the table.) In the table, you can see that participants in the intervention and control groups were similar with respect to sex (39.1% and 40.3% male, in the intervention and unmatched control groups respectively). However, participants in the intervention group were more likely than those

BOX 6-6. Z Approximation and Confidence Interval Approach

Imagine that an investigator is interested in whether an experimental medication reduces the mortality rate among patients with a specific type of cancer. The investigator enrolls 150 people with the type of cancer under investigation and gives 100 the experimental drug and 50 the placebo. Study findings are shown below. What do you conclude?

	Outcome		
Group	**Survive**	**Die**	**Marginals**
Experimental drug	60	40	100
Placebo	10	40	50
Marginals	70	80	150

First, we need to calculate the proportion of patients who survived in each group.

$$P_{ExperimentalDrug} = \frac{60}{100} = 0.60; P_{Placebo} = \frac{10}{50} = 0.20$$

Next, we need to determine if we meet the sample size requirements to use a z approximation test. These calculations show:

$$(P_{ExperimentalDrug})n_{ExperimentalDrug} = (0.60) * 100 = 60;$$

$$(1 - P_{ExperimentalDrug})n_{ExperimentalDrug} = (0.40) * 100 = 40$$

and

$$(P_{Placebo})n_{Placebo} = (0.20) * 50 = 10;$$

$$(1 - P_{Placebo})n_{Placebo} = (0.80) * 50 = 40$$

All four values exceed 5. Therefore, the sample size is adequate to use the z approximation.

The formula for the z approximation test for differences in proportions is:

$$z = \frac{p_1 - p_2}{SE_{Difference}}, \text{ where } SE_{Difference} = \sqrt{\frac{p_1(1-p_1)}{n_1} + \frac{p_2(1-p_2)}{n_2}}$$

Plugging the values from the example into this formula yields:

$$z = \frac{0.6 - 0.2}{\sqrt{\frac{(0.6)(0.4)}{100} + \frac{(0.2)(0.8)}{50}}} = \frac{0.4}{\sqrt{0.0056}} = \frac{0.4}{0.075} = 5.33$$

With alpha set at 0.05, the critical value (CV) for the z test is 2.0. Because the z we calculated (i.e., 5.33) is greater than the CV, we reject the null hypothesis and conclude that the experimental medication improved patients' chances of survival.

Because the sample size requirements for the z approximation test are met, the investigators could compute a confidence interval (CI) for the difference between proportions. The formula for the CI is $CI = (p_1 - p_2) \pm CV(SE_{Difference})$. For a 95% CI, the CV is 2.0.

Plugging the values from the example into the CI formula yields:

$$CI = (0.6 - 0.2) \pm 2(0.075) = (0.4) \pm 0.15 = 0.25 \text{ to } 0.55$$

Because the CI does not include 0, the expected value under the null hypothesis when evaluating difference scores, we conclude that exposure to the experimental medication is associated with an increased chance of survival.

BOX 6-7. Telephone Call Reminder Study

Table 1
Baseline comparisons of MTM intervention and control groups

Baseline characteristic	Unmatched			Propensity score matched[a]		
	Intervention group (n = 563)	Control group (n = 9188)	*P* value[b]	Intervention group (n = 563)	Matched control group (n = 563)	*P* value[c]
Age (y), mean (SD)	76.1 (8.3)	75.0 (9.0)	0.146	76.1 (8.3)	76.3 (8.0)	0.486
Sex, n (%), male	220 (39.1)	3701 (40.3)	0.595	220 (39.1)	201 (35.7)	0.195
County, n (%)						
Broward County	345 (61.3)	4766 (51.9)	<0.001	345 (61.3)	327 (58.1)	0.105
Miami-Dade County	218 (38.7)	4422 (48.1)		218 (38.7)	236 (41.9)	
Rx Treatment						
No. antihypertensive prescriptions, mean (SD)	7.0 (4.4)	7.6 (4.2)	0.001	7.0 (4.4)	6.9 (3.9)	0.804
No. non-antihypertensive prescriptions, mean (SD)	5.7 (3.6)	5.8 (3.7)	0.633	5.7 (3.6)	5.9 (3.7)	0.286
Days of supply, mean (SD)	43 (20.6)	45 (20.1)	0.037	43 (20.6)	44 (19.7)	0.568
Proportion of days covered						
Mean (SD)	63.1 (29.9)	70.6 (27.59)	<0.001	63.1 (29.9)	62.3 (29.4)	0.285
No. patients <80%, n (%)	338 (60.0)	4700 (51.2)	<0.001	338 (60.0)	349 (62.0)	0.266

MTM, medication therapy management; SD, standard deviation.
[a] Intervention and control groups matched on age, sex, county, and baseline proportion of days covered.
[b] χ^2 tests to compare distributions of categorical variables and independent *t* test or Mann-Whitney *U* test between intervention and control groups.
[c] McNemar test to compare distributions of categorical variables and paired *t* test or Wilcoxon signed rank test compare continuous variables between intervention and matched control groups.

Table 2
Change in adherence 6-month postintervention period versus 6-month preintervention period for patients in the intervention and control groups

Proportion of days covered	Intervention group (n = 563)			Matched control group (n = 563)			Difference-in-differences	
	6-month postintervention	Change	*P* value	6-month postintervention	Change	*P* value	Difference-in-differences	*P* value[a]
Mean (SD)	80.5 (22.0)	17.33 (33.56)	<0.001[b]	76.1 (25.9)	13.83 (32.34)	<0.001[b]	3.50 (36.28)	0.022
No. patients ≥80%, n (%)	365 (64.8)	140 (24.9)	<0.001[c]	335 (59.5)	121 (21.5)	<0.001[c]	N/A	

SD, standard deviation; N/A, not available.
[a] *P* values compare the difference-in-differences (Changes in intervention group – Changes in matched control groups) using paired *t* test.
[b] *P* values compare changes between the 6-month preintervention and postintervention using paired *t* tests.
[c] *P* values compare changes between the 6-month preintervention and postintervention using McNemar test.

in the unmatched control group to live in Broward County (61.3% versus 51.9%, respectively). In addition, more patients in the intervention group had PDC values <80% than in the unmatched control group (60.0% versus 51.2%, respectively).

In the **matched analyses**, footnote "c" states that the McNemar test was used to test differences involving categorical variables and that paired t-tests or Wilcoxon signed rank tests were used to compare continuous variables between the intervention and the matched control group. (We have discussed paired t-tests and Wilcoxon signed rank tests in previous chapters.) Note the shift to paired tests given the paired design of this portion of the study. That is, although there were a total of 1,126 participants (i.e., 563 * 2) in this portion of the study, data analyses focused on differences between the 563 matched pairs.

Because the main analyses in this study involved comparisons between the intervention group and the **matched** control group, the primary thing to look at in the first table in Box 6-7 is whether the intervention group and the matched control group were similar at baseline. You can see from the analyses involving the **unmatched** control group that several statistically significant between-group differences are apparent. However, the second set of columns in the first table in Box 6-7 demonstrate that the investigators were able to eliminate these differences in their matched analyses. For example, 39.1% and 35.7% of participants were male in the intervention and matched control groups, respectively. Therefore, it was not necessary to control for differences in baseline characteristics (e.g., number of hypertensive medications used) in the primary analyses. However, the investigators did perform supplemental analyses (not reported in the paper)

TABLE 6-4. McNemar Test for Sex Based on Telephone Call Reminder Study

Intervention Group	Matched Control Group		Marginals
	Male	Female	
Male	103	117	220
Female	98	245	343
Marginals	201	362	563

that controlled for baseline characteristics such as age, sex, county, and PDC at baseline. This type of supplemental analysis is recommended to ensure that the results obtained are consistent with the primary analyses reported in the paper (and described below).

From the first table in Box 6-7, we know that 220 of the 563 patients in the intervention group were male and that 201 of the 563 patients in the matched control group were male. Using this information, I created Table 6-4 to display the data as they would be analyzed by the McNemar χ^2 test. The frequencies shown in Table 6-4 are consistent with the *P* value of 0.195 reported in the paper. From Table 6-4, you can see that of the 563 matched pairs, 103 included two males, 245 included two females, and 215 (i.e., 117 + 98) included one male and one female. Remember that the McNemar test assesses imbalance between the shaded cells in Table 6-4. In this case, the difference between these cells was not statistically significant ($P = 0.195$).

The primary findings from this study are shown in the second table in Box 6-7. Footnote "c" states the following: "*P* values compare changes between the 6-month preintervention and postintervention using McNemar test." This footnote refers to findings in the table where patients were dichotomized as having a PDC value either (1) <80% or (2) ≥80%. You can see in the table that 64.8% of intervention patients (n = 365) had a PDC value ≥80% for the 6-month postintervention period. This was an increase from 40.0% (n = 225) for the 6-month preintervention period. Among the matched controls, 59.5% (n = 335) had a PDC value ≥80% for the 6-month postintervention period. This was an increase from 38.0% (n = 214) for the 6-month preintervention period. Thus, PDC improved significantly from the preintervention to the postintervention period in both groups. In the second table in Box 6-7, the McNemar test was used only to assess change within the intervention and matched control groups. It was not used to assess whether the amount of change was greater in one group than the other. However, results of the paired t-test in the second table in Box 6-7, which treated PDC as a continuous variable, found that PDC improved more among intervention patients than among the matched controls.

The second study examined the impact of California Senate Bill 41, which authorized pharmacists to sell syringes without a prescription.[2] Some of the results from this study were discussed in Chapter 5. Briefly, the study used a cross-sectional research design. Data were collected via an interviewer-administered survey. A total of 404 pharmacists and pharmacy staff, recruited from 212 pharmacies, were interviewed. The primary outcome variable was whether or not the pharmacist stated that he/she would sell syringes to a person who is a known or suspected injection drug user (IDU). Under "Data Analysis," the authors state, "We then conducted a univariate analysis of factors associated with self-reported sales to IDUs by means of Wilcoxon rank sum tests for continuous variables and the Pearson chi-square test for categoric variables. Likert-type scale responses to knowledge, attitudes, and beliefs questions were collapsed to create binary variables (i.e., agree and strongly agree vs. disagree and strongly disagree)" (p. 680). The results of these analyses are shown in Box 6-8. In the top row of the table, you can see that a total of 386 respondents were included in the analyses. (Eighteen respondents were excluded from these analyses, primarily because their pharmacy did not sell syringes at all.) Of the 386 respondents included

BOX 6-8. Nonprescription Syringe Sale Study

Table 2
Factors associated with self-reported nonprescription syringes to IDUs, Fresno and Kern Counties, n (%)

Factor	Total (n = 386)	Sell to IDUs (n = 113)	Do not sell to IDUs (n = 273)	*P* value
Median age, y (IQR)	34 (28–47)	35 (30–43)	34 (28–51)	0.968
Gender				0.283
Male	164 (42.7)	53 (46.9)	111 (40.7)	
Female	220 (57.3)	60 (53.1)	160 (58.6)	
Pharmacist				0.049
Yes	192 (49.7)	65 (57.5)	127 (46.5)	
No	194 (50.3)	48 (42.5)	146 (53.5)	
Pharmacy type				< 0.001
Chain	281 (89.4)	101 (89.4)	180 (65.9)	
Independent and other	105 (27.2)	12 (10.6)	93 (34.1)	
Number of pharmacists at location (IQR)	2 (2–3)	2 (2–3)	2 (2–4)	0.936
Sales policies based on:				< 0.001
Store policy only	172 (45.6)	34 (31.2)	138 (51.5)	
Discretion only	46 (12.2)	12 (11.0)	34 (12.7)	
Both	159 (42.2)	63 (57.8)	96 (35.8)	
Agree or strongly agree that:				
It is legal for IDUs 18 years of age or older to purchase a syringe in a pharmacy without a prescription.	236 (61.1)	94 (83.2)	142 (52.0)	< 0.001
Selling syringes to IDUs prevents infections such as HIV and HCV.	325 (84.2)	101 (89.4)	224 (82.1)	0.072
Only people who have a medical condition such as diabetes should be able to buy syringes.	207 (53.6)	34 (30.1)	173 (63.4)	< 0.001
I am concerned that providing syringes to IDUs encourages drug use.	233 (60.4)	47 (41.6)	186 (68.1)	< 0.001
IDUs are a disruption to my pharmacy.	155 (40.2)	34 (30.1)	121 (44.3)	0.009
Selling syringes to IDUs is not good business for pharmacies like mine.	201 (52.1)	31 (27.4)	170 (62.3)	< 0.001
Pharmacies that sell syringes to IDUs should provide information on how to get drug treatment.	316 (81.9)	91 (80.5)	225 (82.4)	0.662
Pharmacies that sell syringes to IDUs should provide information on how to prevent infection with HIV/HCV.	338 (87.6)	96 (85.0)	242 (88.6)	0.318
Pharmacies can be an important resource for IDUs who may not access health care in the community.	317 (82.1)	100 (88.5)	217 (79.5)	0.036
I am willing to provide information and resources to IDUs who purchase syringes at my pharmacy.	324 (83.9)	104 (92.0)	220 (80.6)	0.005
I am concerned that some people purchasing syringes without a prescription would feel uncomfortable if given HIV-related information and resources.	264 (68.4)	68 (60.2)	196 (71.8)	0.025
I am concerned that some people purchasing syringes without a prescription would feel uncomfortable if given information on how to access drug treatment.	268 (69.4)	68 (60.2)	200 (73.3)	0.011

IDU, injection drug user; HIV, human immunodeficiency virus.
Abbreviations used: IQR, interquartile range; HCV, hepatitis C virus; others as in Table 1.

in the analysis, 113 (29.3%) reported that they would sell syringes to IDUs, and 273 (70.7%) indicated that they would not do so. The Pearson chi-square test was used to assess between group differences for all of the variables in Box 6-8 **except** age and number of pharmacists. I determined this because all of the other variables are measured on a nominal (i.e., categorical) scale.

The primary question that most readers would want to answer when reviewing Box 6-8 is whether respondents with a particular characteristic reported being more (or less) likely than people without the characteristic to sell syringes to IDUs. For example, one might ask, "Are pharmacists more likely than nonpharmacist staff to sell syringes to IDUs?" I abstracted the relevant information to answer this question from the published paper into Table 6-5. The values shown in parentheses are percentages. I added the row labeled "Totals" to the table to show that the published paper reported **column** percentages. That is, the percentages within each column sum to 100%. Unfortunately, these percentages do not directly answer the question of whether pharmacists are more likely than nonpharmacist staff to sell syringes to IDUs. Whenever an explanatory variable (i.e., independent variable) forms the rows in a table, row percentages are needed to answer this type of question. Therefore, in Table 6-6, I replaced the column percentages with row percentages and add a second "Totals" column to emphasize that this table presents row percentages. That is, the percentages within each row sum to 100%. With the data presented in this

TABLE 6-5. Data for Pharmacist Variable From Nonprescription Syringe Sale Study

Factor	Total (n = 386)	Sell to IDUs (n = 113)	Do Not Sell to IDUs (n = 273)	*P* value
Pharmacist				
Yes	192 (49.7)	65 (57.5)	127 (46.5)	0.049
No	194 (50.3)	48 (42.5)	146 (53.5)	
Totals	386 (100%)	113 (100%)	273 (100%)	

IDU, injection drug user.

format, it is easy to see that pharmacists were more likely than nonpharmacists to sell syringes to IDUs (33.9% versus 24.7%, respectively; $P = 0.049$).

The third study assessed the effect of a community pharmacist-led intervention on use of statin therapy among patients with diabetes.[3] Use of statin therapy in this population is endorsed as a performance measure by the Pharmacy Quality Alliance. The study used a randomized controlled trial (RCT) design. Patients between the ages of 40 and 75 who had filled at least two prescriptions for a diabetes medication and who were not currently receiving a statin were eligible for participation. A total of 221 patients were randomly assigned to the intervention group. The primary care providers of patients in this group were contacted by a pharmacist, either by phone or fax, to recommend the prescription of an appropriate statin. A total of 199 patients were randomly assigned to a no-treatment control group. (In a no-treatment control group, individuals receive no intervention but continue to receive usual care.) The primary outcome variables were (1) the proportion of patients for whom a statin was prescribed and (2) the proportion of patients for whom a statin was dispensed. In the statistical analysis section of the paper, the authors state, "It was specified a priori that a 2-sided Fisher exact test would be used to analyze the difference between the intervention and control groups." The term "a priori" means that this decision was made prior to data collection. The authors do not explain why they decided to use the Fisher exact test. Their targeted sample size seems sufficient to meet the requirements for using a chi-square test, which would usually be the preferred statistic given the design of this study.

As shown in Figure 6-1, 46 patients in the intervention group (20.9%) compared to 17 (8.5%) in the control group ($P < 0.001$) were prescribed a statin during the time frame of the study. In addition, a statin was dispensed for 34 patients in the intervention group (15.4%) compared to 15 (7.5%) in the control group ($P < 0.001$). I replicated these analyses using chi-square tests to evaluate the statistical significance of the differences reported rather than Fisher's exact tests. These analyses yielded virtually identical *P* values to those reported in the paper. Thus, this study demonstrated that pharmacists may be able to help primary care providers meet quality metrics for the care of patients with diabetes.

TABLE 6-6. Row Percentages for Pharmacist Variable Based on Data From Nonprescription Syringe Sale Study

Factor	Total (n = 386)	Sell to IDUs (n = 113)	Do Not Sell to IDUs (n = 273)	Total (n = 386)	*P* value
Pharmacist					
Yes	192 (49.7)	65 (33.9)	127 (66.1)	192 (100%)	0.049
No	194 (50.3)	48 (24.7)	146 (75.3)	194 (100%)	

IDU, injection drug user.

FIGURE 6-1. Statin Use in Diabetes Study

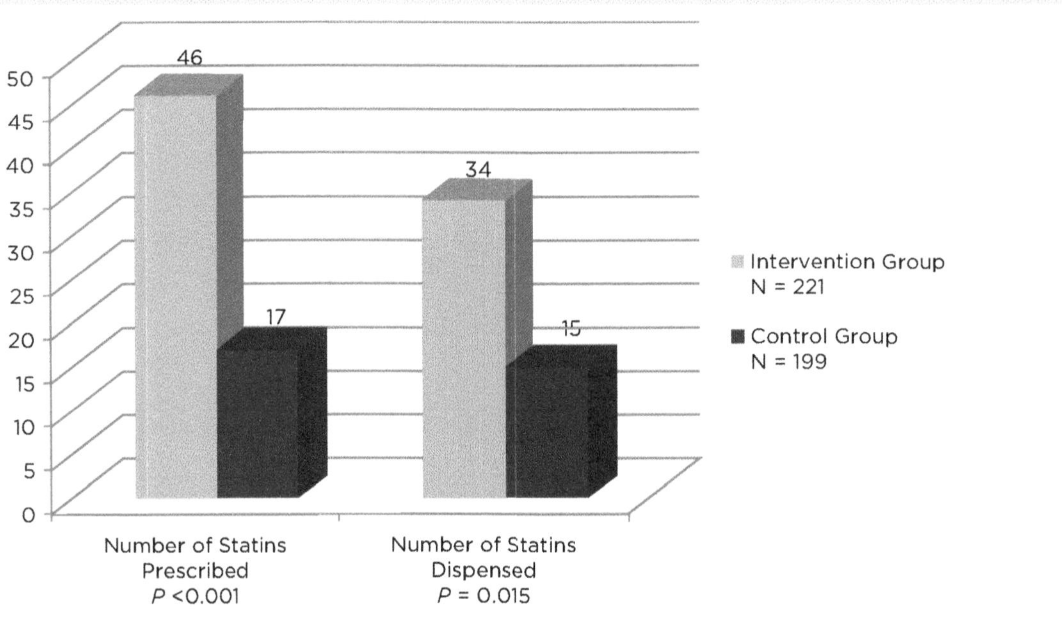

Self-Study Questions

1. Imagine that you are reading a paper. Fifty people with hypertension are given an experimental medication. The investigators want to know whether the medication is effective in controlling blood pressure. Blood pressure is measured before the initiation of therapy and again 2 months later. Assume that, at both time points, blood pressure is dichotomized as either 1 = within normal range or 2 = **not** within normal range. Given that blood pressure was dichotomized, what is the most appropriate statistical test to use to analyze these data?

   A. 1-Sample t-test
   B. Paired t-test
   C. McNemar test
   D. Kappa statistic

2. Imagine that there is a disease that has a 1-year survival rate of 20% with current treatment. In a trial of a new medication, 10 patients took Medication A, and 70% of these patients survived over a year. What statistical test should be used to determine whether the new treatment is more effective than the current one?

   A. 1-Sample t-test
   B. Chi-square test
   C. Binomial test
   D. Z approximation

3. Imagine that you are reading a study in which the investigators examined the effect of an experimental medication on survival following an acute myocardial infarction. Two thousand individuals participated in the study: 1,000 in the experimental group and 1,000 in a placebo control group. Nine hundred people in the experimental group survived compared to 700 people in the control group. Which of the following tests would be most appropriate to use to analyze the results of this study?

   A. Binomial test
   B. Chi-square test
   C. Wilcoxon rank sum test
   D. Wilcoxon signed rank test
   E. Fisher's exact test

4. Is the following statement true or false? The McNemar test is used as an alternative to a chi-square test when you have a small sample size. (True/False)

5. Is the following statement true or false? Probabilities calculated by nonparametric procedures used to analyze nominal data require that raw data be converted to ranks. (True/False)

6. Imagine that a study is conducted to evaluate the effect of a new weight loss medication. A total of 100 people take part in the study. Prior to the initiation of therapy, each participant is classified as either (1) overweight or (2) not overweight. Each participant then is followed for 6 months. At the end of the follow-up period, each participant is again classified as either (1) overweight or (2) not overweight. What type of statistical test would be used to determine if the proportion of participants who were overweight changed over the course of the study?

   A. Fisher's exact test
   B. Paired t-test
   C. McNemar's test
   D. Chi-squared test

7. Imagine that there is a study that assesses the effect of a new weight loss medication. In the study, 50 patients take placebo, and 50 patients take the new medication. If the outcome is measured as whether patients lose weight or not (weight loss: yes/no), what kind of statistical test would be most appropriate for the investigator to use?

   A. Independent group t-test
   B. Chi-square test
   C. Paired t-test
   D. Wilcoxon signed rank test

8. Based on the study described in the previous question, if the outcome had been measured as the number of pounds that a patient lost, which of the following statistical tests would be most appropriate to use?

   A. Independent group t-test
   B. Chi-square test
   C. Paired t-test
   D. Wilcoxon signed rank test

9. What type of statistical test is an alternative to a chi-square test when the sample size requirements for a chi-square test are not met?

   A. Binomial test
   B. Fisher's exact test
   C. Wilcoxon rank sum test
   D. Wilcoxon signed rank test

References

1. Park H, Adeyemi A, Want W, Roane TE. Impact of a telephonic outreach program on medication adherence in Medicare Advantage Prescription Drug (MAPD) plan beneficiaries. *J Am Pharm Assoc.* 2017;57(1):62–6.
2. Pollini RA. Self-reported participation in voluntary nonprescription syringe sales in California's Central Valley. *J Am Pharm Assoc.* 2017;57(6):677–85.
3. Renner HM, Hollar A, Stolpe SF, Marciniak MW. Pharmacist-to-prescriber intervention to close therapeutic gaps for statin use in patients with diabetes: a randomized controlled trial. *J Am Pharm Assoc.* 2017;57(3S):S236–S42.

CORRELATION AND REGRESSION

7

Correlation and Linear Regression

After reading this chapter, you should be able to do the following:

1. Describe the situations in which correlations and linear regression analyses are used.
2. Describe the type of situation in which it would be appropriate to use a Spearman versus a Pearson correlation coefficient.
3. Differentiate between the type of information conveyed by regression coefficients versus correlation coefficients.
4. Differentiate between the type of information conveyed by raw versus standardized regression coefficients.
5. Describe the type of information that is captured by the R^2 for a regression model.
6. Explain how variables are selected for inclusion in a regression model.
7. Given a scatterplot of two variables, describe the nature of the observed relationship.

In Chapters 4, 5, and 6 of this book, we discussed statistical tests used to evaluate between group differences. The independent (predictor) variables in these analyses were measured on a nominal scale indexing membership in a particular group (e.g., male/female, type of medication used). However, investigators are often interested in research questions where at least some of the independent variables are measured on numerical scales. For example, an investigator might want to know if age at onset of a disease is associated with variation in disease outcomes. In addition, with the exception of factorial analysis of variance (ANOVA), all of the procedures covered thus far only permit the examination of the relationship between an outcome variable and a single independent variable. This chapter introduces statistical procedures that can handle **numerical independent variables** and can assess the relationship between an outcome variable and **multiple independent variables** simultaneously. This chapter focuses on situations where the outcome variable is assessed on a numerical scale; Chapter 8 focuses on situations where the outcome variable is assessed on a nominal scale.

Bivariate Correlations

Pearson Correlation Coefficient

The simplest statistic used to assess the relationship between **two variables** when both are measured on a numerical scale is a Pearson correlation coefficient. In addition to requiring that both variables be measured on a numerical scale, Pearson correlation coefficients require that both variables are **normally distributed**. In published papers, Pearson correlation coefficients are denoted by the symbol "r." Pearson correlation coefficients capture the strength of the **linear association** between two variables. Consider the graph shown in Figure 7-1. This type of graph is called a scatterplot. Each small circle corresponds to one person and plots his/her weight against his/her height. For example, the four circles on the far left of the graph depict four people who are 60 inches tall and weigh between 95 and 120 pounds. Just eyeballing this scatterplot suggests that there is an association between weight and height: taller people tend to weigh more than shorter people. If the relationship between weight and height was perfect and linear, all of the points in the scatterplot would fall on a straight line and you would be able to tell how much a person weighed just by knowing his/her height. Obviously, the relationship shown in the graph is not a perfect one. Still, the scatterplot suggests that there is some association between height and weight. Now, we need a way to quantify the strength of that relationship. That is what Pearson correlations do. Trying to avoid as much math as possible, just recognize that if all of the points in the scatterplot fell on a straight line, the relationship between the two variables depicted in the scatterplot would be perfect. The closer the points are to forming a straight line, the stronger the relationship; the more the points diverge from a straight line, the weaker the relationship.

Pearson correlations can range from –1.0 to +1.0. The larger the absolute value of the correlation, the stronger the association. Thus, correlations of both –1.0 and +1.0 indicate perfect linear associations. In the scatterplot shown in Figure 7-1, r = 0.85, a pretty strong association. If r is greater than 0, the association is called a "positive" relationship. If r is less than 0, the association is called a "negative" or "inverse" relationship. For example, an inverse association might exist between experience as a pharmacist and dispensing errors. One would expect the number of dispensing errors to decrease as experience increases. This type of relationship is depicted in the scatterplot in Figure 7-2. The scatterplot depicts a strong inverse relationship (r = –0.90). (Note: The data presented are fictitious and are intended for illustration only.)

It is important to recognize that Pearson correlations only capture the strength of the **linear relationship** between two variables. If there is a **nonlinear relationship** between the variables, the Pearson correlation coefficient will underestimate the strength of this relationship. Figure 7-3 shows this type of nonlinear relationship. In this chart, the line connecting the dots in the scatterplot shows a perfect, inverse but nonlinear relationship between experience and dispensing errors. These data (again, fictitious) suggest that pharmacists with little experience make quite a few errors but that there is a fairly steep decrease in errors as experience is gained. After a certain point, however, few errors are being made, and additional experience is not associated with a further decrease in errors. Although the relationship shown is a perfect one (i.e., every dot lies on the line), r is not –1.0. It is only –0.78, demonstrating that the Pearson correlation

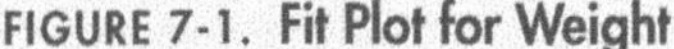

FIGURE 7-1. Fit Plot for Weight

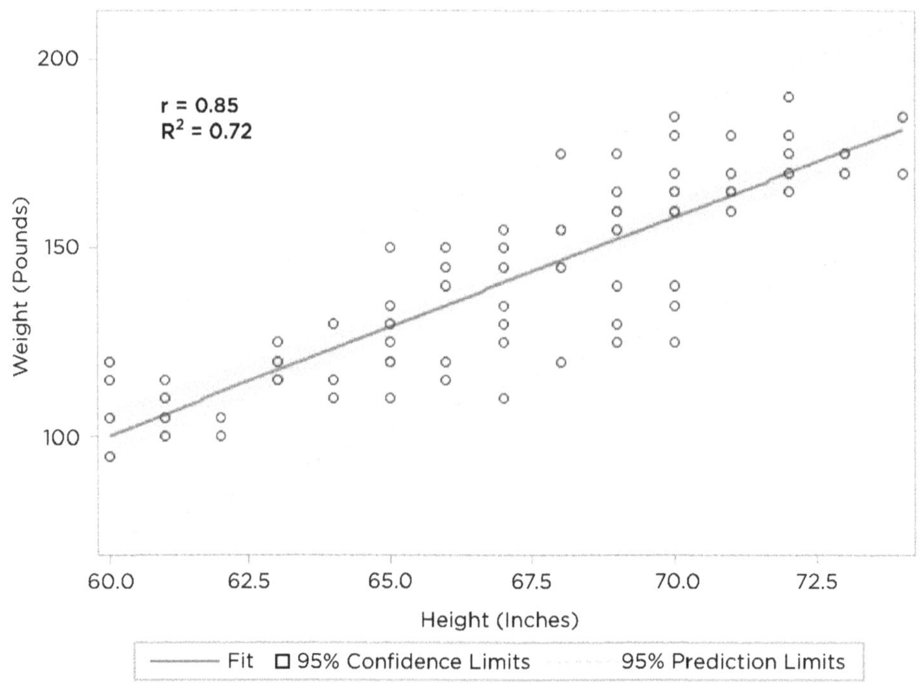

FIGURE 7-2. Fit Plot for Errors

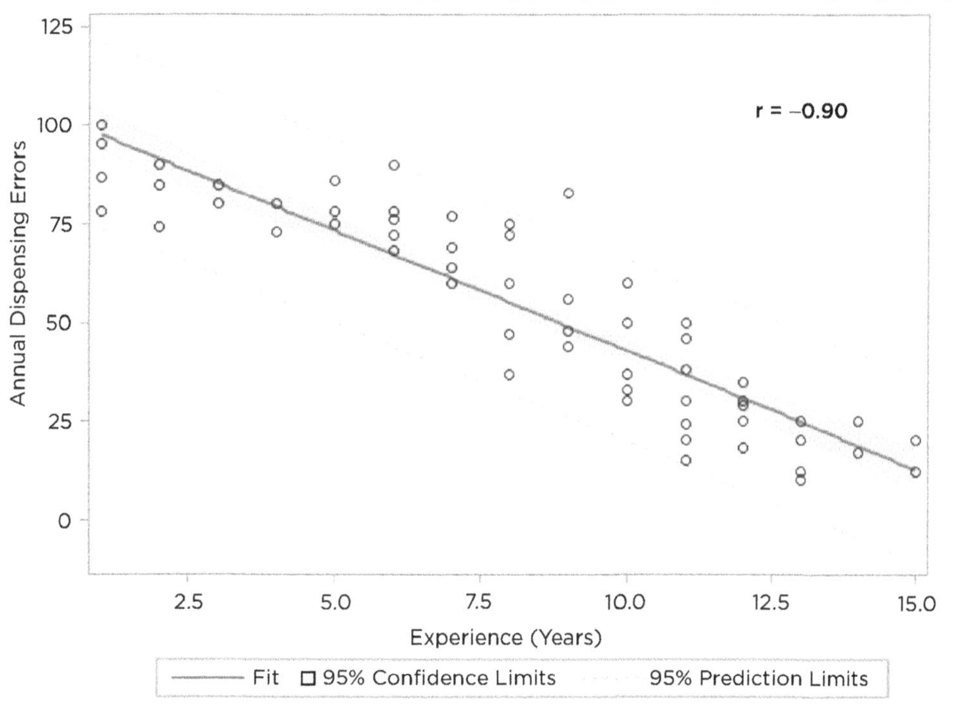

coefficient underestimates the strength of nonlinear relationships. The reason that this occurs is because the Pearson correlation coefficient is trying to put all of the observations (i.e., the dots in the scatterplot) on a **straight** line. Because this is not possible, the Pearson correlation coefficient (which only assesses the strength of the linear association between variables) fails to detect the perfect nonlinear relationship.

Finally, it is important to recognize that Pearson correlation coefficients are sample statistics. We use them only to estimate underlying population parameters. **As is always the case, our true interest is in the relationships that exist in the population from which the subjects in a study were drawn.** Thus, a Pearson r has a standard error (SE), and the SE can be used to compute a confidence interval (CI) in much the

FIGURE 7-3. Nonlinear Relationship

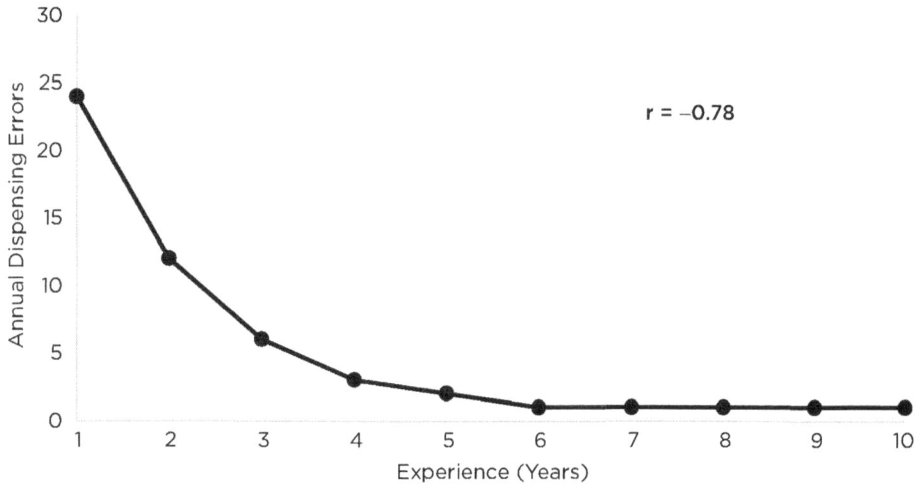

same way that we computed CIs for means in Chapter 3. The SEs for a Pearson r can be used to determine if a correlation is statistically significant. When evaluating a Pearson r for statistical significance, the null hypothesis is that there is no association between the variables. Thus, the expected value for a Pearson r if the null hypothesis is true is 0. When r = 0, there is no association between the variables (at least no linear association). If the *P* value resulting from the hypothesis test is low (e.g., usually less than 0.05), it is unlikely that the null hypothesis is true, and the correlation is considered statistically significant.

Spearman Correlation Coefficient

The Spearman correlation coefficient is similar to the Pearson correlation coefficient described previously. However, it is used when (1) the variables of interest have been measured on ordinal scales; (2) the assumption of normality is not met; or (3) a monotonic, but not straight line, relationship is hypothesized. (The relationship between two variables is monotonic if it always progresses in one direction, either upward [i.e., the value of one variable always increases when the value of the other variable increases] or downward [i.e., the value of one variable always decreases when the value of the other variable increases]. Note that curves that reverse directions [e.g., U-shaped curves] are not monotonic.) Like many other statistics used to analyze ordinal data, Spearman correlation coefficients are computed by converting the raw scores on the variables to ranks and then analyzing the ranks. Spearman correlation coefficients can range from −1.0 to +1.0 and are interpreted in the same manner as Pearson correlation coefficients.

Linear Regression Analysis

Linear regression analysis extends the ideas that underlie correlation analysis. However, one difference is that in regression analysis, investigators must identify one variable as the independent variable and one variable as the outcome variable. (When discussing correlations, I did not do this. I simply talked about the relationship between two variables.) Another difference is that investigators usually have multiple **independent** variables in the same regression model. In some cases, they may have multiple **outcome** variables included in the same regression model as well.

As when one performs ANOVA, regression analysis involves examining the extent to which the independent variable(s) of interest explain variation in the outcome variable. In regression analysis, this is done by determining the linear combination of independent variables that best explain variation in the outcome variable. The formula for the linear model is:

$$Y = B_0 + b_1x_1 + b_2x_2 + b_3x_3 + \cdots + Error,$$

where each x represents an observed value of the independent variables and Y represents observed values of the outcome variable. In the formula, "b_1," "b_2," and "b_3" are **regression coefficients**. Regression coefficients indicate how much the outcome variable is expected to change for each 1-unit change in the independent variable (i.e., the slope of the regression line). Regression coefficients can be either positive or negative. Positive regression coefficients indicate that as the independent variable increases, the outcome variable increases as well. Negative regression coefficients indicate that as the independent variable increases, the outcome variable decreases. B_0 is the Y-intercept. This is the estimated value of the outcome variable if all of the independent variables were "0." A regression analysis also yields an R^2 statistic. The R^2 statistic indicates the amount of variance in the outcome variable that is explained by the independent variables included in the regression model. R^2 has a possible range from 0 to +1.0. If $R^2 = 0$, the independent variables do not explain any of the variance in the outcome variable; if $R^2 = 1.0$, the independent variables explain all of the variance in the outcome variable. More generally, the larger the R^2 is, the greater the variance in the outcome variable that is explained by the independent variables in the model. Box 7-1 provides an example of a simple linear regression analysis involving only one independent variable. Box 7-2 provides output from this analysis generated by PC-SAS, a powerful statistical analysis software package.

BOX 7-1. Simple Linear Regression Example

The table below shows the weights of eight people before they began a clinical trial evaluating a fictitious medication for weight loss (i.e., X42) and after 6 months of treatment with the medication. The outcome variable in the study is weight after treatment.

Subject	1	2	3	4	5	6	7	8	Mean
Group	X42	X42	X42	X42	X42	X42	X42	X42	—
Sex	M	M	M	M	F	F	F	F	—
Weight (before)	341	353	354	361	291	300	305	311	327
Weight (after)	326	333	349	351	281	285	285	286	312

One would expect weight after treatment to be associated with weight prior to the initiation of therapy. Therefore, the investigators wanted to **control statistically** for differences in weight before the trial began when evaluating the effect of the experimental medication on weight at the end of the trial. This can be accomplished using linear regression.

The first step in a linear regression analysis involves fitting a straight line through the observed values of the independent and dependent variables in such a way that the observed values fall as close to the line as possible. In that way, error variance is minimized.

To determine how to position the line so that error is minimized, one must solve the linear model for the values of B_0 and each b in a way that minimizes the *Error* term in the model. If all of the observed values fell on the line defined by the model, the independent variable would explain all of the variation in the outcome variable, and the error term in the model would be "0." In the real world, the error term will almost never be "0." So, more generally, the closer the observed values are to the line, the smaller the error term. The further away the observed values are from the line, the larger the error term.

Because there is only one independent variable in this example, the linear model reduces to:

$$Y = B_0 + b_1x_1 + Error$$

I analyzed the data shown previously using Proc GLM in PC-SAS. From the output of this analysis presented in Box 7-2, you can see that the line that produced the best model fit had a Y-intercept (B_0) of −38.69 pounds and slope (b_1) of 1.07. This information can be used to calculate how much each participant in the study would be predicted to weigh at the end of the study based on his or her weight at the beginning of the study. The values calculated are called **predicted values**.

Box 7-2 also indicates that R^2 for the regression model is 0.959, indicating the weight at the start of the study explains nearly 96% of the variance in weight at the end of the study. Thus, one would expect the predicted values to correspond pretty closely to participants' actual weight at the end of the study.

To calculate the predicted value for each participant's weight at the end of the study, I simply plugged each participant's weight at the start of the study into the linear model equation with B_0 set at −38.69 and b_1 set at 1.07. Thus, for Subject 1, I calculated:

$$\hat{Y} = -38.69 + 1.07(341) = 326.18$$

In this formula, Y is replaced by $\hat{Y}$ to denote that we are calculating predicted values of Y.

To calculate the amount of error associated with each predicted value, I subtracted each participant's predicted weight at the end of the study from their actual weight at the end of the study. Thus, for Subject 1, I calculated:

$$Error = Y - \hat{Y} = 326 - 326.18 = -0.18$$

(continued)

BOX 7-1. Simple Linear Regression Example *(Continued)*

The table below shows the predicted value and error for each of the eight study participants.

Subject	1	2	3	4	5	6	7	8
Group	X42	X42	X42	X42	X42	X42	X42	X42
Sex	M	M	M	M	F	F	F	F
Weight (before)	341	353	354	361	291	300	305	311
Weight (after)	326	333	349	351	281	285	285	286
Weight (after) (predicted)	326.18	339.02	340.09	347.58	272.68	282.31	287.66	294.08
Error	–0.18	–6.02	8.91	3.42	8.32	2.69	–2.66	–8.08

Each participant's before and after weight are depicted by the small circles in the scatterplot below. For example, the fourth small circle from the left depicts the data for Subject 8, who weighed 311 pounds at the start of the study and 286 pounds after. By convention, scatterplots plot the independent variable along the x-axis and the dependent variable along the y-axis.

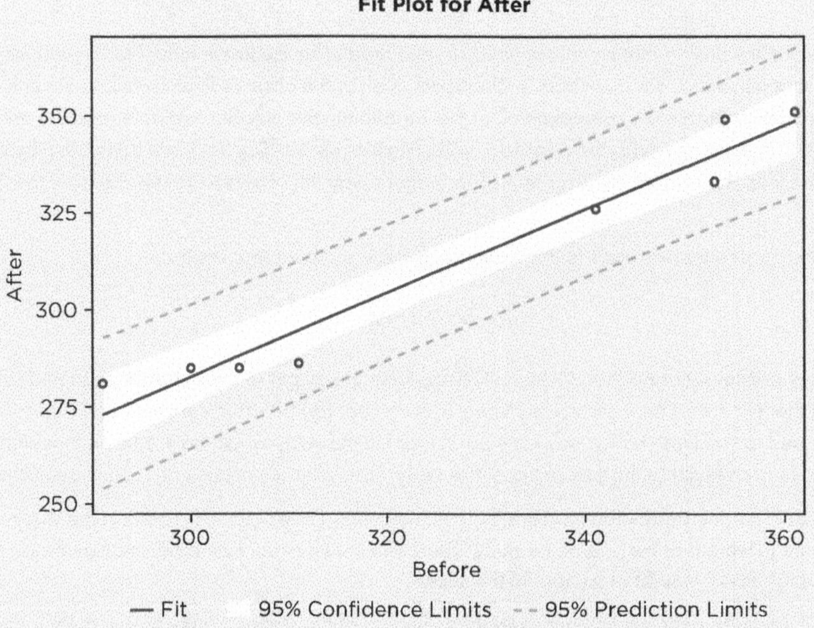

The predicted values for each study participant fall on the blue line, drawn using the values of B_0 and b_1 derived from the analysis.

The distance between the line and each observation corresponds to the error terms calculated previously. For example, Participant 8 weighed about 8 pounds less at the end of the study than predicted. Although none of the observations fall exactly on the straight line, they are all pretty close, reflecting the model R^2 of 0.959.

BOX 7-2. SAS Output for Simple Linear Regression Example

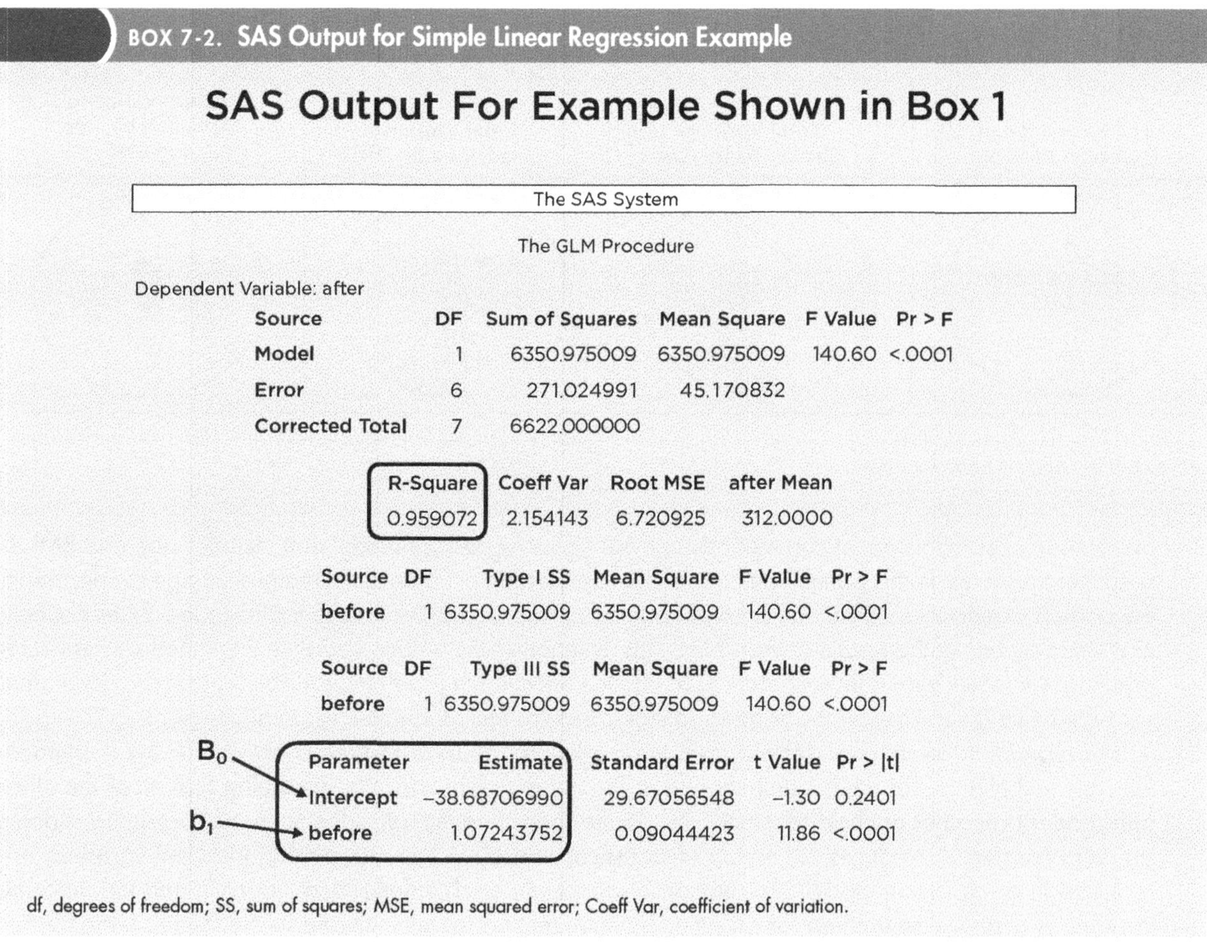

SAS Output For Example Shown in Box 1

The SAS System

The GLM Procedure

Dependent Variable: after

Source	DF	Sum of Squares	Mean Square	F Value	Pr > F
Model	1	6350.975009	6350.975009	140.60	<.0001
Error	6	271.024991	45.170832		
Corrected Total	7	6622.000000			

R-Square	Coeff Var	Root MSE	after Mean
0.959072	2.154143	6.720925	312.0000

Source	DF	Type I SS	Mean Square	F Value	Pr > F
before	1	6350.975009	6350.975009	140.60	<.0001

Source	DF	Type III SS	Mean Square	F Value	Pr > F
before	1	6350.975009	6350.975009	140.60	<.0001

Parameter	Estimate	Standard Error	t Value	Pr > |t|
Intercept	−38.68706990	29.67056548	−1.30	0.2401
before	1.07243752	0.09044423	11.86	<.0001

df, degrees of freedom; SS, sum of squares; MSE, mean squared error; Coeff Var, coefficient of variation.

Multiple Linear Regression

Depending on the sample size, a regression model can include multiple independent variables. In general, regression analysis requires a minimum of 60 subjects and at least 5 to 10 observations for each independent variable in the model. Thus, a sample of at least 100 would be needed to support a regression model with 10 independent variables. In smaller samples, the parameter estimates (i.e., the intercept term and regression coefficients) will be unstable. Therefore, when reading reports of studies reported in the literature, beware of the use of multiple regression in studies with very small samples.

Multiple regression allows investigators to determine how much of the total variance in an outcome variable is explained by the set of independent variables included in the model. In addition, investigators can determine the amount of **unique variance** in the outcome variable that is explained by each independent variable. Perhaps most important, multiple regression allows investigators to measure the association between each independent variable and the outcome variable, predicting how much the outcome variable will change for each 1-unit change in an independent variable while controlling for all of the other independent variables in the model.

The term "unique variance" refers to variance in the outcome variable that cannot be explained by any of the other independent variables in the model. This is depicted diagrammatically in Figure 7-4. In the figure, diastolic blood pressure (DBP) is the outcome variable of interest. The first panel in Figure 7-4 represents the total variance of DBP among the people in the sample. If everyone in the sample had the same DBP, there would be no variance to explain. The second panel shows the portion of the variance in DBP that can be explained by age. The third panel shows the portion of the variance in DBP that can be explained by body mass index (BMI), which is a measure of obesity. The final panel shows the portion of variance in DBP that can be explained by age and BMI taken together. The total area covered by the

FIGURE 7-4. Unique Variance

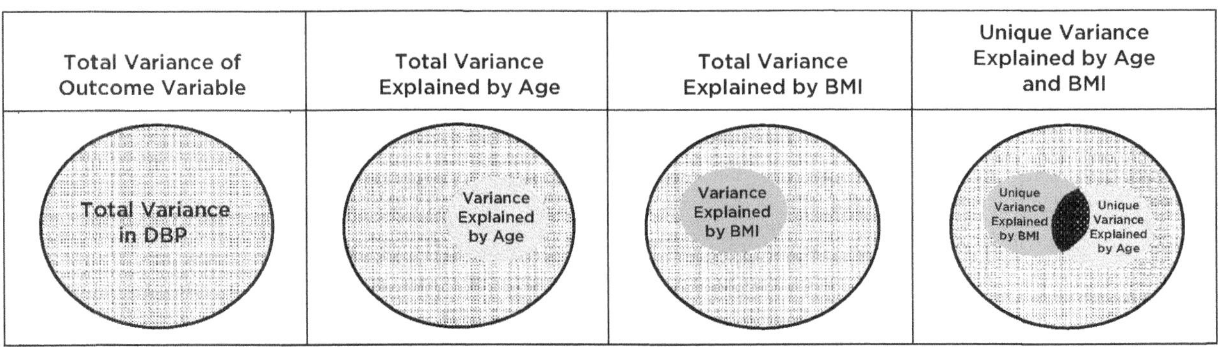

DBP, diastolic blood pressure; BMI, body mass index.

two inner circles in this panel corresponds to the R^2 for a regression model that includes age and BMI as predictor variables. In this panel, you can see that the portion of variance explained by age overlaps with the portion explained by BMI. The area of nonoverlap represents the unique variance in DBP that is only explained by one of the predictor variables. This isolation of the unique variance explained by individual predictor variables allows investigators to assess the effect each predictor variable has on the dependent variable while controlling for the other predictor variables included in the regression model.

The regression coefficients derived from the model can be used to predict how much the dependent variable will change for each 1-unit change in the independent variable, **assuming that all of the other independent variables are held constant**. The phrase "assuming that all of the other independent variables are held constant" introduces the notion of **statistical control**. When multiple independent variables are included in a regression model, the relationship between each independent variable and the outcome variable is assessed **controlling for** all other independent variables included in the model. Imagine, for example, that an investigator was concerned that a medication had the unwanted effect of increasing DBP. She might collect a sample that includes some people who use the medication and others who do not. She could then determine if people who used the medication had higher DBP than people who did not use the medication. As just described, this could be accomplished via an independent groups t-test. However, the investigator knows that DBP tends to increase with age and BMI. Therefore, if people who used the medication tended to be older and more obese than people who did not use the medication, a t-test would likely suggest that DBP is higher among people taking the medication compared to those not taking it. However, this observed difference might be totally explained by differences in age and BMI between medication users and nonusers. Thus, age and BMI are potential **confounders**. Before the investigator can examine the relationship between DBP and medication use, she really needs to control for age and BMI. Conceptually, this is accomplished by first removing all variation in DBP that can be explained by differences in participant age and BMI and then solving the linear model focusing only on the residual variance (i.e., the variance that cannot be explained by age and BMI). This is depicted diagrammatically in Figure 7-5. The total variance in DBP is depicted by the large circle. When age is added to the regression model, it explains a portion of the total variance in DBP. When BMI is added to the model, it explains an additional portion of the variance. This leaves only the remaining area (i.e., the residual variance) that could be explained by medication use.

In this example, age and BMI are a special type of independent variable: control variables. In general, investigators are not particularly interested in the relationship between the control variables included in their regression models and the outcome variable. However, control variables are included to eliminate the type of potential confounding described previously. As a reader of the literature, one of your primary responsibilities is to determine whether the investigators have included in their models all of the variables that could potentially confound the relationships of primary interest. For the most part, identification of appropriate control variables does not require statistical expertise; it requires clinical expertise. If you are

FIGURE 7-5. **Statistical Control**

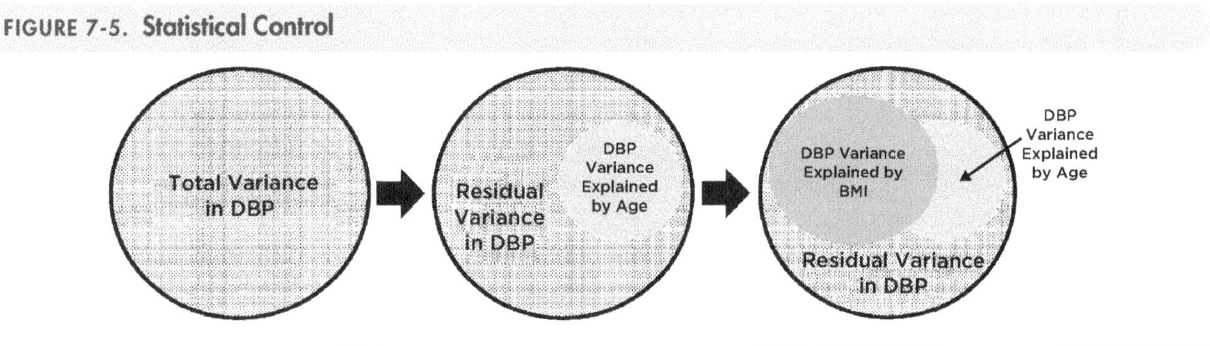

DBP, diastolic blood pressure; BMI, body mass index.

a student, you will become better at being able to identify the control variables that should be included in analyses designed to answer different research questions as you gain clinical expertise. If you read an article and an important potential confounder was not included in the regression model, you cannot rule out the possibility that any relationship observed was due to the potential confounder, which makes it difficult to interpret the findings reported.

Model Building

The procedures that investigators follow to determine which variables to include in a regression model are often referred to as "model building." The most common **statistical procedures** are forward regression, backward regression, and stepwise regression.

In forward regression, the initial regression model does not include any predictor variables. The investigator sets a criterion level of statistical significance (i.e., *P* value) that candidate predictor variables (i.e., those being considered for addition to the model) must meet to be entered into the model. This *P* value typically ranges from $P<0.05$ to $P<0.20$. To identify the first variable to enter the model, one must examine the association between the outcome variable and each candidate predictor variable. If any of the predictor variables have *P* values less than the criterion set by the investigator, the variable with the smallest *P* value is selected for entry. To identify the second variable to enter the model, one must examine the association between the outcome variable and each of the remaining candidate predictor variables, controlling for the first variable entered into the model. If any of these variables has a *P* value less than the criterion set by the investigator, the variable with the smallest *P* value is selected for entry. This process continues until none of the candidate predictor variables has a *P* value that meets the criterion for entry.

In backward regression, the initial model includes all of the candidate predictor variables. The investigator sets a criterion level of statistical significance (i.e., *P* value) that the candidate variables must meet to remain in the model. As before, this *P* value typically ranges from $P<0.05$ to $P<0.20$. To identify the first variable to eliminate from the model, the association between the outcome variable and each candidate predictor variable is examined, controlling for all of the other predictor variables in the model. If any of the candidate variables has a *P* value greater than the criterion set by the investigator, the variable with the largest *P* value is selected for elimination. To identify the second variable to eliminate from the model, the association between the outcome variable and each of the remaining candidate variables is examined. Again, if any of the candidate variables has a *P* value larger than the criterion set by the investigator, the variable with the largest *P* value is selected for elimination. This process continues until all of the predictor variables remaining in the model have *P* values that meet the criterion set by the investigator.

Stepwise regression can be performed in either a forward or backward manner, with no predictor variables entered initially (forward method) or all predictor variables entered initially (backward manner). Unlike forward or backward regression, however, in stepwise regression, variables may enter the model in one step and be eliminated from the model in a subsequent step. This can occur when the association between the outcome variable and a predictor variable becomes statistically nonsignificant after controlling for another predictor variable.

All of these statistical strategies for model building are criticized because decisions about what variables to include in the final model are based entirely on statistical criteria. As a result, variables that clinicians believe are important may not be included simply because a fairly arbitrary statistical criterion was not met. In addition, because so many relationships are evaluated, the potential inflation of Type I (α) error is a major concern.

Alternatively, investigators can select the variables to include in a regression model (as well as the order in which they are added to the model) based on scientific and clinical knowledge. This is referred to as "hierarchical regression." Hierarchical regression has the advantage of allowing investigators to use their clinical expertise when building models. However, beware of papers that state hierarchical regression was used when, in reality, the investigators used a model-building strategy guided only by statistical criteria. Preferably, model building is guided by scientific/clinical knowledge and statistical criteria to identify the best-fitting model.

Regardless of the model-building strategy used, when you are reading a paper that uses regression analyses, be sure that the investigators considered all potential confounding factors. Be wary of study findings when potentially important confounders are not included in a regression model only because they failed to meet a statistical criterion.

Summary of Important Points

Below, I summarize important things to understand concerning the interpretation of the results of correlation and regression analyses:

1. **Unstandardized Regression Coefficients.** The *b*s in a regression model are called **regression coefficients**. They are also sometimes called **beta coefficients**. These coefficients indicate how much the outcome variable is expected to change for every 1-unit change in the independent variable, controlling for all of the other independent variables in the model. Expected change is expressed in raw units, corresponding to the measurement scales of the variables involved (e.g., pounds, mmHg).

   If a predictor variable is dichotomous (e.g., male versus female, experimental medication versus placebo), investigators typically assign a value of "0" to the people in one group and "1" to the people in the other group. The regression coefficient then indicates the difference between the groups on the outcome variable. For example, imagine that a randomized controlled trial (RCT) is conducted investigating the effect of a new medication on low-density lipoprotein (LDL). People assigned to the placebo group were coded as "0" and people assigned to the experimental medication group were coded as "1." Results of a regression analysis indicate that the regression coefficient for the variable indexing treatment group is –3.2 (95% CI: –1.2 to –5.2). This indicates that LDL was 3.2 points (mg/dL) lower among people who took the experimental medication compared to those who took the placebo. Further, because the 95% CI does not include 0, one would conclude that the difference between the placebo and experimental medication groups was statistically significant.

   If a predictor variable is measured on a nominal (i.e., categorical) scale but has more than two levels (i.e., it is **not** dichotomous), investigators often convert the variable into multiple dichotomous variables. This is accomplished via "dummy" coding. For example, imagine that in the RCT described previously, the investigators were examining two different medications (Medications A and B) and wanted to compare the effects of each medication to a placebo. To do this, they would create two "dummy" variables. Because they want to compare each medication to a placebo, people assigned to the placebo group would form the "reference" group. The variable "Medication A" would be coded "1" for patients who took Medication A and "0" for patients who took either a placebo or Medication B. The variable "Medication B" would be coded "1" for patients who took Medication B and "0" for patients who took either a placebo or Medication A. Note that people in the reference group receive a 0 for both dummy variables.

Results of a regression analysis indicate that the regression coefficient for Medication A is –3.2 (95% CI: –1.2 to –5.2), identical to that reported previously, and that the regression coefficient for Medication B is –0.8 (95% CI: –2.8 to 1.2). As before, the regression coefficient for Medication A indicates that LDL was 3.2 points (mg/dL) lower among people who took Medication A compared with those who took the placebo and that this difference was statistically significant. The regression coefficient for Medication B indicates that LDL was –0.8 points lower among people who took Medication B compared to those who took the placebo. However, this difference was not statistically significant. Notice that with this type of coding scheme, people reading a paper reporting study findings cannot directly compare the effectiveness of Medication A to Medication B. It is only possible to compare the effectiveness of each medication to placebo. Moreover, because the CIs for Medications A and B overlap, it is impossible for readers to determine whether Medication A is more effective than Medication B. However, readers can calculate the difference in the means for Medication A and Medication B by taking the difference between the two betas, such that (Medication A – Placebo) – (Medication B – Placebo) = Medication A – Medication B = –3.2 – (–0.8) = –2.4. Thus, Medication A decreases LDL by an additional 2.4 points as compared to Medication B. The lack of an SE for this difference score prevents one from determining if the difference is statistically significant.

Finally, remember that regression coefficients are estimates of population parameters based on data from a sample. Thus, they have SEs that reflect sampling variability, and it is possible to evaluate them for statistical significance using either CIs or hypothesis tests. In most cases, the null hypothesis is that change in the independent variable is not associated with any change in the outcome variable. Thus, the expected value of a regression coefficient under the null hypothesis is usually "0."

2. **Standardized Regression Coefficients.** Regression coefficients can be standardized so that change is expressed in standard deviation (SD) units. Thus, standardized regression coefficients indicate how many SDs the outcome variable is expected to change for every one SD increase in the independent variable. This can make it easier to compare the effects of different predictor variables included in a model. Standardized regression coefficients are sometimes denoted by "βs" rather than "*bs*," but this convention is not followed routinely in the literature. When you are reading a paper, be sure to determine whether standardized or unstandardized regression coefficients are being reported. This will determine whether you interpret the "βs/*bs*" in raw units (e.g., pounds, mmHg) or SD units.
3. The **R^2** for a regression model indicates the proportion of variance in the outcome variable that is explained by the independent variables in the model. R^2 is sometimes referred to as the coefficient of determination.
4. **Correlation Coefficients (r).** Correlation coefficients capture the strength of the linear relationship between two variables. They are sample statistics used to estimate the correlation between the variables in the population of interest. Correlation coefficients have SEs that reflect sampling variability and can be evaluated for statistical significance using either CIs or hypothesis tests. In most cases, the null hypothesis is that the correlation between the variables is "0" in the population. Thus, the expected value of a correlation coefficient under the null hypothesis is usually "0."
5. **Regression Coefficients Versus Correlation Coefficients.** It is important to recognize the distinction between regression and correlation coefficients because they provide quite different information. Regression coefficients provide information about the expected change in the outcome variable for each 1-unit increase in the independent variable. As a regression coefficient increases, the slope of the straight line becomes steeper. However, the observed values do not necessarily get closer to the line. Thus, the independent variable may still explain little of the variance in the outcome variable. Correlation coefficients, in contrast, provide information about how close the observed values are to a straight line. As the absolute value of a correlation coefficient increases, the observed values fall closer to a straight line and more of the variance in the outcome variable is explained by the independent variable. However, the slope of the line does not necessarily

become steeper. Thus, changes in the independent variable may still result in little change in the outcome variable.

6. **Statistical Control.** A major advantage of regression analysis is the ability to control for potential confounders. Obviously, the model can only control for variables that are measured and included in the model. When you read a paper, always ask yourself whether the investigators included all of the relevant control variables in their models.

Extensions of the Linear Model

Regression techniques are incredibly versatile. They can be used to answer a wide variety of research questions using data derived from many different study designs. In this section, I briefly describe some of the extensions of the linear model that you are most likely to encounter when reading the medical literature.

Polynomial regression is a special type of regression model used to capture **curvilinear relationships** between the independent and outcome variables. As the name suggests, polynomial regression models include independent variables that are raised to a power of "x." Thus, if the outcome variable is blood pressure, age^2 might be included as an independent variable if the investigators believe that there is a curvilinear relationship between age and blood pressure. Squared variables (e.g., age^2) are referred to as "quadratic terms." Models can also include cubic (e.g., age^3) terms. More generally, polynomial regression is subsumed within the general linear model: $Y_i = b_0 + \Sigma b_i\ f(X_i)$, where $f(X_i)$ indicates that each term in the model is a mathematical function of the predictor variables (i.e., *X*s).

Analysis of covariance (ANCOVA) is used when an investigator is interested in differences between two or more groups but needs to control for a numerical variable. For example, in a study comparing the effectiveness of two medications for weight loss, ANCOVA might be used to control for baseline (pre-intervention) weight.

In **mixed models,** one of the assumptions of linear regression is that the observations in the sample are independent of one another. This assumption is often violated in studies where participants are assessed multiple times. For example, in a study evaluating the effectiveness of a weight loss medication, participants might be weighed at monthly intervals over a 12-month follow-up period. Clearly, participants' weight for 1 month would not be independent of their weight at other months. When this type of design is used, investigators can incorporate predictor variables into their regression models to control for variation in the outcome variable **within** each study participant across the multiple assessments. This is called "within person" variance. Thus, each participant might be given a unique identification (ID) number and this ID number would be entered into the regression model as a **random effect**. In regression models, random effects are used when one collects data from a sample of the possible levels of a predictor variable but wants to generalize findings to other levels. This will almost always be the case with variables included to control for within-person variation because investigators want to make inferences about everyone in the population from which study participants were drawn. In contrast, **fixed effects** are used when the investigator wants to make inferences only about the levels of the variable included in the study. For example, if an investigator wanted to determine if Medication A is more effective than placebo, treatment (i.e., Medication A/placebo) would be considered a fixed effect. In case you have not guessed, mixed models derive their name from the fact that they include both fixed and random effects, which is due to the fact that they include effects that vary between subjects as well as effects that vary within subjects. Thus, a mixed model combines an x-way ANOVA with a repeated measures ANOVA.

In **generalized estimating equations,** one assumption that the observations in a sample are independent of one another is also violated in multicenter studies where people recruited from one site may be more similar to others recruited from that site than they are to people recruited from other sites. It is also violated in studies where multiple patients are recruited from the same physician because patients seen by the same physician may be more similar to one another than they are to people seen by other doctors. In this latter example, patients are said to be **nested** within physicians. Generalized estimating equations is a group of methods that can accommodate these types of complex designs and is now frequently used in the literature. Conceptually, these procedures control statistically for any variation in the outcome variable that may be explained by the similarity among people within clusters (e.g., the patients seen by a particular physician or recruited from a particular site).

Examples from the Literature

We will now review selected findings from three recent studies that have used some of the tests described in this chapter to analyze study data. The first study examined the effect of a device called a "talking pill bottle" on medication self-efficacy, knowledge, adherence, and blood pressure among hypertensive patients with low health literacy.[1] This device allows pharmacists to record a message up to 60 seconds in length that patients can replay at home on an as-needed basis. The study used an RCT design with two groups. In the intervention group, participants received their hypertension medications in "talking pill bottles." In the control group, participants received standard care. A total of 134 patients were recruited from two community pharmacies. Each participant was assessed four times: at baseline and at 1 month, 2 months, and 3 months following baseline. The primary outcome variables were antihypertensive medication knowledge; self-efficacy, assessed by the Self-Efficacy for Appropriate Medication Use Scale (SEAMS); medication adherence, assessed by the Morisky Medication Adherence Scale (MMAS-8), and blood pressure. In the data analysis section of the paper, the investigators state, "For our primary study outcomes, we used the between-groups t test to compare end points at the 3-month (T90) mark" (p. 23). Although it is appropriate to focus on between group differences, the study might have had more power to detect clinically meaningful between-group differences if the investigators had used regression analysis to control for baseline values of the outcome variables. They might also have used a mixed models approach that would have allowed them to incorporate data from all four time points into their primary analyses. The investigators go on to state, "We also used the repeated-measures t test to look for change scores within each arm between baseline (T0) and the 3-month exit point (T90)" (p. 23). **The results of these within-group changes should be considered exploratory given that the study was designed as an RCT.** However, rather than reporting the results of their primary analyses in the abstract for the paper (see Box 7-3), the abstract states, "Blood pressure decreased significantly in the intervention arm." The abstract fails to mention that all of the analyses assessing between group differences were not statistically significant, as reflected in the excerpts from the text of the paper shown in Box 7-3. This example illustrates why readers of the literature should only take the information in the abstract of a paper as a starting point. The primary analyses in any RCT should focus on differences **between** the groups. Type I (α) error can increase dramatically as investigators move beyond these primary analyses.

Box 7-3 also presents a figure from the "talking pill bottle" study that the investigators used to reach their conclusion that the intervention had a positive effect on blood pressure. The figure shows the mean change from baseline and 95% CIs for diastolic and systolic blood pressure **within each group** at the three follow-up assessments. In their discussion of this figure, the investigators focused on the fact that the 95% CIs for the standard care group spanned "0," whereas the 95% CIs for the intervention group did not. Although this is true, one can also see from the figure in Box 7-3 that most of 95% CIs for the intervention group contained the mean observed in the standard care group. Thus, one cannot rule out the possibility (with 95% confidence) that the true population means are the same, a conclusion that is consistent with the results of the between group t-tests. The take home message is that, while some of the differences reported in this paper are interesting, it would be premature to declare that the "talking pill bottle" can help patients with hypertension and low literacy better control their blood pressure. Notably, the investigators identified this study as a pilot study in the title of the paper, suggesting that a larger study may follow.

Finally, the analysis section of the "talking pill bottle" study also states, "Pearson product-moment correlation coefficients were computed to assess the association between self-reported medication adherence

BOX 7-3. Talking Pill Bottle Study

ABSTRACT

Objectives: To test the effect of "Talking Pill Bottles" on medication self-efficacy, knowledge, adherence, and blood pressure readings among hypertensive patients with low health literacy and to assess patients' acceptance of this innovation.
Design: Longitudinal nonblinded randomized trial with standard treatment and intervention arms.
Setting and participants: Two community pharmacies serving an ethnically diverse population in the Pacific Northwest. Participants were consented patients with antihypertension prescriptions who screened positive for low health literacy based on the Test of Functional Health Literacy Short Form. Participants in the intervention arm received antihypertensive medications and recordings of pharmacists' counseling in Talking Pill Bottles at baseline. Control arm participants received antihypertensive medications and usual care instructions.
Main outcome measures: Comparison and score changes between baseline and day 90 for medication knowledge test, Self-Efficacy for Appropriate Medication Use Scale (SEAMS), Morisky Medication Adherence Scale (MMAS-8), blood pressure, and responses to semi-structured exit interviews and Technology Acceptance Model surveys.
Results: Of 871 patients screened for health literacy, 134 eligible participants were enrolled in the trial. The sample was elderly, ethnically diverse, of low income, and experienced regarding hypertension and medication history. In both arms, we found high baseline scores in medication knowledge test, SEAMS, and MMAS-8 and minimal changes in these measures over the 90-day study period. Blood pressure decreased significantly in the intervention arm. Acceptability scores for the Talking Pill Bottle technology were high.
Conclusion: Our results suggest that providing audio-assisted medication instructions in Talking Pill Bottles positively affected blood pressure control and was well accepted by patients with low health literacy. Further research involving newly diagnosed patients is needed to mitigate possible ceiling effects that we observed in an experienced population.

Excerpts from text

At T90, in the between-group analysis, the overall mean knowledge score of the standard treatment arm (M = 0.93; SD = 0.11) was not significantly different from that of the intervention arm (M = 0.93; SD = 0.09): t(159) = –0.07; *P* = 0.948. (p. 24)

At T90, the between-group mean self-efficacy score of the standard treatment arm (M = 33.00; SD = 5.38) was not significantly different from that of the intervention arm (M = 32.76; SD = 6.71): t(109) = 0.21; *P* = 0.838. (p. 24)

Comparing between groups at T90, the Morisky Medication Adherence Scale score was not significantly different between the standard treatment arm (M = 7.07; SD = 1.25) and the intervention arm (M = 7.06; SD = 1.27): t(108) = 0.46; *P* = 0.496. (p. 24)

The overall mean cumulative medication gap score based on 90-day refill history for the intervention arm (M = 6.57; SD = 7.93) showed slightly higher adherence than the standard treatment arm (M = 8.85; SD = 11.71), but it was not significantly different: t(127) = 1.30; *P* = 0.197. (p. 24)

In the between-group analysis, the BP readings at T90 between the standard treatment arm (SBP: M = 139.63, SD = 15.29; DBP: M = 75.23, SD = 10.52) and the intervention arm (SBP: M = 138.89, SD = 19.37; DBP: M = 74.71, SD = 13.00) were not significantly different (SBP: t(127) = 0.24, *P* = 0.810; DBP: t(127) = 0.25, *P* = 0.801). (p. 25)

BOX 7-3. Talking Pill Bottle Study *(Continued)*

Figure From Paper

Figure With Annotations

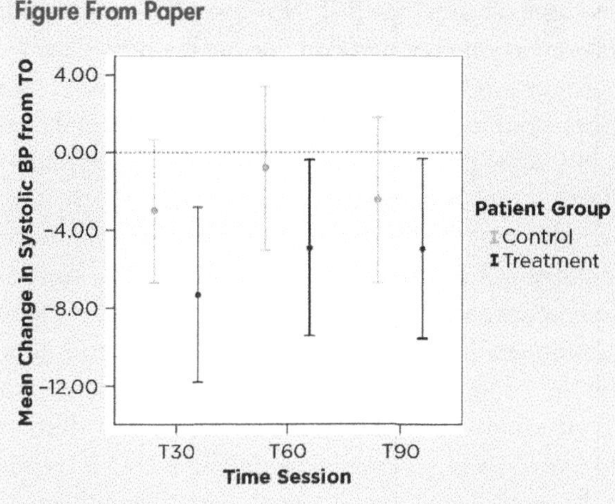

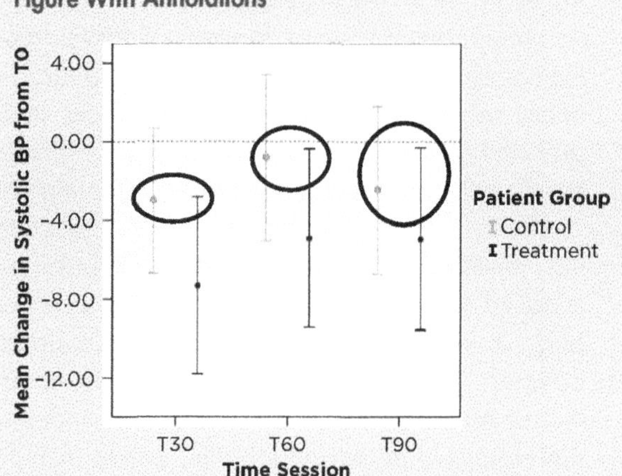

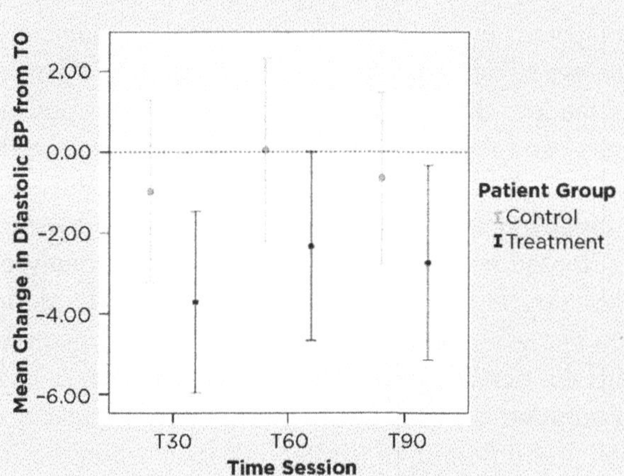

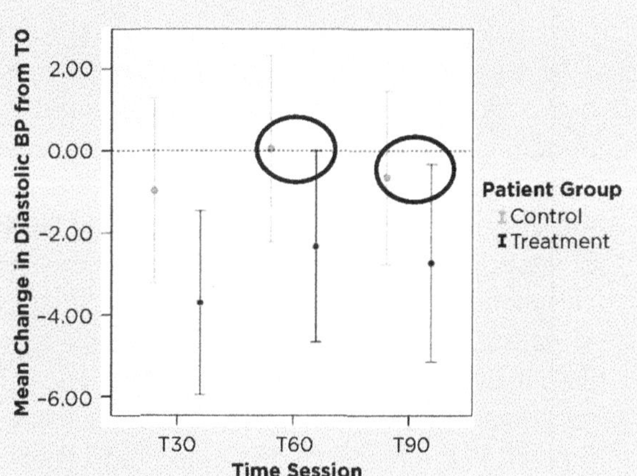

Table 5
Correlation between medication self-efficacy, adherence, and diastolic blood pressure

Measurement 1	Measurement 2	Standard treatment		Intervention	
		Pearson coefficient	*P* value	Pearson coefficient	*P* value
Mean MMAS-8 score	Mean DBP	−0.168	0.012	−0.259	<0.001
Mean SEAMS	Mean DBP	−0.132	0.048	−0.145	0.029
Mean SEAMS	Mean MMAS-8 score	−0.490	<0.001	−0.539	<0.001

Abbreviations as in Tables 3 and 4.

rates (SEAMS and the MMAS-8) and diastolic blood pressures" (p. 23). Higher scores on the SEAMS and MMAS-8 reflect greater medication self-efficacy and adherence, respectively. As shown in the table in Box 7-3, all of the correlations are negative and statistically significant at $P < 0.05$. Thus, greater adherence and self-efficacy were associated with lower DBP. However, the negative correlation shown in the table between self-efficacy and medication adherence, which indicates that higher levels of self-efficacy are associated with lower levels of medication adherence, is surprising. It may be a typo because in the text of the paper the investigators state, "A positive association also was found between mean MMAS and mean SEAMS for both arms" (p. 25). In the text of the paper, the investigators also state, "A negative correlation between the adherence and self-efficacy variables and mean DBP readings of the 2 arms was identified, with a stronger relationship found in the intervention arm" (p. 25). However, the investigators do not appear to have performed a statistical test to determine whether one can rule out the possibility that the correlations in the intervention and standard care groups are the same. In general, when making inferences about any between group differences, investigators need to perform a statistical test to determine the probability that any differences in point estimates (in this case, point estimates of population correlation coefficients) are simply the result of sampling variability.

The second study examined factors associated with pharmacists' perceptions of the ease with which they could find a different position with specific characteristics.[2] As described in Chapter 4, this variable is called "perceived job alternatives" and includes four separate dimensions: environmental conditions (e.g., lower workload, less stress), professional opportunities (e.g., more intellectual challenge, more patient contact), compensation (e.g., better pay, better benefits), and coworkers (e.g., better pharmacist and technician coworkers). The independent variables used to predict scores on the different dimensions of perceived job alternatives include demographics (e.g., age, sex), practice characteristics (e.g., primary work setting), and worklife attitudes (e.g., work–home conflict, professional commitment). Data were collected via a cross-sectional survey completed by a nationally representative sample of 1,574 practicing pharmacists. In Chapter 4, we reviewed findings from this study reporting bivariate associations between the independent variables and the four dimensions of perceived job alternatives. In addition to the bivariate analyses, the investigators used multiple linear regression to examine the unique association between each independent variable and each of the four dimensions of perceived job alternatives **while controlling for all of the other independent variables**. In the data analysis section of the paper, the investigators state that they used a "forced entry method" in the regression analyses. This means that they included all of the independent variables in the regression models without regard to statistical significance. Findings from the regression analyses are shown in Box 7-4. I have annotated the table with numbers to facilitate reference. Toward the bottom of the table (see [1]), the adjusted R^2 for each model is reported. In contrast to the R^2, the adjusted R^2 takes into consideration the number of predictor variables included in the regression model. The adjusted R^2 is often reported when a fairly large number of predictor variables are included in a regression model because the addition of predictor variables into a model can only increase R^2 (i.e., R^2 cannot become smaller with the addition of predictor variables). In contrast, the adjusted R^2 can decrease with the addition of predictor variables that explain little variance in the outcome variable. From the adjusted R^2s shown in Box 7-4, you can see that model explains the most variance in the "professional opportunities" dimension of perceived job alternatives (17.7%). The first footnote at the bottom of the table (see [2]) explains that the table reports standardized regression coefficients that allow readers to more easily compare the relative impact of the various independent variables on the outcome variable. From the regression coefficients, you can see that of the 14 independent variables, organizational commitment was the most strongly associated with three of the four dimensions of perceived job satisfaction (see [3]). Because the regression coefficients for organizational commitment are negative, the findings indicate that higher scores on the measure of organizational commitment were associated with greater perceived difficulty finding a different job with better environmental conditions, professional opportunities, and coworkers. Notably, organizational commitment was not associated with perceived difficulty finding a different job with better compensation. For categorical variables such as sex (see [4]), regression coefficients cannot be interpreted unless one knows how the variable was scored. For example, for the variable "male," we need to know whether males were

BOX 7-4. Perceived Job Alternatives Study

Table 5

Standardized regression coefficients from multivariate results of the 4 perceived job alternatives dimensions[a]

Characteristics		Environmental conditions	Professional opportunities	Compensation	Coworkers
Demographic variables					
Male		0.070	0.091[*]	−0.002	0.069
White		0.096[*]	0.055	0.157[*]	−0.047
Age	4	−0.119[†]	−0.136[†]	−0.058	−0.062
Married or partnered		0.015	−0.005	−0.051	0.008
Divorced or widowed		−0.019	−0.047	−0.057	−0.008
Practice variables					
Primary work setting					
Hospital		0.052	−0.055	0.035	−0.056
Other patient care	5	−0.042	−0.039	0.002	−0.020
Other nonpatient care		0.024	−0.007	−0.006	−0.007
Work status					
Full-time		−0.016	−0.021	−0.086[*]	0.001
Job position					
Management		0.055	0.010	−0.031	0.029
Worklife attitudes					
Environmental stress[b]		0.125[†]	0.085	0.030	0.027
Control in work environment[c]		0.036	−0.130[†]	0.012	0.008
Professional commitment[d]		0.097[†]	0.001	0.073	0.026
Work-home conflict[e]	3	0.063	−0.099[†]	−0.077	−0.010
Organizational commitment[e]		−0.239[†]	−0.272[†]	−0.066	−0.282[†]
Future employment plan[f]		0.134[†]	0.144[†]	0.166[†]	0.094[†]
Model summaries					
Adjusted R^2	1	0.119	0.177	0.050	0.083
Standard error of the estimate		3.811	3.086	2.370	1.564
F-statistic		5.688	8.485	2.863	4.199

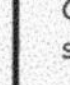

Coefficients are standardized regression coefficients. Reference category for the independent variables is female, nonwhite, single, working in community setting, part-time status, and staff position.

[a] Perceived job alternative dimensions measured with the use of a 5-point Likert-type scale (1 = very difficult to 5 = very easy). Coefficients are standardized regression coefficients. Reference category for the independent variables is female, nonwhite, single, working in community setting, part-time status, and staff position.

[b] Environmental stress was rated on a 4-point scale (0 = not at all stressful to 3 = highly stressful).

[c] Control in the work environment was rated on a 5-point scale (0 = no control to 4 = total control).

[d] Professional commitment was rated on a 5-point scale (1 = strongly disagree to 5 = strongly agree).

[e] Work-home conflict and organizational commitment were rated on a 7-point scale (1 = strongly disagree to 7 = strongly agree).

[f] Future employment plan of working with a different employer but within the same work type was rated on a 4-point scale (1 = very unlikely to 4 = very likely).

[*] Statistically significant difference at $P < 0.05$.

[†] Statistically significant at $P < 0.05$ is for all the continuous variables, namely, age, and worklife attitude variables.

coded as 1 or 0. In this case, because the variable is labeled "male," it is usually safe to assume that males were coded as 1 and that females were coded as 0. Conversely, if the variable had been labeled "female," it would usually be safe to assume that females were coded as 1 and males were coded as 0. However, the investigators remove all doubt by explaining it in the first footnote: "Reference category for the independent variables is female, nonwhite, single, working in community setting, part-time status, and staff position." Individuals in the reference category are always coded as 0. Now that we know how the categorical predictor variables were scored, we can look at whether the regression coefficients are positive or negative to interpret the statistically significant relationships observed. For example, the positive correlation coefficient for the variable "male" in the model predicting professional opportunities indicates that higher values on one variable are associated with higher values on the other variable. Recalling that higher scores on the perceived job alternatives measure indicate greater ease finding a new position, it follows that males reported that it would be easier to find a different position with better professional opportunities compared to females ($\beta = 0.091$). Similarly, white pharmacists reported that it would be easier to find a different position with better environmental conditions and compensation compared to nonwhite pharmacists ($\beta s = 0.096$ *and* 0.157, respectively). Because age was measured as a numerical variable, the negative regression coefficients indicate that younger pharmacists reported that it would be easier to find a different position with better environmental conditions and professional opportunities. Finally, only one of the regression coefficients involving the predictor variables reflecting practice characteristics is statistically significant (see 5). This negative coefficient indicates that full-time pharmacists reported greater difficulty finding a different position with better compensation compared to part-time pharmacists ($\beta = 0.086$). A final caution. When interpreting information presented in tables similar to that in Box 7-4, readers should keep in mind that when a large number of relationships are examined, the probability of making one or more Type I (α) errors increases dramatically.

The third study examined the effect of a pharmacist-run intervention using low health literacy flashcards and a smartphone-activated quick response (QR) barcoded educational video designed to increase medication adherence and disease state understanding among patients taking medications for heart failure, hypertension, and type 2 diabetes.[3] The QR code to access the educational video was attached to patients' prescription bottles. Participants in the intervention group were recruited from an outpatient clinic that had established clinical pharmacy services. To be eligible to participate, patients had to be at least 18 years old, speak either English or Spanish as their primary language, have a baseline measure of medication adherence (assessed by the proportion of days covered [PDC]) of less than or equal to 50% for the previous 6 months. Patients were excluded from the study if they used insulin, had filled prescriptions outside of the health care system from which they were recruited, or were pregnant. The criterion of PDC ≤ 50% was used to ensure that participants had the potential to benefit from the intervention. If participants with high adherence at baseline had been enrolled, the investigators may have encountered "ceiling effects," which occur in intervention studies when many participants are doing so well at baseline that there is little room for improvement. The exclusion of patients who filled prescriptions at outside pharmacies ensured that the investigators would have access to the prescription refill records needed to calculate PDC. Control participants were recruited from an outpatient clinic within the same health care system that did not have established clinical pharmacy services. Control participants were matched to intervention participants on comorbid conditions, number of targeted medications, and medication class. A total of 34 intervention and 34 matched control participants were enrolled. The primary outcome variable was the difference in PDC between intervention and control participants 6 months after intervention implementation.

The first table in Box 7-5 shows the characteristics of participants in the intervention and control groups. (Because participants were not randomly assigned to treatment, it would be more appropriate to refer to the "control" group as a "comparison" group.) Despite the matching procedures employed, several differences between intervention and control participants are evident. For example, participants in the intervention group were more likely than those in the control group to speak English as their primary language. Participants in the control group also used more over-the-counter medications but had fewer clinic visits than participants in the intervention group. Readers need to keep these differences in mind when interpreting study findings.

The primary findings from the study are reported in the second table in Box 7-5. Given the matched design of the study, the investigators use the Wilcoxon signed rank test to evaluate between group differences when PDC was used as a numerical variable. They used the McNemar test when PDC values were used to create dichotomous, secondary outcome variables (i.e., PDC improved at least 25%, yes/no; PDC at least 80%, yes/no). As shown in the second table in Box 7-5, PDC was significantly higher in the intervention group than in the control group for both the 90-day and 180-day periods following intervention implementation. However, the between group differences were not statistically significant for the dichotomous measures derived from the PDC. This is not surprising because collapsing continuous measures into dichotomous ones results in a loss of precision and power.

The investigators also used linear regression to examine between group differences when controlling for age, race, and total number of medications used. They reported that "Linear regression revealed that the intervention group PDC remained significantly higher when adjusted for confounders (beta coefficient = –0.34; $P = 0.003$; $r^2 = 0.17$)" (p. 34). The small sample size limited the investigators' ability to include more than just a few control variables in their regression model. Nonetheless, it is a bit surprising that they chose to control for age, which did not differ between the groups, and did not control for number of clinic visits, which did differ.

Nonetheless, the findings reported in this study seem quite promising and support the need for a larger study evaluating the intervention using an RCT design.

BOX 7-5. Low Health Literacy Flashcard and QR Video Study

Table 2
Baseline characteristics

Characteristic	Intervention (n = 34)	Control (n = 34)	*P* value
Mean age in years	51.8 ± 8.4	53.8 ± 9.4	0.27
Female sex, n (%)	21 (61.8)	18 (53)	0.25
Race, n (%)			0.12
White, Non-Hispanic	4 (11.8)	1 (3.0)	
White, Hispanic	17 (50)	23 (67.6)	
African American	13 (38.2)	8 (23.5)	
Asian	0	2 (5.9)	
Language, n (%)			0.06
English	22 (64.7)	17 (50)	
Spanish	12 (35.3)	17 (50)	
Number of clinic visits	2.9 ± 1.3	2.0 ± 1.1	0.003
Payor, n (%)			0.12
Charity funding	30 (88.2)	31 (91.2)	
Medicare	4 (11.7)	3 (8.8)	
Total number of prescription medications	6.7 ± 3.3	7.0 ± 3.4	0.51
Total number of OTC medications	0.6 ± 0.8	1.2 ± 1.0	0.003
Medication indications, n (%)			
DM and HTN	27 (79.4)	27 (79.4)	
DM only	1 (3.0)	1 (3.0)	
CHF	3 (8.8)	3 (8.8)	
HTN only	3 (8.8)	3 (8.8)	
Nonadherent medications, n (%)			
Metformin	21 (61.8)	21 (61.8)	
ACEi/ARB	20 (58.8)	20 (58.8)	
Secretagogue	11 (32.4)	11 (32.4)	
Beta blocker	6 (17.6)	6 (17.6)	
Loop diuretic	4 (11.8)	5 (14.7)	
Thiazolidinedione	4 (11.8)	4 (11.8)	
Nitrate	2 (5.9)	1 (2.9)	
Hydralazine	2 (5.9)	1 (2.9)	
Spironolactone	0	1 (2.9)	
Overall baseline PDC, range (%)	38 (17–50)	34 (13–50)	

Abbreviations used: OTC, over-the-counter; ACEi, angiotensin-converting-enzyme inhibitor; ARB, angiotensin II receptor blockers; PDC, proportion of days covered; DM, type 2 diabetes mellitus; HTN, hypertension; CHF, congestive heart failure.

Table 4
Primary and secondary outcomes

Outcomes	Intervention (n = 34)	Control (n = 34)	*P* value
Primary outcome			
180-day PDC, %	71	44	0.007
Secondary outcomes			
90-day PDC, %	67	38	0.01
Increase of 25% in PDC, n (%)	22 (64.7)	16 (47.1)	0.17
Final PDC greater than 80%, n (%)	12 (35.3)	5 (14.7)	0.09

Abbreviation used: PDC, proportion of days covered.

Self-Study Questions

1. In a multiple regression analysis, R^2 is:

    A. The proportion of variance in the dependent variable explained by the independent variables
    B. The proportion of variance in the dependent variable **not** explained by the independent variable(s)
    C. The proportion of variance in the independent variable explained by the dependent variable
    D. Greater if error variance is greater

2. A paper states that the correlation between two variables is 0.34 with a standard error of 0.08. This correlation is based on a sample size of 500. If alpha were set at 0.05, would this correlation be considered statistically significant?

    A. Yes, it would be considered statistically significant.
    B. No, it would not be considered statistically significant.
    C. Statistical significance cannot be determined from the information provided.

3. In linear regression analysis, calculation of error variance is based on:

    A. The difference between individual observations and predicted values on the regression line
    B. The difference between individual observations and the overall mean
    C. The difference between predicted values and the overall mean
    D. None of the above

4. In linear regression analysis, the regression line is drawn in a way that:

    A. Maximizes the slope of the regression line
    B. Minimizes the slope of the regression line
    C. Minimizes error variance
    D. Maximizes error variance

5. In linear regression analysis, the regression coefficient:

    A. Indexes the magnitude of the effect of the independent variable on the dependent variable
    B. Indexes the slope of the regression line
    C. Increases as the regression sums of squares increases
    D. Both A and B
    E. A, B, and C

6. Is the following statement true or false? The possibility of confounding can be controlled through the use of multivariate statistical methods **after** data for a study have been collected. (True/False)

Use Question Table 7-1 to answer Questions 7–9.

QUESTION TABLE 7-1. Regression Analysis Predicting Diastolic Blood Pressure (mmHG)

Predictor Variable	Regression Coefficient (SE)	95% CI
Intercept	30.82 (12.45)	5.92 to 55.72
Female	3.31 (1.12)	1.07 to 5.55
Body mass index (BMI)	0.34 (0.07)	0.2 to 0.48
Smoker	5.78 (2.95)	–0.12 to 11.68

Data in this table are fictitious. Regression coefficients are unstandardized. The reference groups for sex and smoking status are male and nonsmoker, respectively.

7. Question Table 7-1 shows the results of a linear regression analysis predicting diastolic blood pressure. How do you interpret the regression coefficient for "Female"?

    A. Controlling for BMI and smoking status, the average blood pressure of females is 3.31 points higher than males.
    B. Controlling for BMI and smoking status, the average blood pressure of males is 3.31 points higher than females.
    C. Controlling for BMI and smoking status, the relationship between sex and blood pressure is not statistically significant.
    D. A and C
    E. B and C

8. How do you interpret the regression coefficient for BMI in Question Table 7-1?

A. On average, controlling for sex and smoking status, for every 1-unit increase in blood pressure, BMI goes up 0.34 units.
B. On average, controlling for sex and smoking status, for every 1-unit increase in BMI, blood pressure goes up 0.34 units.
C. On average, controlling for sex and smoking status, for every 1-unit increase in blood pressure, BMI goes down 0.34 units.
D. On average, controlling for sex and smoking status, for every 1-unit increase in BMI, blood pressure goes down 0.34 units.

9. Based on the data reported in Question Table 7-1, is the relationship between "Smoker" and blood pressure statistically significant?

A. Yes, it is statistically significant.
B. No, it is **not** statistically significant.

Imagine that you are a pharmacist working in an ambulatory care clinic. A 62-year-old white female with newly diagnosed hypertension and diabetes asks you about treatment options for her elevated blood pressure. After counseling her about antihypertensive therapy, she asks whether she should take a new drug called Notapril. The woman heard about the drug while listening to a cardiologist on a morning news show. During the show, the cardiologist described results from a recent clinical trial that was published in the current issue of the *New England Journal of Medicine*. You tell the woman that you will find out more about Notapril and discuss it with her before she leaves the clinic. While the patient is having her blood drawn, you go online and retrieve the article. It contains Question Table 7-2.

Use Question Table 7-2 to answer Questions 10–12.

QUESTION TABLE 7-2. Effect of Notapril on Systolic Blood Pressure (mmHg)

Predictor Variable	Regression Coefficient	*p*
Intercept	47.44	0.01
Male	3.25	0.02
Smoking status		
1 pack/day	2.57	0.03
>2 pack/day	4.22	0.01
Age (yr)	0.56	0.04
Presence of diabetes	15.32	0.03
Weight (lb)	0.97	0.01
Notapril	−9.53	0.02

Regression coefficients are unstandardized. Reference groups are females, nonsmokers, and patients who took a placebo.

10. Based on Question Table 7-2, how is the coefficient for sex interpreted?

A. Controlling for the other variables in the model, the average blood pressure of men is 3.25 points higher than women.
B. Controlling for the other variables in the model, the average blood pressure of women is 3.26 points higher than men.
C. Controlling for the other variables in the model, the difference in blood pressure between men and women is not statistically significant if alpha is set at 0.05.

11. Based on Question Table 7-2, how is the coefficient for diabetes interpreted?

A. After adjusting for other factors, diabetics require 15.32 mg more Notapril to obtain the same effect as nondiabetics.
B. After adjusting for other factors, the blood pressure of diabetics is 15.32 mmHg higher than nondiabetics.
C. After adjusting for other factors, the blood pressure of diabetics is 15.32 mmHg lower than nondiabetics.
D. After adjusting for other factors, diabetics require 15.32 mg less Notapril to obtain the same effect as nondiabetics.
E. After adjusting for other factors, the relationship between diabetes and systolic blood pressure is not statistically significant if alpha is set at 0.05.

12. The woman in the scenario in Question Table 7-2 is concerned that, because she has diabetes, Notapril may have less effect on her blood pressure than it has on the blood pressure of people without diabetes. Is there any information contained in Question Table 7-2 that would support her concern?

    A. Yes, there is information in Question Table 7-2 that supports her concern.
    B. No, there is no information in Question Table 7-2 that supports her concern.

References

1. Lam AY, Nguyen JK, Parks JJ, et al. Addressing low health literacy with "Talking Pill Bottles": a pilot study in a community pharmacy setting. *J Am Pharm Assoc.* 2017;57(1):20–9.
2. Rojanasarot S, Gaither CA, Schommer JC, et al. Exploring pharmacists' perceived job alternatives: results from the 2014 National Pharmacist Workforce Survey. *J Am Pharm Assoc.* 2017;57(1):47–55.
3. Yeung DL, Alvarez KS, Quinones ME. Low-health literacy flashcards and mobile video reinforcement to improve medication adherence in patients on oral diabetes, heart failure, and hypertension medications. *J Am Pharm Assoc.* 2017;57(1):30–7.

Logistic Regression

8

After reading this chapter, you should be able to do the following:

1. Describe the types of situations in which it would be appropriate to use logistic regression.
2. Given the results of a study that used logistic regression, interpret observed relationships in terms of statistical significance and magnitude of effect.

In Chapter 7 of this book, we focused on situations where the outcome of interest was a numerical variable and the investigator wanted to examine the relationship between the outcome variable and multiple independent variables simultaneously. In those situations, investigators would probably use **linear regression** or a variant of linear regression based on the general linear model. However, if the outcome of interest is measured on a nominal or ordinal scale, investigators must turn to **logistic regression**.

Logistic regression is among the analytic procedures most frequently used in the medical literature. In most cases, the outcome variable in a logistic regression analysis is dichotomous. Thus, it will have only two levels (e.g., lived/died, developed side effect/did not develop side effect). Medical researchers seem to love logistic regression because it provides odds ratios (ORs)—a measure of risk. In many cases, even if researchers have a numerical outcome variable, they will dichotomize the variable to create two groups so that they can use logistic regression. For example, rather than use bone density assessed in g/cm^2, the investigators might use bone density scores to classify study participants as (1) has osteoporosis or (2) does not have osteoporosis. They will then use this dichotomous variable (i.e., osteoporosis: yes/no) as the outcome variable in a logistic regression.

As was the case for linear regression, logistic regression models can incorporate many independent variables. Also as was the case for linear regression, the independent variables in a logistic regression can be measured on any scale of measurement. Again, investigators often turn numerical independent variables into dichotomous variables to facilitate the interpretation of ORs. However, they should only do this if it makes clinical sense.

Comparison of the Linear and Logistic Models

Remember that the goal in **linear regression** is to develop a prediction equation that best explains variance in a **numerical** outcome (i.e., dependent) variable. Because the outcome variable is numerical, values can lie anywhere along the plausible range of the variable. For example, a linear regression model examining the relationship between weight and systolic blood pressure (SBP) using fictitious data yielded the regression equation: $\hat{Y} = 63.53 + 0.4(\mathit{Weight})$. Thus, the predicted value of SBP for a person weighing 120 pounds would be $\hat{Y} = 63.53 + 0.4(120) = 111.53$, whereas the predicted value of SBP for a person weighing 180 pounds would be $\hat{Y} = 63.53 + 0.4(180) = 135.53$. These predicted values can be used to draw the blue line in Figure 8-1. The closer participants' actual SBP (depicted by the small circles in the figure) fall to the line, the greater the variance in SBP that is explained by weight.

The goal in **logistic regression** is also to explain variation in the outcome variable. However, in logistic regression, the outcome variable is usually dichotomous. Any given individual in a study can only have one of two values on a dichotomous variable. That is, they either experience the outcome or they do not. Therefore, when using logistic regression, investigators are trying to predict which people in the study will experience the outcome and which people will not experience the outcome. Examples of outcomes that might be examined using logistic regression include survives (yes/no), experiences an adverse event (yes/no), and develops a disease (yes/no). In most cases, dichotomous variables are scored such that: 0 = *individual did **not** experience event* and 1 = *individual experienced event.*

The probability that an individual will experience an event (i.e., the predicted probability) can range only from 0 to 1, just like any probability. Therefore, when trying to predict which individuals will experience a particular outcome (and which will not), investigators need a regression model that yields predicted values that range only from 0 to 1. This can be accomplished using a logistic transformation: $Pr(Y|Z) = \frac{1}{1+e^{-Z}}$. This transformation predicts the probability that Y will occur given a specific value of Z. As shown in Figure 8-2, this transformation produces an S-shaped curve that yields a predicted probability of 0.5 when Z is 0. The predicted probabilities quickly drop to 0 as Z decreases from 0. Similarly, the predicted probabilities quickly rise to 1 as Z increases from 0.

FIGURE 8-1. Fit Plot for SBP

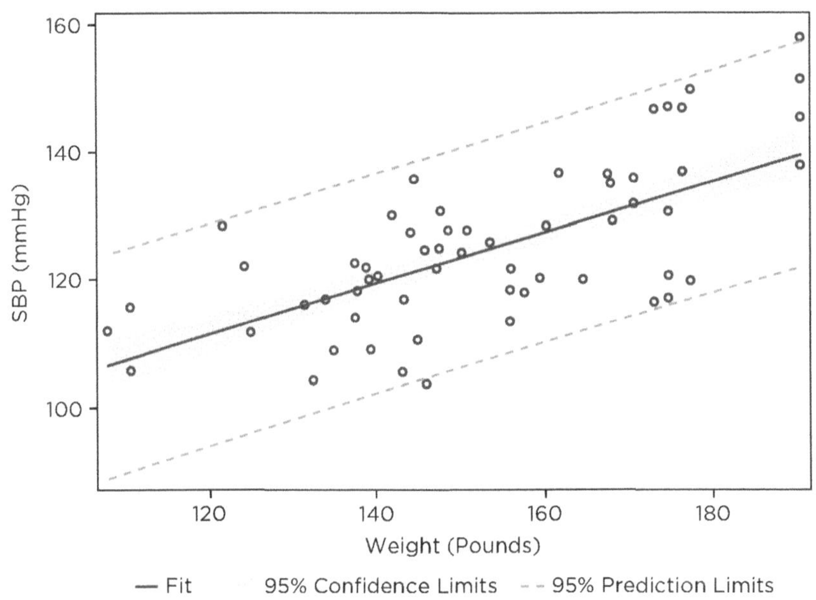

SBP, systolic blood pressure.

FIGURE 8.2. Logistic Function

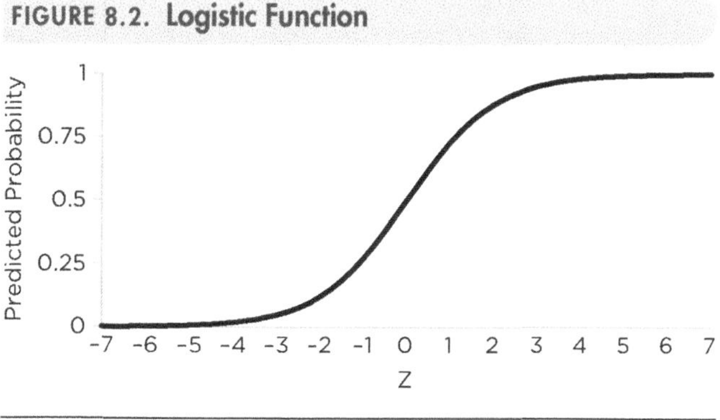

Values of Z can be derived from the linear model and then converted into predicted probabilities using the logistic transformation, such that: $p_{Y|Z} = \frac{1}{1 + exp^{[-(b_0+b_1X_1+b_2X_2+\cdots)]}}$. Without going into the math, this formula can be used to derive the **logistic regression model**:

$$log\frac{y}{(1-y)} = b_0 + b_1X_1 + b_2X_2 + \cdots + Error,$$

where $log\frac{y}{(1-y)}$ is called the logit function of y.

Interpreting Logistic Regression Findings

In logistic regression, investigators want to minimize the difference between (1) each participant's predicted probability of experiencing the outcome of interest and (2) the variable indicating whether or not the participant actually experienced the outcome. Thus, for participants who experience the outcome, the predicted probabilities should be close to 1.0; for participants who do **not** experience the outcome, the predicted probabilities should be close to 0. Box 8-1 provides an example of the computations required to compute predicted probabilities using the logistic model.

The parameter estimates obtained by solving the logistic model can also be converted into ORs as shown in Box 8-2. This box also shows, for each predictor variable in the model, the 95% confidence interval (CI) for the OR and the probability (*P*) of observing an OR as large or larger than the one observed **if** the null hypothesis was true.

An important aside. Whenever you are assessing the statistical significance of a ratio (OR, relative risk ratio), the expected value under the null hypothesis is "1." That is because ratios are formed by dividing the value obtained in one group by the value obtained in another group. When two numbers are the same, if you divide one number by the other, you obtain "1." For example, if 20% of people who took a placebo died and 20% of people who took an experimental drug died, $\frac{20\%}{20\%} = 1$. This is in contrast to statistical procedures, such as t-tests, that compare means in two groups using subtraction. In those types of analyses, the expected value under the null hypothesis is "0." That is because when two numbers are the same and you subtract one from the other, you obtain "0." For example, if the mean weight in one group is 130 pounds and the mean weight in another group is 130 pounds, 130 pounds – 130 pounds = 0. As simple as this distinction may seem, many learners struggle with it. Hopefully, you will now be able to explain it to them!

BOX 8-1. Deriving Predicted Probabilities From a Logistic Regression Model

Imagine that an investigator wanted to determine if an experimental drug reduces the risk of 1-year mortality among patients with hypertension who are at high risk of heart attack. The investigator enrolled 100 people into the study. Participants are randomly assigned to receive either a placebo ($n = 50$) or the experimental drug ($n = 50$). The investigator collects baseline data on each participant's age, systolic blood pressure (SBP), low-density lipoproteins (LDL), and body mass index (BMI). All participants are followed for 1 year. During the 1-year follow-up period, a total of 22 people died, 15 of whom received the placebo and 7 of whom received the experimental drug.

The table below provides data for the independent variables in the study (i.e., treatment group, age, SBP, LDL, and BMI) and the outcome variable (died during follow-up period) for 10 of the 100 study participants.

Person	Treatment Group	Age	SBP	LDL	BMI	Died During Follow-Up Period
1	Placebo	87	130	205	31	1
2	Placebo	77	133	188	30	1
3	Placebo	80	128	181	33	1
4	Placebo	75	137	169	33	0
5	Placebo	73	141	112	29	1
6–50	Placebo	***	***	***	***	***
51	Experimental drug	87	130	205	31	1
52	Experimental drug	76	117	183	32	1
53	Experimental drug	79	117	183	27	0
54	Experimental drug	73	136	151	26	0
55	Experimental drug	71	137	146	32	0
56–100	Experimental drug	***	***	***	***	***

The investigator used logistic regression to estimate the coefficients for the regression model:

$$\log\frac{y}{(1-y)} = B_0 + b_1(Age) + b_2(SBP) + b_3(LDL) + b_4(BMI) + b_5(Treatment\ Group).$$

The estimates derived from the regression analysis are shown below.

Parameter	Estimate
Intercept (B_0)	−45.5663
Age (b_1)	0.2086
SBP (b_2)	0.1504
LDL (b_3)	0.0457
BMI (b_4)	0.0834
Treatment group (b_5) (Reference group: placebo)	−1.6684

The estimates were used to calculate Z for each study participant. For example,

$$Z_{(Person\ 1)} = -45.5663 + 0.2086(87) + 0.1504(130) + 0.0457(205) + 0.0834(31) + (-1.6684)(0) = 4.09$$

$$Z_{(Person\ 53)} = -45.5663 + 0.2086(79) + 0.1504(117) + 0.0457(183) + 0.0834(27) + (-1.6684)(1) = -2.54$$

BOX 8-1. Deriving Predicted Probabilities From a Logistic Regression Model *(Continued)*

The Zs calculated were then plugged into the logistic transformation to predict the probability of death for each participant in the study. For example,

$$P_{Death\ Person\ 1} = \frac{1}{1+exp^{[-(4.09)]}} = 0.98;\ P_{Death\ Person\ 53} = \frac{1}{1+exp^{[-(-2.54)]}} = 0.07$$

The Zs and predicted probabilities are shown in the table below with the variable they are trying to predict (died during follow-up period; 0 = no, 1 = yes). Six of the 10 participants shown died during the follow-up period. The predicted probability of death for four of these six participants was 0.80 or greater, indicating pretty accurate predictions. However, two of the six participants who died (Participants 5 and 52) had predicted probabilities below 0.20. Thus, their deaths were not predicted by the model. Among the four participants shown in the table who survived, three had very low predicted probabilities (i.e., below 0.10), indicating pretty accurate predictions. However, one participant (Participant 4) defied the odds by surviving despite a predicted probability of death of 0.76.

Person	Treatment Group	Z	Predicted Probability of Death	Died During Follow-Up Period
1	Placebo	4.09	0.98	1
2	Placebo	1.59	0.83	1
3	Placebo	1.40	0.80	1
4	Placebo	1.16	0.76	0
5	Placebo	−1.60	0.17	1
6–50	Placebo	***	***	***
51	Experimental drug	2.42	0.92	1
52	Experimental drug	−2.75	0.06	1
53	Experimental drug	−2.54	0.07	0
54	Experimental drug	−2.48	0.08	0
55	Experimental drug	−2.48	0.08	0
56–100	Experimental drug	***	***	***

BOX 8-2. Deriving Odds Ratios from a Logistic Regression Model

The final step in the analysis is to convert the parameter estimates obtained from the logistic model into odds ratios via exponentiation. For example, $OR_{Age} = e^{b_1} = e^{0.2086} = 1.232$.

Parameter	Estimate	OR	95% CI	*P*
Intercept (B_0)	−45.5663	—	—	<0.0001
Age (b_1)	0.2086	1.232	1.097, 1.383	0.004
SBP (b_2)	0.1504	1.162	1.052, 1.284	0.0030
LDL (b_3)	0.0457	1.047	1.01, 1.085	0.0113
BMI (b_4)	0.0834	1.087	0.921, 1.283	0.3240
Treatment group (b_5) (Reference group: placebo)	−1.6684	0.189	0.047, 0.763	0.0194

BMI, body mass index; LDL, low-density lipoprotein; OR, odds ratio; SBP, systolic blood pressure; CI, confidence interval; —, not applicable.

Back to Box 8-2. From the *P* values shown in Box 8-2, you can see that all of the predictor variables in the logistic regression model, with the exception of body mass index (BMI), are statistically significant. Looking at BMI, you can see that the 95% CI (i.e., 0.921 to 1.283) crosses "1," the expected value under the null hypothesis. This tells you that BMI was not a significant predictor of death during the 1-year follow-up period after controlling for other variables included in the model. This conclusion is confirmed by the nonsignificant *P* value for BMI (i.e., 0.3240). You can also see in Box 8-2 that none of the CIs for the other predictor variables cross "1."

For numerical predictor variables, ORs indicate the amount of change in risk for each 1-unit change in the predictor variable. Thus, each 1-year increase in age is associated with a 23.2% increase in the odds of dying during the follow-up period. Similarly, each 1-unit change in LDL is associated with a 4.7% increase in the odds of dying during the follow-up period.

For dichotomous predictor variables, ORs indicate the change in risk associated with going from **not having** to **having** the characteristic indexed by the independent variable (e.g., taking an experimental medication rather than a placebo). For example, results of the fictitious study shown in Box 8-2 indicate that the odds of dying during the follow-up period among participants who took the experimental drug was about one-fifth of that experienced by those who took a placebo (OR = 0.189).

Model Building and Evaluating Model Fit

Investigators use the same types of procedures for building logistic regression models that they use for building linear regression models. Several tests can be used to test the global null hypothesis that the regression coefficients for all of the predictor variables are equal to zero. These tests include: the likelihood ratio test, the efficient score test, and the Wald chi-square statistic. For the model described in Box 8-1, all of these tests were statistically significant at $P < 0.01$, indicating that one or more of the predictor variables in the model had regression coefficients that were not equal to zero.

To assess model fit, investigators can examine classification tables such as the one shown in Box 8-3, derived from the regression model introduced in Box 8-1. The rows in the table indicate whether participants were predicted to die, dichotomized at a predicted probability of 0.5. The columns indicate whether the participant actually died during the follow-up period (yes/no). The shaded boxes show the number of participants who were correctly classified by the model (i.e., participants were predicted to die and died; people were not predicted to die and did not die). If you add the numbers in these two boxes together, you can see that 85% of the participants were classified correctly by the model. However, if you look more closely, you can see that the model did a better job of predicting who would **not** die than who would die. Of the 78 study participants who did not die, 74 (94.9%) were classified correctly. In contrast, of the 22 study participants who died, 11 (50.0%)

BOX 8-3. Logistic Regression Classification Table

	Died		
Predicted Probability	**Yes**	**No**	**TOTALS**
Greater than or equal to 0.5	11	4	15
Less than 0.5	11	74	85
TOTALS	22	78	100

were classified correctly. These two values are called the specificity and sensitivity of the model. We will return to these terms in Chapter 10 on measurement.

The Hosmer–Lemeshow test is also often used to evaluate how well a logistic regression model fits the data. The null hypothesis for this test is that the model does fit the data. Therefore, investigators usually want the test to be nonsignificant (e.g., $P > 0.05$), indicating that the model fits the data reasonably well. For the model described previously, the Hosmer–Lemeshow test yielded a P value of 0.95.

Examples From the Literature

We will now review selected findings from three recent studies that have used logistic regression to analyze study data. The first study examined the impact of California Senate Bill 41, which authorized pharmacists to sell syringes without a prescription.[1] Some of the results from this study have been discussed in previous chapters. Briefly, the study used a cross-sectional research design, which means that data were collected at one point in time. Data were collected via an interviewer-administered survey. A total of 404 pharmacists and pharmacy staff, recruited from 212 pharmacies, were interviewed. The primary outcome variable was whether or not the pharmacist stated that he/she would sell syringes to a person who is a known or suspected injection drug user (IDU). The investigators performed univariate analyses to identify factors that were associated with the outcome variable. In the "data analysis" section of the paper, the author sates, "Variables significant at $P < 0.10$ in the univariate analysis were manually entered into a multiple logistic regression model in a forward stepwise fashion to identify factors independently associated with the outcome variable at a significance level of $P < 0.05$" (p. 680). The results of the logistic regression are shown in Box 8-4. Note that the abbreviation AOR in the table stands for adjusted OR, indicating that the ORs are adjusted for all of the other variables included in the logistic regression model. The findings in Box 8-4 indicate the following:

1. Respondents at independent or other pharmacies were less likely to report selling syringes to IDUs compared to staff at chain pharmacies (AOR: 0.29, 95% CI: 0.14–0.59),

BOX 8-4. Nonprescription Syringe Sale Study

Table 3
Factors associated with self-reported nonprescription syringe sales to IDUs, Fresno and Kern Counties

Factor	AOR (95% CI)
Pharmacy type	
Chain	1.00
Independent/other	0.29 (0.14-0.59)
Sales policies based on:	
Store policy only	1.00
Discretion only	1.37 (0.59-3.20)
Both	3.08 (1.75-5.40)
It is legal for IDUs 18 years of age or older to purchase a syringe in a pharmacy without a prescription.	3.38 (1.83-6.26)
Only people who have a medical condition like diabetes should be able to buy syringes.	0.44 (0.25-0.76)
Selling syringes to IDUs is not good business for pharmacies like mine.	0.36 (0.21-0.63)

Abbreviations used: IDU, intravenous drug user; AOR, adjusted odds ratio; CI, confidence interval.

2. Respondents at pharmacies that had policies regarding nonprescription syringe sale **and** allowed staff discretion regarding sales were more likely to report selling syringes to IDUs compared to staff in pharmacies that did not allow discretion (AOR: 3.08, 95% CI: 1.75–5.40).
3. Respondents who agreed with the statement "It is legal for IDUs 18 years of age or older to purchase a syringe in a pharmacy without a prescription" were more likely to report selling syringes to IDUs compared to those who disagreed (AOR: 3.38, 95% CI: 1.83–6.26).
4. Respondents who agreed with the statement "Only people who have a medical condition like diabetes should be able to buy syringes" were less likely to report selling syringes to IDUs compared to those who disagreed (AOR: 0.44, 95% CI: 0.25–0.76).
5. Respondents who agreed with the statement "Selling syringes to IDUs is not good business for pharmacies like mine" were less likely to report selling syringes to IDUs compared to those who disagreed (AOR: 0.36, 95% CI: 0.21–0.63.)

In interpreting these results, keep in mind that these relationships are statistically significant after controlling for all of the other variables in the model. Thus, for example, the association between pharmacy type and nonprescription syringe sales is not due to differences in store policies (i.e., allowing staff discretion) or staff attitudes. Also note that several of the attitude variables that were significant in the bivariate analyses, discussed in a previous chapter (e.g., "I am concerned that providing syringes to IDUs encourages drug use," $P<0.0001$ in the bivariate analyses), did not make it into the final model. This is because any variance in syringe sales that these variables explained was also explained by one of the variables shown in Box 8-4. Finally, what is the strongest relationship shown in Box 8-4? This might surprise you. It is easy to see that the strongest association involving the predictor variables that have an OR greater than 1 is the attitude item "It is legal for IDUs 18 years of age of older to purchase a syringe in a pharmacy without a prescription" (AOR = 3.38). However, the OR for pharmacy type (AOR = 0.29) is actually stronger. If independent or other pharmacies had been the reference group rather than chain pharmacies, this AOR would have been: $\frac{0.29}{1} = \frac{1}{X}; 0.29X = 1; X = \frac{1}{0.29}; 3.45$, narrowly beating out the AOR for the attitude item. Thus, staff at chain pharmacies were more likely to report selling syringes to IDUs compared to staff at independent or other pharmacies (OR = 3.45). Remember that if you have trouble visualizing the strength of an OR (or AOR) that lies between 0 and 1, you can always flip the reference group in this manner.

The second study used data from two national studies to examine the association between caregiver: (1) involvement in helping a family member manage his or her medications and (2) seeking information, training, and support regarding caregiving.[2] The study used a cross-sectional research design. Data were derived from the 2011 National Health and Aging Trends Study (NHATS) and its supplement, the National Study of Caregiving (NSOC). The NHATS involves data collection from a nationally representative sample of community-dwelling adults aged 65 or older. In the NSOC, family caregivers of participants in NHATS are interviewed. The final data set analyzed included information collected from a total of 1,367 caregivers and 1,367 care recipients. To assess caregiver involvement in the management of the care recipient's medications, caregivers were asked two questions: (1) whether they had helped the care recipient keep track of his or her medications in the past month and (2) whether they helped the care recipient take shots or injections. To assess caregiver information seeking, caregivers were asked if they ever looked for information, training, or services to help them with their caregiving role. In the "Data Analysis" section of the paper, the investigators state, "A multivariate logistic regression model was developed to examine the association between caregivers' assistance with keeping track of medications and their information-seeking behavior, while controlling for caregivers' age, sex, and education as well as care recipients' age, sex, race, and education. Additional control variables included caregiving items, such as duration of caregiving (≤1 year or >1 year); living arrangement; involvement in activities of daily living (ADLs), instrumental ADLs (IADLs), and medical tasks; and care recipient health conditions. A similar model was developed examining the association between caregivers' involvement in injecting medications and their information-seeking behavior with the same control variables. Both caregiver and care recipient factors are likely to play a role in caregivers' information-seeking behavior, based on information-seeking literature." Thus, the investigators appear to have made a substantial effort to control for as many potential confounders as possible when examining the relationships of primary interest. However, in the description of their analyses, they should have stated that they developed a **multiple** logistic regression model rather than a **multivariate** one. Multivariate models include **multiple dependent (outcome) variables**. The model the investigators developed included only one dependent variable.

The findings from these analyses are shown in Box 8-5. The table shows the regression coefficients for two separate logistic regression models. In both models, the outcome variable was whether caregivers reported seeking information, training, or support to help them with their caregiving activities (yes/no). The primary predictor variable in the middle column is whether caregivers reported helping the care recipient keep track of his or her medications (yes/no). I will refer to this as Model 1. The primary predictor variable in the far right column is whether caregivers reported helping the care recipient take shots or injections (yes or no). I will refer to this as Model 2. I have annotated the table for ease of reference. The investigators used the adjusted Wald chi-square statistic (see [1]) to evaluate the global null hypothesis that

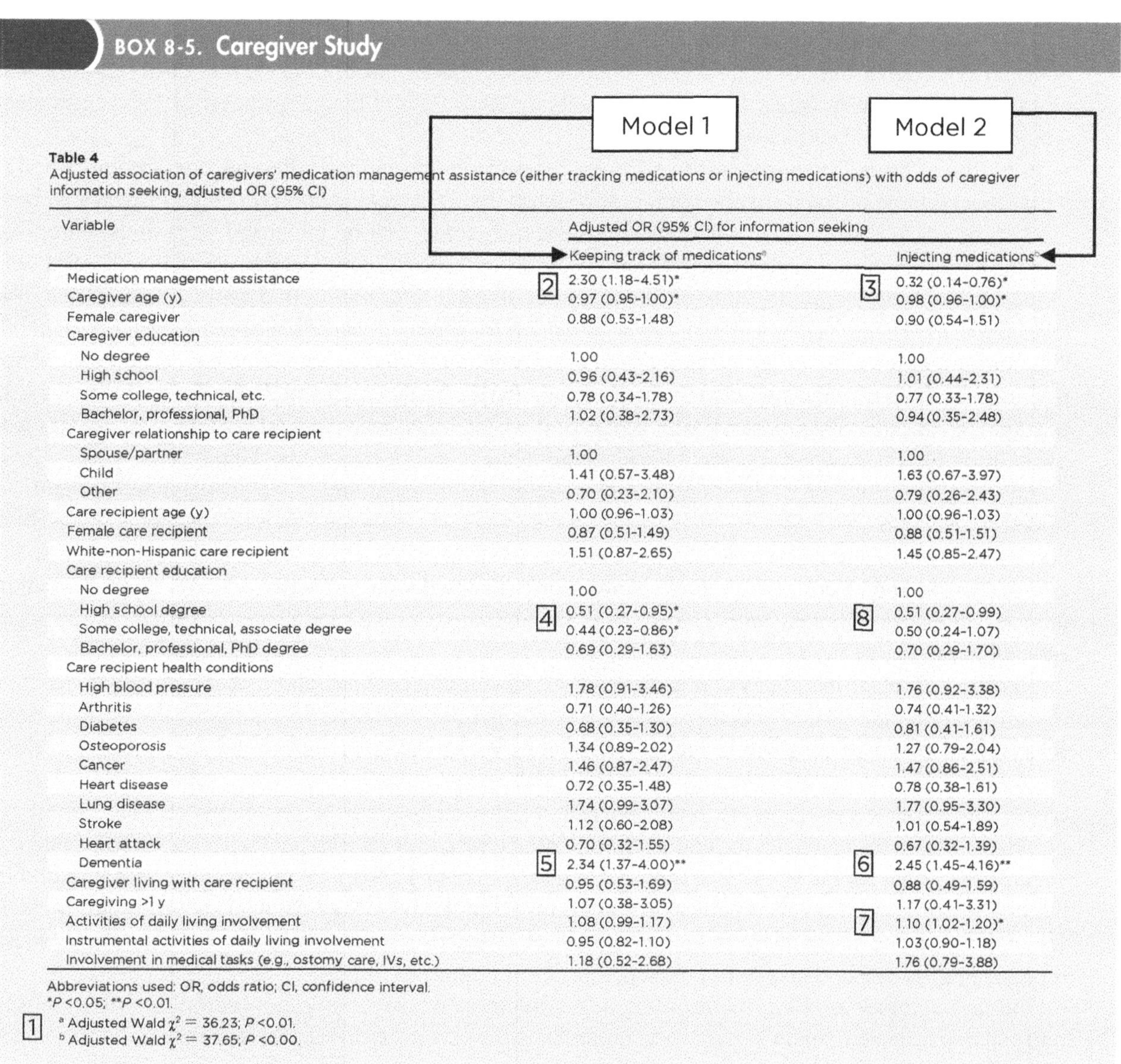

BOX 8-5. Caregiver Study

Model 1 Model 2

Table 4
Adjusted association of caregivers' medication management assistance (either tracking medications or injecting medications) with odds of caregiver information seeking, adjusted OR (95% CI)

Variable		Adjusted OR (95% CI) for information seeking		
		Keeping track of medications[a]		Injecting medications[b]
Medication management assistance	[2]	2.30 (1.18-4.51)*	[3]	0.32 (0.14-0.76)*
Caregiver age (y)		0.97 (0.95-1.00)*		0.98 (0.96-1.00)*
Female caregiver		0.88 (0.53-1.48)		0.90 (0.54-1.51)
Caregiver education				
No degree		1.00		1.00
High school		0.96 (0.43-2.16)		1.01 (0.44-2.31)
Some college, technical, etc.		0.78 (0.34-1.78)		0.77 (0.33-1.78)
Bachelor, professional, PhD		1.02 (0.38-2.73)		0.94 (0.35-2.48)
Caregiver relationship to care recipient				
Spouse/partner		1.00		1.00
Child		1.41 (0.57-3.48)		1.63 (0.67-3.97)
Other		0.70 (0.23-2.10)		0.79 (0.26-2.43)
Care recipient age (y)		1.00 (0.96-1.03)		1.00 (0.96-1.03)
Female care recipient		0.87 (0.51-1.49)		0.88 (0.51-1.51)
White-non-Hispanic care recipient		1.51 (0.87-2.65)		1.45 (0.85-2.47)
Care recipient education				
No degree		1.00		1.00
High school degree	[4]	0.51 (0.27-0.95)*	[8]	0.51 (0.27-0.99)
Some college, technical, associate degree		0.44 (0.23-0.86)*		0.50 (0.24-1.07)
Bachelor, professional, PhD degree		0.69 (0.29-1.63)		0.70 (0.29-1.70)
Care recipient health conditions				
High blood pressure		1.78 (0.91-3.46)		1.76 (0.92-3.38)
Arthritis		0.71 (0.40-1.26)		0.74 (0.41-1.32)
Diabetes		0.68 (0.35-1.30)		0.81 (0.41-1.61)
Osteoporosis		1.34 (0.89-2.02)		1.27 (0.79-2.04)
Cancer		1.46 (0.87-2.47)		1.47 (0.86-2.51)
Heart disease		0.72 (0.35-1.48)		0.78 (0.38-1.61)
Lung disease		1.74 (0.99-3.07)		1.77 (0.95-3.30)
Stroke		1.12 (0.60-2.08)		1.01 (0.54-1.89)
Heart attack		0.70 (0.32-1.55)		0.67 (0.32-1.39)
Dementia	[5]	2.34 (1.37-4.00)**	[6]	2.45 (1.45-4.16)**
Caregiver living with care recipient		0.95 (0.53-1.69)		0.88 (0.49-1.59)
Caregiving >1 y		1.07 (0.38-3.05)		1.17 (0.41-3.31)
Activities of daily living involvement		1.08 (0.99-1.17)	[7]	1.10 (1.02-1.20)*
Instrumental activities of daily living involvement		0.95 (0.82-1.10)		1.03 (0.90-1.18)
Involvement in medical tasks (e.g., ostomy care, IVs, etc.)		1.18 (0.52-2.68)		1.76 (0.79-3.88)

Abbreviations used: OR, odds ratio; CI, confidence interval.
$^*P<0.05$; $^{**}P<0.01$.

[1] [a] Adjusted Wald $\chi^2 = 36.23$; $P<0.01$.
[b] Adjusted Wald $\chi^2 = 37.65$; $P<0.00$.

all of the parameter coefficients are zero. The *P* values for both models are less than 0.01, indicating that, in both models, at least some of the coefficients are not zero. In the table, you can see that caregivers who reported helping the care recipient keep track of his or her medications (see [2]) were more likely to report seeking caregiving information and support compared to caregivers who did not provide this type of assistance (AOR: 2.30, 95%CI: 1.18–4.51). In contrast, caregivers who reported helping the care recipient take injected medications (see [3]) were less likely to report having sought caregiving information and support compared to caregivers who did not provide assistance with injected medications (AOR: 0.32, 95% CI: 0.14–0.76). The investigators had difficulty interpreting this latter finding. As stated in the "Discussion" section of the paper, "On the other hand, caregivers who were helping to inject medications had significantly lower odds of looking for information. It is not clear why there is an inverse relationship between these 2 caregiving behaviors" (p. 174). They also note the need for more research before generalizing the findings from the study to other caregivers.

Turning to the control variables included in the logistic regression models, one would expect to see a similar pattern of relationships with information seeking in both models. Remember that the only difference between the two models is the manner in which the variable "medication management assistance" is operationalized. In Model 1, this variable indexes whether the caregiver helps the care recipient keep track of his or her medications; In Model 2, it indexes whether the caregiver helps the care recipient take injected medications. In both models, the odds of seeking caregiving information and support decreases by 2%–3% with every 1-year increase in caregiver age (see [2] and [3]). Note that although "1" is included in the CI in Model 2, this has to be due to rounding error. Thus, if the confidence had been reported with more precision, it likely would have been something like 0.996. If the CI included "1," the coefficient would not have been statistically significant.

In Model 1, caregivers were less likely to report seeking information when the care recipient had a high school degree or some college compared to when the care recipient had no degree (see [4]). In both models, having a care recipient with dementia was associated with an increased odds of the caregiver seeking information and support (see [5] and [6]). In Model 2 only, providing assistance with ADLs was associated with an increased odds of the caregiver seeking information and support (see [7]). Finally, there appears to be a typo in the information provided for Model 2 (see [8]). Based on the CI, it appears that care givers were less likely to report seeking information when the care recipient had a high school degree compared to when the care recipient had no degree (AOR = 0.51, 95% CI: 0.27–0.99). If this is accurate, it is statistically significant at $P<0.05$ and should have been marked with an asterisk. This is a trivial error. However, when you see things like this in the literature, do not let them confuse you.

An important limitation of this study is described by the investigators in the "Discussion" section: "In addition, owing to the cross-sectional nature of the survey data, only associations between the variables can be highlighted and no causality can be demonstrated" (p. 176). Thus, for example, although helping care recipients keep track of their medications **was associated with** an increased odds of seeking information, we cannot infer that helping care recipients keep track of their medications **caused** caregivers to seek information.

The objective of the third study was to examine the relationship between pharmacist density (i.e., number of licensed pharmacists in a county/population of county) and influenza vaccination.[3] The analytic data set included variables assessed at the county level as well as the individual level. Individual-level data were obtained from the 2008–2012 Behavioral Risk Factor Surveillance System (BRFSS). Data for the BRFSS are collected via telephone interviews with a nationally representative sample of adults (aged 18 or older). The BRFSS interviews include a question asking respondents whether they have had an influenza vaccination within the previous 12 months. Data from a total of 1,696,119 respondents were included in the analytic data set. County-level attributes were obtained from the Area Health Resources Files (AHRF). The AHRF includes information about the number of licensed pharmacists in the counties where BRFSS respondents resided and county population.

The investigators used logistic regression to examine the relationship between pharmacist density and influenza immunization status while controlling for several individual-level and county-level attributes. The results of the logistic regression predicting immunization status are shown in Box 8-6. I have

BOX 8-6. Influenza Immunization Study

Table 3

Survey-weighted multivariable logistic regression predicting effects of individual attributes, neighborhood attributes, and pharmacist per 1000 population on influenza vaccination status, AOR (95% CI)

	Variable	Entire sample (n = 1,696,119)
	Individual-level attributes	
	Gender (male as reference group)	
	Female	1.20[a] (1.18-1.22)
	Race (non-Hispanic white as reference group)	
	Non-Hispanic black	0.79[a] (0.77-0.81)
	Non-Hispanic Asian	1.03 (0.98-1.08)
	Hispanic	0.91[a] (0.89-0.94)
	Non-Hispanic other race	0.94[a] (0.90-0.97)
	Marital status (never married as reference group)	
	Married	1.11[a] (1.08-1.14)
	Unmarried couple	0.95[b] (0.91-1.00)
	Widowed or divorced or separated	1.02 (0.99-1.05)
	Age (y, 18-29 as reference group)	
	30-39	1.01 (0.98-1.05)
	40-49	1.03[c] (1.00-1.06)
5	50-64	1.63[a] (1.58-1.68)
	65 and older	3.45[a] (3.33-3.57)
	Employment status (out of work as reference group)	
	Wage employment	1.22[a] (1.18-1.26)
	Self-employment	0.77[a] (0.74-0.80)
	Homemaker	1.03 (0.98-1.07)
	Student	1.25[a] (1.17-1.33)
	Retired	1.56[a] (1.51-1.62)
	Unable to work	1.58[a] (1.52-1.65)
	Education attainment (less than high school as reference)	
	Some college	1.12[a] (1.10-1.14)
	College or post baccalaureate	1.42[a] (1.39-1.44)
	Household income (less than $10,000 as reference group)	
	$10,000-$14,999	1.08[a] (1.03-1.13)
	$15,000-$19,999	1.12[a] (1.07-1.17)
	$20,000-$24,999	1.12[a] (1.07-1.17)
	$25,000-$34,999	1.13[a] (1.09-1.18)
	$35,000-$49,999	1.14[a] (1.09-1.18)
	$50,000-$74,999	1.16[a] (1.11-1.21)
	$75,000 or above	1.31[a] (1.26-1.37)
3	Insurance status (none as reference group)	
	Insured	1.67[a] (1.62-1.72)
4	Access to care (none as reference group)	
	Personal doctors or health care providers	1.87[a] (1.82-1.91)
	Health status (excellent and very good as reference group)	
	Good	1.12[a] (1.10-1.14)
	Fair or poor	1.32[a] (1.29-1.34)
	County-level attributes	
1	Number of pharmacists per 1000 population	1.13[a] (1.11-1.15)
	Rural and urban categories (metropolitan as reference)	
	Urban but nonmetropolitan	1.08[a] (1.06-1.10)
	Rural	1.08[a] (1.03-1.13)
	Health professional shortage areas (none as reference)	
	Part	0.99 (0.97-1.02)
	All	0.99 (0.97-1.01)
	Median household income level	1.003[a] (1.002-1.003)
2	Number of primary care physicians per 1000 population	1.05[a] (1.02-1.07)
	Survey year	
	2009	1.08[a] (1.05-1.10)
	2010	1.17[a] (1.15-1.20)
	2011	1.08[a] (1.06-1.10)
	2012	1.02[c] (1.00-1.04)

All adjusted odds ratios and confidence intervals are weighted with the use of the Stata command "svy: logit" to account for the sample design. The complete models for subgroups based on race and ethnicity are available in Appendix Table 2 (available online at japha.org).

Abbreviations used: OR, odds ratio; CI, confidence interval; AOR, adjusted odds ratio.

[a]$P<0.01$; [b]$P<0.05$; [c]$P<0.1$.

annotated the table with numbers for ease of reference. The results indicate that for each additional pharmacist per 1,000 population, the odds of having received an influenza vaccination within the previous 12 months increases by 13% (see [1], AOR: 1.13, 95% CI: 1.11–1.15). Among the control variables, the odds of having received a vaccination also increases as the number of primary physicians in the county increases (see [2]). Compared to individuals without health insurance, the odds of having had a vaccination were 67% higher among individuals with health insurance (see [3]). Compared to individuals without a personal health care provider, the odds of having had a vaccination were 87% higher among individuals who had a personal health care provider (see [4]). The strongest association shown in the table involves age. Compared to individuals aged 18–29, the odds of having had a vaccination were 3.45 times greater (i.e., 245% greater) among individuals aged 65 or older (see [5]).

A final word of caution. You can see that almost all of the relationships examined in Box 8-6 are statistically significant. This is not surprising for a study with over 1.5 million participants. Remember that in large samples, even very small differences that are not clinically meaningful may be statistically significant. Therefore, when readers interpret findings from studies with large sample sizes, it is especially important for them to consider whether the magnitude of differences reported are clinically meaningful, not only whether they are statistically significant.

Self-Study Questions

1. Which of the following statements are true with respect to logistic regression?
   - **A.** The goal is to predict the probability that individuals in the sample will experience the outcome of interest.
   - **B.** In a well-fitting model, most predicted probabilities will be close to either 1 or 0.
   - **C.** In a well-fitting model, the difference between expected and observed probabilities will be small.
   - **D.** All of the above

Use Question Table 8-1 to answer Questions 2–5.

QUESTION TABLE 8-1. Logistic Regression Predicting Development of Lung Cancer (Data Fictitious)

Variable	Regression Coefficient	OR	95% CI
Age (yr)	0.1521	1.16	1.06–1.89
Female	–0.3001	0.74	0.64–0.96
White	0.5489	1.73	0.92–3.11
Smoker	1.578	4.85	3.82–6.74

Reference groups: male, nonwhite, nonsmoker.

2. What is the outcome variable in this study?
   - **A.** Racial classification
   - **B.** Average age
   - **C.** Development of lung cancer
   - **D.** A and B
   - **E.** None of the above

3. In what way is race associated with lung cancer risk?
   - **A.** The odds of lung cancer are 1.73 times higher among individuals who are nonwhite compared to those who are white.
   - **B.** The odds of lung cancer are 1.73 times higher among individuals who are white compared to those who are nonwhite.
   - **C.** The relationship between race and the development of lung cancer is not statistically significant.

4. How is the OR for age interpreted?
   - **A.** The risk of developing lung cancer increases 16% for each 1-year increase in age.
   - **B.** The risk of developing lung cancer decreases 16% for each 1-year increase in age.
   - **C.** People over the age of 65 are 16% more likely to develop lung cancer than younger people.
   - **D.** The relationship between age and development of lung cancer is not statistically significant.

5. Is the following statement true or false? After controlling for age, sex, and race, the relationship between smoking and development of lung cancer is not statistically significant. (True/False)

Use Question Table 8-2 to answer Questions 6–10.

Reference: Qato DM, Wilder J, Zenk S, Davis A, Makelarski J, Lindau ST. Pharmacy accessibility and cost-related underuse of prescription medications in low-income Black and Hispanic urban communities. *J Am Pharm Assoc.* 2017;57:162–9.

QUESTION TABLE 8-2. Logistic Regression Examining Individual and Pharmacy Characteristics of Cost-Related Medication Underuse

Table 3

Individual and pharmacy characteristics associated with cost-related underuse among prescription medication users on Chicago's South Side (n = 169)

Characteristic	Estimated prevalence, % (95% CI)	Unadjusted OR (95% CI)	Adjusted OR (95% CI)
Pharmacies			
Primary pharmacy type			
Retail independent (n = 12)	15.5 (3.5-47.8)	Reference	Reference
Retail chain (n = 109)	11.2 (6.4-18.7)	0.69 (0.12-3.8)	1.3 (0.19-8.5)
CHC or clinic (n = 23)	9.2 (3.2-23.5)	0.55 (0.08-3.9)	0.42 (0.04-4.1)
Distance traveled to primary pharmacy		0.21 (0.16-0.27)*	1.1 (0.94-1.2)
<1 mile (n = 95)	8.7 (4.9-15.2)	Reference	Reference
≥1 mile (n = 58)	14.3 (6.4-28.9)	1.7 (0.59-5.2)	2.1 (0.62-6.9)
Individuals			
Household income			
25k/y (n = 66)	14.4 (7.9-27.2)	Reference	Reference
≥25k/y (n = 77)	9.1 (4.5-17.5)	0.55 (0.20-1.5)	0.90 (0.26-3.1)
Insurance status			
Uninsured (n = 31)	18.9 (7.4-40.4)	Reference	Reference
Private insurance (n = 64)	5.0 (1.7-13.6)	0.22 (0.05-1.0)	0.13 (0.02-0.68)*
Medicare (n = 50)	13.4 (6.3-26.3)	0.67 (0.17-2.6)	0.46 (0.10-2.2)
Medicaid (n = 18)	10.4 (3.0-30.2)	0.50 (0.09-2.7)	0.29 (0.05-1.8)
Other Insurance (n = 4)	0 (0-0)	—	—

CI, confidence interval; CHC, community health clinic; OR, odds ratio.
Logistic regression was used to examine individual and pharmacy characteristics associated with cost-related underuse. Adjusted model includes pharmacy and individual charateristics plus age and number of prescription medications.
* Statistically significant difference at $P < 0.05$.

6. What is the prevalence of cost-related medication underuse among people who used retail independent pharmacies, retail chain pharmacies, and community health clinics (CHCs)?

   A. 18.9%, 5.0%, 13.4%, respectively
   B. 15.5%, 11.2%, 9.2%, respectively
   C. 14.4%, 9.1%, 18.9%, respectively
   D. Prevalence cannot be determined from the information provided.

7. Is the difference in the prevalence of cost-related medication underuse among people who used CHCs versus those who used retail independent pharmacies statistically significant?

   A. Yes, it is statistically significant in both the adjusted and the unadjusted models.
   B. No, it is not statistically significant in either model.
   C. It is statistically significant in the adjusted model but not the unadjusted one.
   D. It is statistically significant in the unadjusted model but not the adjusted one.

8. In the adjusted model, which of the following is true?

   A. Individuals with private insurance were significantly less likely than those with no insurance to experience cost-related medication underuse.
   B. Individuals with Medicare were significantly less likely than those with no insurance to experience cost-related medication underuse.
   C. Individuals with Medicaid were significantly less likely than those with no insurance to experience cost-related medication underuse.
   D. All of the above

9. In the unadjusted model, which of the following is true?

   A. Individuals with private insurance were significantly less likely than those with no insurance to experience cost-related medication underuse.
   B. Individuals with Medicare were significantly less likely than those with no insurance to experience cost-related medication underuse.
   C. Individuals with Medicaid were significantly less likely than those with no insurance to experience cost-related medication underuse.
   D. None of the above

10. How is the adjusted OR for private insurance interpreted?

   A. The odds of cost-related medication underuse is 13% lower among those with private insurance compared to those with no insurance.
   B. The odds of cost-related medication underuse is 87% lower among those with private insurance compared to those with no insurance.
   C. The odds of cost-related medication underuse is 13% lower among those with private insurance compared to those with Medicaid.
   D. The odds of cost-related medication underuse is 87% lower among those with private insurance compared to those with Medicaid.

References

1. Pollini RA. Self-reported participation in voluntary nonprescription syringe sales in California's Central Valley. *J Am Pharm Assoc.* 2017;57(6):677–85.
2. Noureldin M, Murawski MM, Mason HL, et al. The association between family caregivers' involvement in managing older adults' medications and caregivers' information-seeking behavior. *J Am Pharm Assoc.* 2017;57(2):170–7.
3. Gai Y, Feng L. Relationship between pharmacist density and adult influenza vaccination after controlling for individual and neighborhood effects. *J Am Pharm Assoc.* 2017;57(4):474–82.

9 Survival Analysis

After reading this chapter, you should be able to do the following:

1. Describe the types of situations in which it would be appropriate to use survival analysis and the Cox proportional hazards model.
2. Explain the type of information conveyed by hazard ratios.
3. Given the results of a study that used survival analysis or the Cox proportional hazards model, interpret observed relationships in terms of statistical significance and magnitude of effect.
4. Interpret a Kaplan–Meier curve.

Survival analysis is used in situations where the outcome of interest is the length of time that elapses until an event (i.e., outcome) occurs. For example, investigators might assess (1) the length of time until death following diagnosis with a specific illness or (2) the length of time until death following the initiation of therapy with different medications. Although the outcome of interest in a survival analysis may be death, survival analysis can be used to analyze a wide variety of different outcomes. Examples of negative (bad) outcomes include time to first fall, time to first fracture, time to illness relapse, time to onset of end-stage renal disease, and time to second myocardial infarction. Examples of positive (good) outcomes include time to illness remission, time to hospital discharge, and time to return to work following an illness. As clinicians, we are often looking for therapies that delay the occurrence of bad outcomes and hasten the occurrence of good outcomes.

Analytic Challenges

Three methodological issues make it difficult to measure "time to event" in a study. **First,** people often enter a study at different times. In many studies, it can take a year or more to recruit all the participants needed to achieve adequate power. Consequently, participants who enter the study the day recruitment begins have the potential to be followed for a longer period of time than people who enter on the last day of recruitment. The longer participants are followed, the more likely they are to experience the outcome of interest. Therefore, it is necessary to adjust for variation in length of follow-up. This issue is depicted diagrammatically in Figure 9-1 where, patients 3 and 4 entered well after the initiation of recruitment and, therefore, could not be followed for the full 6 years of the study.

Second, every study has to end at some point. Therefore, it is not possible to follow all participants until they experience the outcome of interest. Some study participants may experience the outcome the day after follow-up ends. Others may not experience the outcome for 20 years.

FIGURE 9-1. Methodological Challenges When Measuring Time to Event

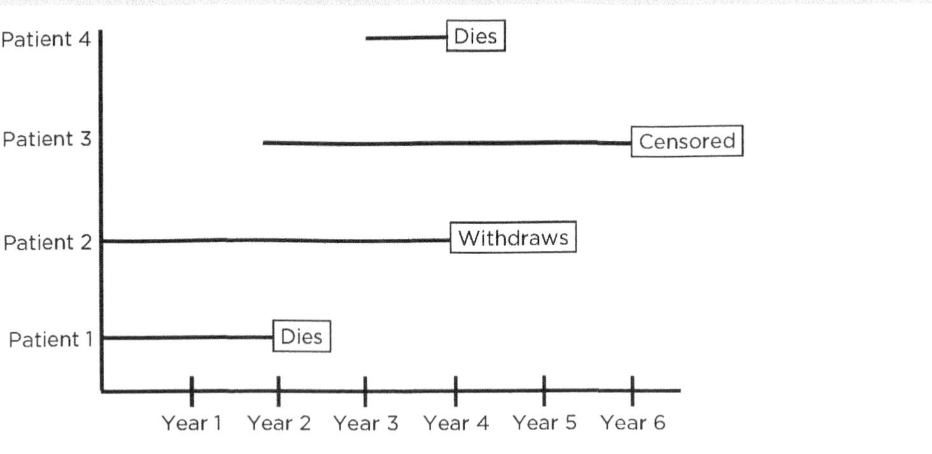

The study investigators will never know because no data are collected once the follow-up period ends. People who are still in the study when it ends but who have not yet experienced the outcome of interest are referred to as "censored." Papers might say that the observations were "right censored." This issue is depicted in Figure 9-1 where Patient 3 was still being followed when the study ended.

Third, people sometimes withdraw from studies or are lost to follow-up (e.g., move with no forwarding address). Therefore, as noted previously, the study investigators have no way to determine when (or if) they experience the outcome of interest. This issue is depicted in Figure 9-1, where patient 2 withdrew from the study before experiencing the outcome of interest.

To overcome these three analytic challenges, investigators perform some statistical "magic." They begin by pretending that everyone entered the study at the same time. Thus, in Figure 9-2, all four patients are backed up as though they had entered the study on the first day of participant recruitment. As long as a person remains in the study **and** does **not** experience the outcome of interest (in this example, dies), that person is considered "at risk" for experiencing the outcome. Individuals are removed from the "at risk" pool when (1) they experience the outcome of interest **or** (2) they withdraw from the study or are otherwise lost to follow-up. It is then possible to calculate how long each person was "at risk" (i.e., the length of follow-up

FIGURE 9-2. Conceptual Design of Studies Measuring Time to Event

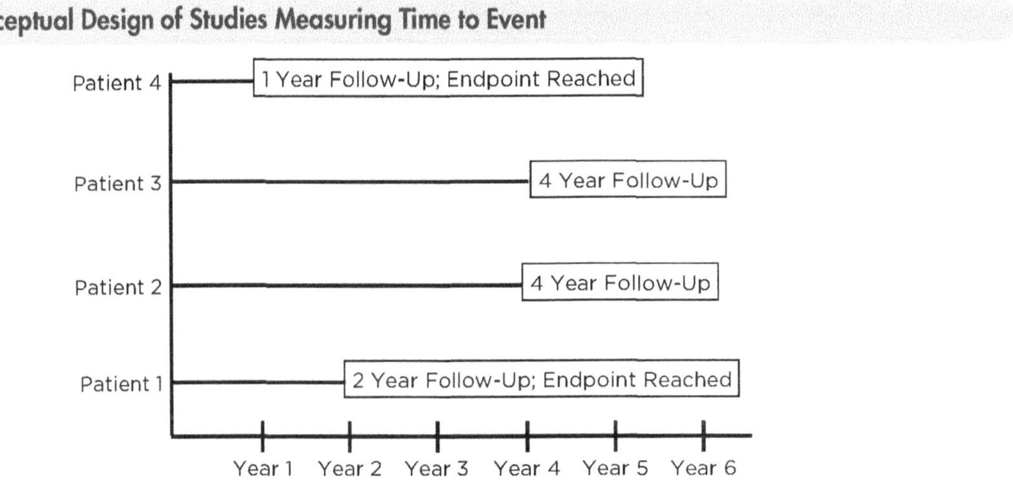

prior to experiencing the outcome of interest) **and** whether they experienced the outcome of interest. In Figure 9-2, the term "endpoint reached" indicates that the person experienced the outcome of interest (in this example, death) while being followed.

Life Table Analysis

The information depicted diagrammatically in Figures 9-1 and 9-2 can be used to create a survival table such as the one shown in Table 9-1. Each row in the table shows what happened during a particular study year. In the table, each participant is assumed to enter at the same time. Thus, data from all four participants are available in the first year of follow-up (i.e., year 1). There was one death during that year (patient 4). Thus, Patient 4 was removed from the "at risk" group, leaving three participants being followed in the second year of follow-up (i.e., year 2). There was one more death during the second year of follow-up (Patient 1). Thus, Patient 1 was removed from the "at risk" group, leaving two participants being followed in the last 2 years of the study. Both of these participants were followed for 2 additional years at which time they were lost to follow-up; Patient 2 was lost because he or she withdrew and Patient 3 because the study ended.

Within each time period, the probability of death during the time period, **given that a person has survived up to the beginning of the time period**, is calculated by the following formula: $Hazard = q_i = \dfrac{D_i}{R_i - \frac{L_i}{2}}$, where D_i is the number of people who died during the time interval, R_i is the number of people at risk at the beginning of the time period, and L_i is the number of people lost to follow-up during the time period. In the formula, L_i is divided by 2 because it is assumed that the investigators do not know exactly when the participants were lost to follow-up. Dividing by 2 assumes that, on average, people were lost to follow-up halfway through the time interval. The probabilities calculated by the hazard formula are shown in Table 9-1 in the column labeled "Probability of Death." These probabilities represent the **hazard function**.

Within each time period, the probability of surviving through the time period, **given that a person has survived up to the beginning of the time period**, is calculated as $p_i = 1 - q_i$. Finally, the cumulative probability of survival from entry into the study through the time interval of interest is calculated by $S_{t+1} = (p_{t+1})\, S_t$. For year 1–2, $p_{t+1} = 0.67$ and $S_t = 0.75$. Therefore, $S_{Year\ 1\text{–}2} = (0.67)(0.75) = 0.50$. For year 2–3, $p_{t+1} = 1$ and $S_t = 0.50$. Therefore, $S_{Year\ 2\text{–}3} = (1)(0.50) = 0.50$. The probabilties calculated by the cumulative survival formula are shown in Table 9-1 in the column labeled "Cumulative Probability of Survival." These probabilities represent the **survival function**.

The results of a survival analysis can be presented diagrammatically by plotting the survival function in a "survival curve," such as the one shown in Figure 9-3. This figure simply shows the cumulative probability

TABLE 9-1. Survival Table

Study Year	Number at Risk	Number of Deaths	Number Lost to Follow-Up	Probability of Death	Probability of Survival	Cumulative Probability of Survival
1	4	1	0	0.25	0.75	0.75
2	3	1	0	0.33	0.67	0.50
3	2	0	0	0	1	0.50
4	2	0	2	0	1	0.50

FIGURE 9-3. Survival Curve

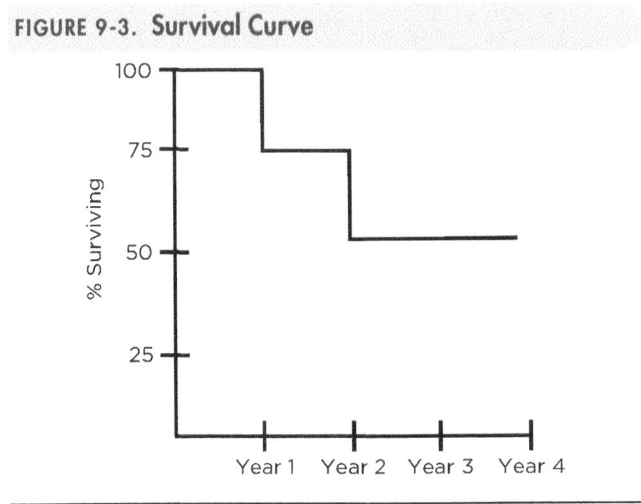

of surviving to the end of each time period. If everyone were followed until they reached the end point of interest, the survival curve would drop to the x-axis.

Comparing Survival Curves

Survival analysis can be used to determine if the risk of experiencing a particular event (e.g., death, return to work) over a specified period of time differs between groups. In the medical literature, a common application of survival analysis involves comparing event risk across treatment groups (i.e., intervention versus control groups). The logrank test can be used to determine if the difference between two survival curves is statistically significant. The logic underlying this test is similar to the logic that underlies Pearson chi-square tests discussed in Chapter 6. Briefly, the follow-up period is divided into intervals of equal length (e.g., 1 year), and the number of events observed **during each interval** is compared to the number of events expected **given the number of people at risk during the interval**. The larger the difference between observed and expected values, the more likely it is that the logrank test will be statistically significant, indicating that risk differs across the groups. Box 9-1 provides an example of the computations for the logrank test.

Hazard Ratio

As described previously, the logrank test simply allows one to determine whether the risk of a particular event differs between groups. However, it does not assess the direction (i.e., which group is at higher risk) or the magnitude of the difference that exists. This information is conveyed by the hazard ratio. Remember that a hazard reflects the probability that a person will experience the event of interest during a specific time interval, given that the person has not already experienced the event (i.e., they are still in the at-risk pool). The hazard ratio (HR) is simply the ratio of the hazard in one group divided by the hazard in the other group, such that $HR = \frac{Hazard_{Group1}}{Hazard_{Group2}}$. Hazard ratios are usually interpreted in the same manner as relative risk (RR). However, hazard ratios have a time element. Thus, hazard ratios convey the RR of experiencing an event at a given point in time, given that the event has not been experienced previously. As with all ratios, the expected value under the null hypothesis is that the hazard ratio is "1," which occurs when the hazard in the two groups is the same. Because hazard ratios are estimates of population parameters based on data collected from a sample, they have standard errors (SEs). Investigators use these SEs to compute confidence intervals (CIs) within which they can have a desired level of confidence (e.g., 95%, 99%)

BOX 9-1. Calculation of Logrank Test and Hazard Ratios

Imagine that a study is conducted to evaluate the effectiveness of an experimental drug that has shown promise in preventing cancer relapse. A total of 350 people are enrolled in the study; 100 are randomly assigned to receive the experimental drug, and 250 are randomly assigned to receive standard care. Participants are followed for up to 15 years. During the follow-up period, there were a total of 61 deaths in the experimental group and 76 deaths in the standard care group. Data for the first 3 years of the study are summarized below.

Study Year	Experimental Drug Group		Standard Care Group	
	# at Risk	# of Deaths	# at Risk	# of Deaths
1	100	5	250	0
2	93	4	248	3
3	85	5	240	5
4–15	***	***	***	***
Totals	***	61	***	76

To calculate the logrank test, each time interval is examined one at a time. This is done by using the data from each time interval to construct a contingency table, as you would do if you were calculating a chi-square test. The contingency tables for Years 1 and 2 are shown below. Note that the row totals reflect the number of people at risk during the time interval.

Year 1				Year 2			
Group	Died	Survived	Row Totals	Group	Died	Survived	Row Totals
Experimental	5	95	100	Experimental	4	89	93
Standard care	0	250	250	Standard care	3	245	248
Column totals	5	345	350	Column totals	7	334	341

Next, the number of expected deaths within each group is calculated just as would be done if a chi-square statistic were being calculated. Thus, in year 1, the expected number of deaths in the experimental group is $\frac{5*100}{350} = 1.43$. Similarly, in year 1, the expected number of deaths in the control group is $\frac{5*250}{350} = 3.57$.

The total number of expected deaths in the two groups are calculated by summing the values in each column, yielding a total of 28.06 expected deaths in the experimental group and 108.93 expected deaths in the standard care group. These computations are summarized below.

Study Year	Experimental Drug Group		Standard Care Group	
	# of Deaths	# of Expected Deaths	# of Deaths	# of Expected Deaths
1	5	1.43	0	3.57
2	4	1.91	3	5.09
3	5	2.62	5	7.38
4–15	***	***	***	***
Totals	61	28.06	76	108.93

(continued)

BOX 9-1. Calculation of Logrank Test and Hazard Ratios *(Continued)*

The logrank statistic can then be computed using the chi-square formula. Thus,

$$\sum\frac{(Observed - Expected)^2}{Expected} = \chi^2(1) = \frac{(61-28.06)^2}{28.06} + \frac{(76-108.93)^2}{108.93} = 48.62$$

As with any other test statistic, if this value is greater than the critical value (CV) determined by alpha, the null hypothesis is rejected. In this case, the CV for a chi-square test with 1 degree of freedom (alpha = .05) is 3.84. Therefore, we would reject the null hypothesis. This is equivalent to saying that the difference between the survival curves is statistically significant.

We now know that the risk of death during the follow-up period differs between the experimental and standard care groups. However, we still do not know two very important things: (1) how much the risk differs between the groups (i.e., the magnitude of the difference) and (2) whether the risk is higher in the experimental or the standard care group (i.e., the direction of the difference). For that, we need the hazard ratio.

Hazard ratios can be interpreted as the magnitude of risk in one group relative to another group. The formula for the hazard ratio (HR) is:

$$HR = \frac{Observed_{Group1}/Expected_{Group1}}{Observed_{Group2}/Expected_{Group2}}$$

Plugging the values calculated above into this formula gives us:

$$\frac{Observed_{Experimental}/Expected_{Experimental}}{Observed_{StandardCare}/Expected_{StandardCare}} = \frac{61/28.06}{76/108.93} = 3.12$$

These findings indicate that the risk of death was over 3 times greater in the experimental drug group than in the standard care group. Not good news for the pharmaceutical company that manufactures the experimental drug!

that the true population parameter lies. A hazard ratio is considered statistically significant if "1" is not contained within the CI.

Kaplan–Meier Method and Cox Proportional Hazards Model

In the simple examples presented previously, I assumed that we did not know exactly when each participant experienced the outcome of interest. However, if this information is known, investigators can use the Kaplan–Meier Method to perform survival analysis. The main difference between this approach and the survival table analysis approach described previously is that because the exact date participants experience the outcome of interest is known, it is not necessary to lump events into arbitrary time intervals (e.g., number of deaths in study year 1). This makes the math a bit more complex. However, the underlying concepts remain the same.

The Cox proportional hazards model extends the general approach used in survival analysis by allowing investigators to include control variables in the regression model. The outcome is still "time to event." A Cox proportional hazards model can include a large number of predictor variables, just like linear and logistic regression. When one interprets the hazard ratios from a Cox proportional hazards model, each hazard ratio is adjusted for all other predictor variables included in the model. Box 9-2 presents an example using the Cox proportional hazards model to evaluate the effectiveness of a fictitious experimental medication.

BOX 9-2. Example of Cox Proportional Hazards Model

This example is based on the fictitious study described in Chapter 8. You may remember being asked to imagine that an investigator wanted to determine if an experimental drug reduces the risk of 1-year mortality among patients with hypertension at high risk of heart attack. Participants were randomly assigned to receive either a placebo (n = 50) or the experimental drug (n = 50). All participants were followed for 1 year. A total of 22 people died during the follow-up period: 15 who took the placebo and 7 who took the experimental drug. Now, imagine that the investigator recorded the date each participant died, allowing him to use time-to-death as the primary outcome variable.

The table below provides data for the 22 people who died during the follow-up period. The next-to-last column on the right indicates how long each participant was followed. For the people who died, this is the time from study entry to date of death. I assumed that no one was lost to follow-up. Therefore, the people who did not die during the 1-year follow-up period were assumed to be censored after participating in the study for 365 days.

Ref #	Treatment Group	Age	SBP	LDL	BMI	Time (Days)	Censored
1	Placebo	87	130	205	31	17	0
2	Experimental drug	77	133	188	30	22	0
3	Placebo	77	133	188	30	38	0
4	Placebo	80	128	181	33	69	0
5	Experimental drug	87	130	205	31	93	0
6	Placebo	76	117	183	32	95	0
7	Placebo	79	117	183	27	132	0
8	Placebo	87	138	148	28	164	0
9	Experimental drug	76	117	183	32	178	0
10	Placebo	78	134	182	26	198	0
11	Placebo	88	134	141	29	257	0
12	Placebo	82	159	114	33	276	0
13	Experimental drug	88	134	141	29	277	0
14	Placebo	76	132	171	30	289	0
15	Experimental drug	68	142	142	37	303	0
16	Placebo	78	145	113	27	311	0
17	Placebo	74	133	169	37	327	0
18	Experimental drug	60	150	139	29	337	0
19	Placebo	73	141	112	29	346	0
20	Experimental drug	82	159	114	33	348	0
21	Placebo	71	143	150	30	352	0
22	Placebo	68	142	142	37	360	0
23+	***	***	***	***	***	365	1

To analyze the data from this fictitious study, I ran two regression models using Proc Phreg in SAS. In Model 1, I included only a dichotomous variable indexing whether the participant took the placebo or the experimental drug. In Model 2, I added four control variables to the model: age, systolic blood pressure (SBP), low-density lipoprotein (LDL), and body mass index (BMI).

(continued)

BOX 9-2. Example of Cox Proportional Hazards Model *(Continued)*

By default, SAS uses three different tests to evaluate the global null hypothesis that all of the regression coefficients are 0: the likelihood ratio (LR), score, and Wald tests. All of these tests follow a chi-square distribution. In Model 1, the *P* value for each of these three tests is greater than 0.05. Therefore, we cannot conclude that the experimental drug reduced the risk of death. In contrast, in model 2, the *P* value for each test is less than 0.05. Therefore, we can conclude that the regression coefficient for at least one of the variables in Model 2 is statistically significant (i.e., different from 0). However, we still do not know which specific variable(s) account for rejection of the null hypothesis in Model 2.

MODEL 1. Testing Global Null Hypothesis

Test	Chi-Square	df	Pr > ChiSq
LR	3.7660	1	0.0523
Score	3.7056	1	0.0542
Wald	3.4869	1	0.0619

MODEL 2. Testing Global Null Hypothesis

Test	Chi-Square	df	Pr > ChiSq
LR	54.2627	5	<.0001
Score	45.9839	5	<.0001
Wald	35.6984	5	<.0001

df, degrees of freedom.

To determine which variables are statistically significant, one has to look at the parameter estimates, just like in any other type of regression analysis. As shown below, Model 1 only has one predictor variable, (i.e., treatment group). In the model, I called this variable "medication" because the placebo group was the reference group. The significance of each variable is assessed by the Wald chi-square test. Because there is only one predictor variable, the significance of this variable matches the *P* value for the Wald test evaluating the overall global hypothesis.

The parameter estimate for "medication" is –0.85502. This can be converted into a hazard ratio (HR) by calculating the exponent of the parameter estimate such that $HR = \exp(-0.85502) = 0.425$. By itself, this value suggests that the experimental medication reduced the risk of death throughout the follow-up period by more than 50%. But don't be fooled. Because the parameter estimate was not statistically significant, we cannot rule out the possibility that the experimental drug has no effect on the risk of death.

MODEL 1. Analysis of Maximum Likelihood Estimates

Parameter	df	Parameter Estimate	SE	Chi-Square	Pr > ChiSq	Hazard Ratio	95% CI
Medication	1	–0.85502	0.46	3.49	0.0619	0.425	0.17–1.04

Below are the parameter estimates for Model 2. Here, all of the predictor variables except BMI are statistically significant at $P<0.05$. In addition to looking at the *P* values, you can see that none of the 95% CIs for the hazard ratios cross "1," with the exception of BMI.

Note that all of the estimates shown are adjusted for the other variables in the model. Thus, after controlling for other variables in the model, the risk of death during the follow-up period increased about 20% with each 1-year increase in age, 10% with each 1-point increase in SBP, and 5% with each 1-point increase in LDL.

Our primary interest, however, lies with the effect of the experimental drug. Here, we can see that after controlling for the other variables in the model, the experimental drug reduced the risk of death throughout the 1-year follow-up period by over 80% (i.e., relative risk reduction = $|1-0.198| = 0.802$. Remember that this is just a point estimate of risk. However, based on the 95% CI, you can be 95% confident that the experimental drug reduces the risk of death throughout the follow-up period by at least 46% (i.e., $|1 - 0.54|$).

BOX 9-2. **Example of Cox Proportional Hazards Model** *(Continued)*

MODEL 2. **Analysis of Maximum Likelihood Estimates**

Parameter	df	Parameter Estimate	SE	Chi-Square	Pr > ChiSq	Hazard Ratio	95% CI
Medication	1	−1.61765	0.51	9.99	0.0016	0.198	0.07 to 0.54
Age	1	0.19352	0.04	21.97	<.0001	1.214	1.12 to 1.32
SBP	1	0.09807	0.03	9.15	0.0025	1.103	1.04 to 1.18
LDL	1	0.05207	0.01	15.97	<.0001	1.053	1.03 to 1.08
BMI	1	0.06556	0.06	1.04	0.3069	1.068	0.94 to 1.21

Below is the Kaplan–Meier curve showing the probability of surviving throughout the 1-year follow-up period in the two treatment groups. The curves are adjusted for all of the predictor variables in Model 2. The steeper decline of the curve for those taking placebo reflects the greater risk of death in this group throughout the follow-up period.

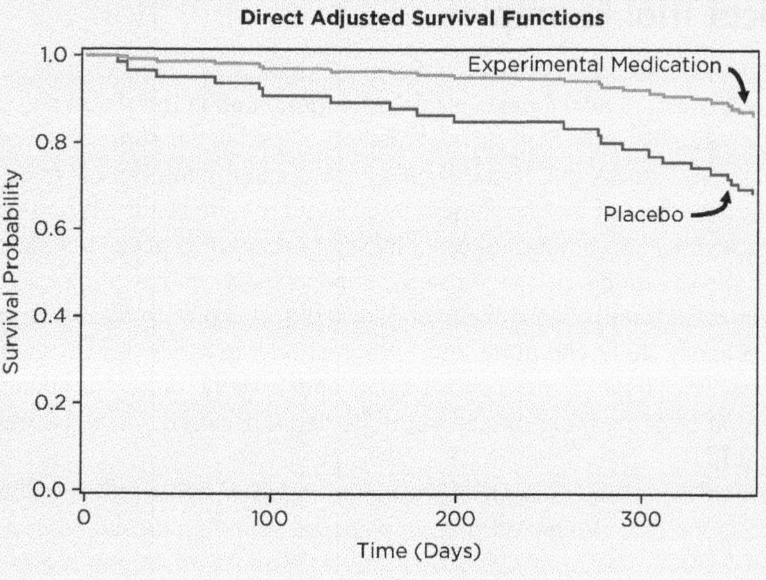

Assumptions of Survival Analysis

Several important assumptions must be met for investigators to use survival analysis. These include:

1. There is an identifiable starting point (e.g., the date that therapy was initiated). This is often a problem if an investigator in interested in studying the natural history of a disease because the date of illness onset may be difficult to determine.
2. The outcome of interest must be well defined and dichotomous. Survival certainly meets this criterion. It is reasonably easy for trained professionals to determine whether someone is alive or dead. However, it is much more difficult to determine if a person has experienced other outcomes of interest. For example, mild strokes may be difficult to diagnose definitively. In papers, you will often read that the primary end points were **adjudicated** by a panel of experts. This is particularly important when some subjective judgment is required to identify individuals who

have experienced the outcome (end point). Reliability of the classification (end point reached or not reached) is enhanced by using a panel of experts, rather than relying on a single individual to make the classifications.

3. Loss to follow-up is not related to the outcome of interest. If people withdraw from a study because they are doing poorly (and at greater risk of experiencing the outcome) or doing well (and at less risk of experiencing the outcome), estimates from the survival analysis can be seriously biased.
4. There are no secular trends. This assumption would be violated, for example, if treatment improved over time or diagnostic practices changed over time resulting in earlier detection. If these types of secular trends are present, it would not be appropriate to "pretend" that everyone entered the study at the same time as is required to create the survival table.
5. For the proportional hazards model, the relative risk associated with predictor variables must be consistent over time. This assumption would be violated, for example, if two medications were equally safe for the first 2 years of therapy but the risk of a serious side effect increased for one of the drugs (but not the other) after 2 years of therapy.

Clinical Trial Examples

In this section, I will use data from three clinical studies described in U.S. Food and Drug Administration–approved drug labels to illustrate how survival analysis is used in the pharmaceutical industry.

The first study, CLEOPATRA (NCT00567190), was a multicenter, double-blind, placebo-controlled trial investigating the effect of adding Perjeta to a regimen of trastuzumab and docetaxel in the treatment of patients with human epidermal growth factor receptor 2–positive metastatic breast cancer.[1] A total of 808 patients participated in the study. Patients were randomly allocated to treatment group (i.e., Perjeta plus trastuzumab and docetaxel versus placebo plus trastuzumab and docetaxel) on a 1:1 basis. The **primary study end point** was "progression-free survival (PFS) as assessed by an independent review facility (IRF). PFS was defined as the time from the date of randomization to the date of disease progression or death (from any cause) if the death occurred within 18 weeks of the last tumor assessment" (p. 25).

The primary analyses found "CLEOPATRA demonstrated a statistically significant improvement in IRF-assessed PFS in the PERJETA-treated group compared with the placebo-treated group [hazard ratio (HR)=0.62 (95% CI: 0.51, 0.75*)*, p < 0.0001] and an increase in median PFS of 6.1 months (median PFS of 18.5 months in the PERJETA-treated group vs. 12.4 months in the placebo-treated group) (see Figure [9-4])" (p. 26).

In the previous paragraph, notice that the CI for the hazard ratio does not include "1," which is consistent with the conclusion that the between group difference in PFS was statistically significant. Because the hazard ratio is **below** 1, one can conclude that the difference favored the Perjeta-treated group. Readers can draw the same inference from the longer median PFS observed in the Perjeta-treated group compared to the placebo-treated group, 18.5 and 12.4 months, respectively.

The Kaplan–Meier curve shown in Figure 9-4 appears on page 28 of the Perjeta package insert. Looking at the x-axis, you can see that approximately 35 months of follow-up time is reported. The proportion of participants who were progression free is shown on the y-axis. If you draw a horizontal line out from 0.5 on the y-axis, you can determine the month at which each curve crosses this line, which corresponds to the median PFS time (i.e., 12.4 months in the placebo-treated group and 18.5 months in the Perjeta-treated group). Along the bottom of the figure, you can see two rows labeled Ptz + T + D and Pla + T + D, denoting the Perjeta- and placebo-treated groups, respectively. These rows show the number of participants who remained at risk at different time points. For example, at Month 0, there were 402 and 406 participants in the Perjeta- and placebo-treated groups, respectively. At Month 20, the number of at-risk participants had dropped to 83 and 42 in the Perjeta- and placebo-treated groups, respectively. This type of information

FIGURE 9-4. Kaplan–Meier Curve of IRF-Assessed Progression-Free Survival for CLEOPATRA

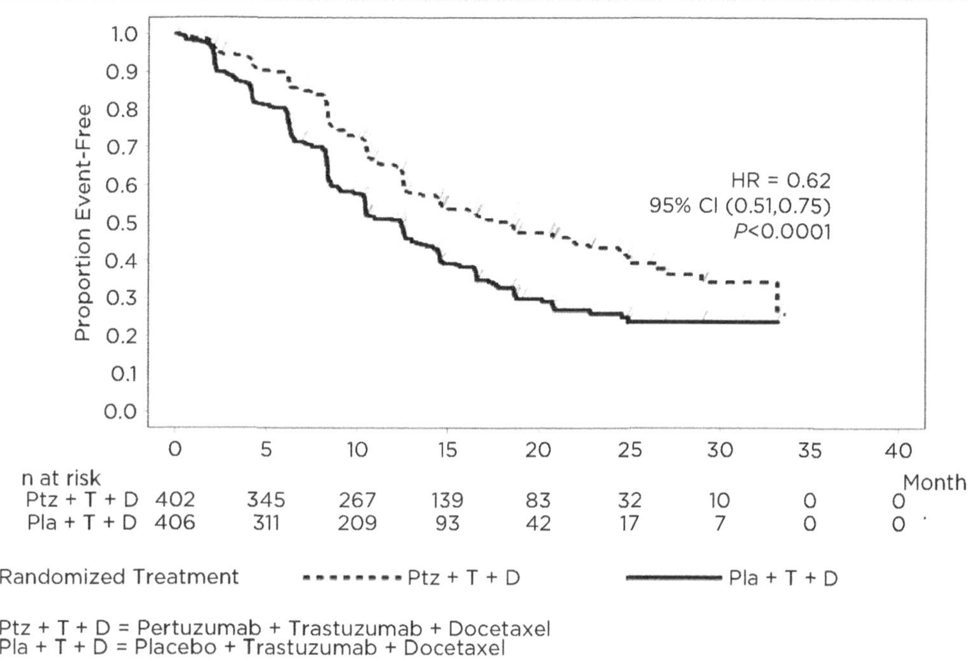

IRF, independent review facility; HR, hazard ratio; CI, confidence interval.

is useful because, as the number of people at risk decreases, parameter estimates become more unstable. When you are reading the literature, if you see a Kaplan–Meier curve that does not contain this information, be sure to read the text carefully to determine the number remaining at risk at various points throughout the follow-up period.

The second study, the Anglo-Scandinavian Cardiac Outcomes Trial, assessed the effect of Lipitor on the risk of fatal and nonfatal coronary heart disease.[2] The study used a double-blind, placebo-controlled, clinical trial design. Participants were patients with hypertension, aged 40–80, who had a total cholesterol level ≤251 mg/dL and at least three cardiovascular risk factors. Patients with a history of a previous myocardial infarction were excluded. Participants were randomly assigned to receive either Lipitor 10 mg daily (n = 5,168) or placebo (n = 5,137). All participants also received antihypertensive therapy. The median follow-up time was 3.3 years. The study found that "Lipitor significantly reduced the rate of coronary events [either fatal coronary heart disease (46 events in the placebo group vs. 40 events in the Lipitor group) or nonfatal [myocardial infarction] (108 events in the placebo group vs. 60 events in the Lipitor group)] with a relative risk reduction [RRR] of 36% [(based on incidences of 1.9% for Lipitor vs. 3.0% for placebo), $p = 0.0005$ (see Figure [9-4])]" (pp. 15–16).

Notice that the incidence rates mentioned in the excerpt of study findings from the package insert reflect the number of events experienced within each group. For example, in the Lipitor group, there were a total of 40 fatal and 60 nonfatal events, for a total of 100 events. Dividing that by the sample size yields an incidence rate of $\frac{100}{5,168} = 0.019 * 100\% = 1.9\%$. Figure 9-5 appears on page 16 of the package insert. It shows the cumulative incidence of nonfatal myocardial infarction or coronary heart disease death. The total follow-up time shown is 3.5 years, corresponding roughly to the median follow-up time. You may notice that the figure does not provide information about the number of people at risk throughout the follow-up period. However, this is not a concern because the sample size was quite large and the number of people experiencing the event was quite small. Thus, relatively few people were being removed from the at-risk pool because they experienced the event. We also know that the median duration of follow-up was 3.3 years. Taken together, it seems likely that over 2,000 people remained in the at-risk group throughout

FIGURE 9-5. Effect of LIPITOR 10 mg/day on Cumulative Incidence of Non-Fatal Myocardial Infarction or Coronary Heart Disease Death (in ASCOT-LLA)

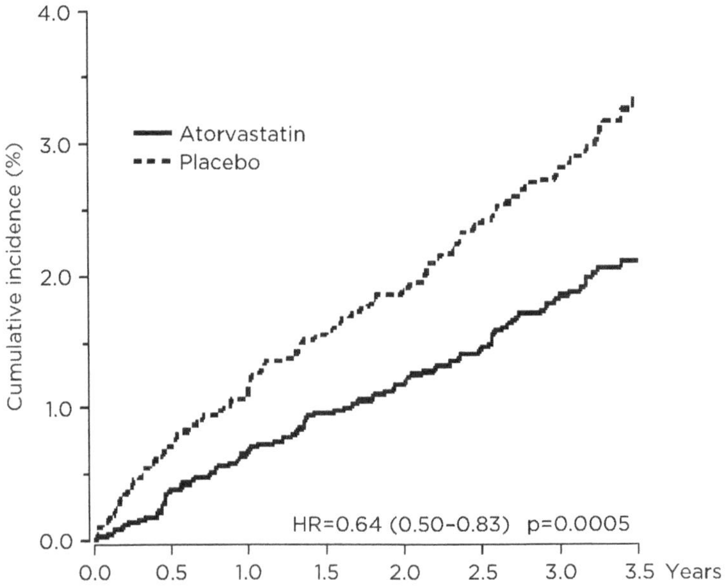

ASCOT-LLA, Anglo-Scandinavian Cardiac Outcomes Trial—Lipid Lowering Arm.

the first 3.5 years of follow-up. The figure also shows the hazard ratio comparing the two groups. It is 0.64, corresponding to the 36% RRR mentioned in the excerpt of study findings from the package insert.

The third study was the Clopidogrel in Unstable Angina to Prevent Recurrent Events (CURE) study. This study enrolled patients with acute coronary syndrome who were hospitalized within 24 hours of onset of chest pain or symptoms consistent with ischemia and who did not display ST-elevation. Participants were randomly assigned to one of two groups. Individuals in one group (n = 6,259) received a 300 mg loading dose of Plavix followed by a regimen of 75 mg/day. Individuals in the second group (n = 6,303) received a placebo. All participants also received aspirin and other standard care. Participants were treated for up to 1 year. The primary outcome was experience of cardiovascular death, myocardial infarction, or stroke. Thus, if a participant experienced any of these three events, he or she was considered to have reached the study's primary end point.

A total of 582 (9.3%) of patients in the Plavix-treated group experienced the primary outcome, compared to 719 (11.4%) in the placebo-treated group, a 20% RRR (95% CI of 10%–28%; P <0.001) in the Plavix-treated group. The package insert states, "Most of the benefit of Plavix occurred in the first two months, but the difference from placebo was maintained throughout the course of the trial (up to 12 months) (see Figure [9-6])" (p. 13).[3] Figure 9-6 appears on page 14 of the package insert dated October 2017. It shows the cumulative incidence of the primary outcome over the 12-month follow-up period. Although the number of participants who remained at risk is not shown under the x-axis, as in Figure 9-4, this is not a major concern because of the large sample size. In addition, this information is provided in a publication of study findings.[4] That publication reported that over 2,000 people in each group remained at risk at the 12-month follow-up.

The package insert also states, "The effect of Plavix did not differ significantly in various subgroups, as shown in Figure [9-7]. The benefits associated with Plavix were independent of the use of other acute and long-term cardiovascular therapies, including heparin/[low molecular weight heparin], intravenous glycoprotein IIb/IIIa (GPIIb/IIIa) inhibitors, lipid-lowering drugs, beta-blockers, and ACE inhibitors. The efficacy of Plavix was observed independently of the dose of aspirin (75–325 mg once daily)" (p. 14).

FIGURE 9-6. Cardiovascular Death, Myocardial Infarction, and Stroke in the CURE Study

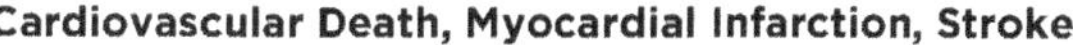

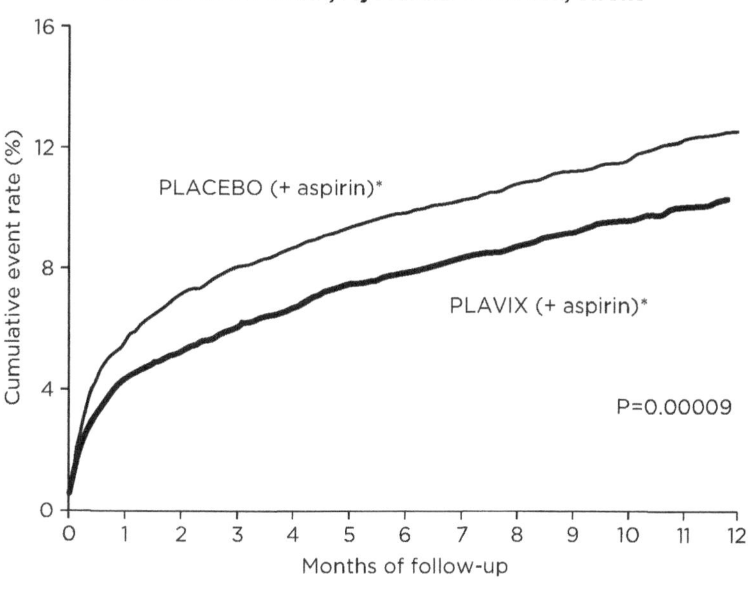

*Other standard therapies were used as appropriate.

FIGURE 9-7. Hazard Ratio for Patient Baseline Characteristics and On-Study Concomitant Medications/Interventions for the CURE Study

Subgroup	N	Plavix n(%)	Placebo n(%)
Age			
<65	5996	154 (5.2)	228 (5.2)
65-74	4136	211 (10.2)	258 (12.4)
75+	2430	217 (17.8)	233 (19.2)
Gender			
Male	7726	351 (9.1)	461 (11.9)
Female	4836	231 (9.5)	258 (10.7)
Race			
Caucas	10308	470 (9.1)	568 (11.0)
Non-Cauc	2250	112 (10.1)	151 (13.2)
Elev Card Enzy			
Yes	3176	169 (10.7)	207 (13.0)
No	9381	413 (8.8)	512 (10.9)
Diabetes			
Yes	2840	200 (14.2)	239 (16.7)
No	9721	382 (7.9)	480 (9.9)
Previous MI			
Yes	4044	253 (12.5)	310 (15.4)
No	8517	329 (7.8)	409 (9.5)
Previous Stroke			
Yes	506	49 (17.9)	52 (22.4)
No	12055	533 (8.9)	667 (11.0)
Overall	12562	582 (9.3)	719 (11.4)

Favors Plavix | Favors Placebo

0.3 0.4 0.5 0.6 0.7 0.8 0.9 1.0 1.1 1.2 1.3 1.4

Hazard Ratio (95% CI)

Subgroup	N	Plavix n(%)	Placebo n(%)
Heparin/LMWH			
Yes	11611	559 (9.7)	682 (11.7)
No	951	23 (4.9)	37 (7.7)
Aspirin(mg)			
<100	1927	80 (8.5)	96 (9.7)
100-200	7428	345 (9.2)	402 (10.9)
>200	3201	157 (9.9)	221 (13.7)
GPIIb/IIIa Antag			
Yes	823	58 (15.7)	87 (19.2)
No	11739	524 (8.9)	632 (10.8)
Beta-Blocker			
Yes	10530	484 (9.2)	594 (11.3)
No	2032	98 (9.9)	125 (12.0)
Ace Inhibitor			
Yes	7749	433 (11.2)	522 (13.5)
No	4813	149 (6.3)	197 (8.1)
Overall	12562	582 (9.3)	719 (11.4)

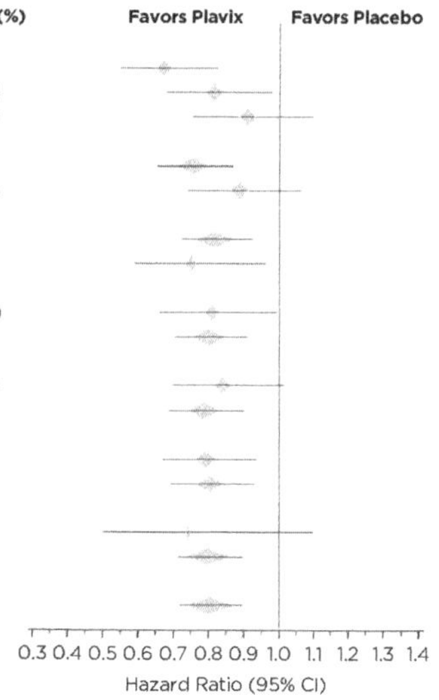

Favors Plavix | Favors Placebo

0.3 0.4 0.5 0.6 0.7 0.8 0.9 1.0 1.1 1.2 1.3 1.4

Hazard Ratio (95% CI)

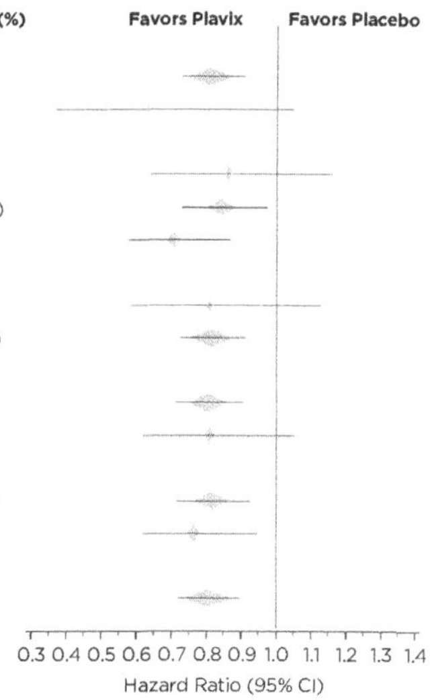

MI, myocardial infarction; CI, confidence interval; LMWH, low molecular weight heparin; Elev Card Enzy, elevated cardiac enzyme.

Figure 9-7, mentioned in the excerpt from the package insert above, appears on pages 15 and 16 of the package insert dated October 2017. Notice that the column labeled "N" shows the number of study participants in each subgroup. The next columns show the number and percentage of participants in the Plavix-treated and placebo-treated groups who reached the primary study end point. On the right side of the figure, the HR (95% CI) comparing the risk of reaching the primary end point in the two study groups is shown, stratified by participant characteristics.

For each subgroup, the horizontal bar depicts the width of the 95% CI and the gray diamond near the center of the bar depicts the point estimate for the HR. Notice that the CIs vary in length. For example, the CI for people who have had a previous stroke is much wider than most of the others. This is primarily because this subgroup is much smaller than the other subgroups. (Remember that CIs become narrower, and more precise, as sample size increases). You might also notice that the diamonds representing the point estimates of the HR vary in size. The size of the diamond corresponds roughly to the sample size in the subgroup. The vertical line rising from a HR of 1.0, divides the figure into two portions. Values that fall to the left of this vertical line indicate that risk was lower in the Plavix-treated group; values that fall to the right of the line indicate that risk was lower in the placebo-treated group. If the CI for an HR crosses the line, the HR would not be considered statistically significant at $P<0.05$. In general, Figure 9-7 shows considerable consistency across the study subgroups. Most notably, all of the point estimates for the HR lie on the side of the figure favoring the Plavix-treated group and all of the 95% CIs include the value of 0.80, the HR observed in the overall sample, supporting the conclusion that the effect of Plavix did not differ significantly in various subgroups.

Self-Study Questions

1. Results of a study involving survival analysis are often depicted diagrammatically using which of the following?

   A. Kaplan–Meier curve
   B. Scatterplot
   C. Box plot
   D. Histogram

2. The outcome of interest in a study examining a new cancer medication is 5-year survival. Patients who are alive 5 years after diagnosis are coded as "1." Patients who die prior to this time are coded as "0." Of the following choices, which type of analysis would be most appropriate to use in analyzing these data?

   A. Logistic regression
   B. Linear regression
   C. Analysis of variance
   D. Survival analysis

3. The outcome of interest in a study examining a new cancer medication is 5-year survival. The primary outcome variable is time to death, measured in days from study enrollment. Of the following choices, which type of analysis would be most appropriate to use in analyzing these data?

   A. Logistic regression
   B. Linear regression
   C. Analysis of variance
   D. Survival analysis

4. When survival analysis is used to analyze between group differences, which of the following tests can be used to assess the statistical significance of differences observed?

   A. McNemar test
   B. Independent groups t-test
   C. Logrank test
   D. F-test
   E. None of the above

5. Which of the following is **not** an assumption of survival analysis?

   A. A dichotomous outcome is being analyzed.
   B. Loss to follow-up is not associated with the outcome.
   C. At least 5% of study participants experience the outcome.
   D. There are no secular trends that affect the probability of the outcome.
   E. This is a trick question; all of the above are assumptions of survival analysis.

6. Is the following statement true or false? It is possible to control for confounding factors when survival analysis is used. (True/False)

References

1. Perjeta [package insert]. South San Francisco, CA; Genentech; revised December 2017. https://www.accessdata.fda.gov/drugsatfda_docs/label/2017/125409s113s118lbl.pdf.
2. Lipitor [package insert]. New York, NY; Parke-Davis; May 2017. https://www.accessdata.fda.gov/drugsatfda_docs/label/2017/020702s067s069lbl.pdf.
3. Plavix [package insert]. Bridgewater, NJ; Bristol-Myers Squibb/Sanofi; revised October 2017. https://www.accessdata.fda.gov/drugsatfda_docs/label/2017/020839s068lbl.pdf.
4. Yusuf S, Zhao F, Mehta SR, et al. Clopidogrel in Unstable Angina to Prevent Recurrent Events Trial Investigators. Effects of clopidogrel in addition to aspirin in patients with acute coronary syndromes without ST-segment elevation [published corrections appear in *N Engl J Med.* 2001;345(20):1506 and *N Engl J Med.* 2001;345(23):1716]. *N Engl J Med.* 2001;345(7):494–502.

FINISHING TOUCHES

Assessing Study Measures 10

After reading this chapter, you should be able to do the following:

1. Differentiate between the reliability, validity, and responsiveness of a measure.
2. Discuss methods that can be used to assess reliability and validity.
3. Define and distinguish between the sensitivity, specificity, positive predictive value, and negative predictive value of a diagnostic test.
4. Calculate the sensitivity, specificity, positive predictive value, and negative predictive value of a diagnostic test.
5. Describe how different cutoff values affect the above measures.
6. Identify factors that affect the clinical importance of higher or lower values of sensitivity and specificity.
7. Explain how the prevalence of a disease affects the above measures.
8. Use information concerning the results of a diagnostic test with a given level of sensitivity and specificity to compute the probability of disease.
9. Critically evaluate the measurement section of a paper to determine the adequacy of the measures used.

Measurement lies at the heart of all scientific inquiry: what cannot be measured, cannot be studied. This leads to the expression "garbage in, garbage out." That is to say, the most sophisticated statistical techniques are of no value if the measures used to collect data on study variables are seriously flawed. As a reader of the literature, one of the first things you should examine when reading a paper is whether the measures of key variables were adequate. Two key characteristics to examine in all studies are the reliability and validity of the measures used. In intervention studies, it is also important to assess the responsiveness of the primary outcome variables to change. These three characteristics are described next.

Reliability. Conceptually, a measure is reliable if it yields the same value upon repeated administrations. For example, imagine that I step on my bathroom scale, record that it reads "210 pounds," step off, wait 1 minute (without eating or drinking anything), step back on, record that it reads "210 pounds" again, step off, and keep repeating this process many times. If every time I step on the scale it reads "210 pounds," the scale would be a reliable measure of weight. In contrast, if each time I step on the scale it provides a different value (sometimes "210 pounds," sometimes "110 pounds," and other times values in between), it would be an unreliable measure. The values obtained would be worthless. If I were conducting a study that involved measuring weight, I would be well advised to find a better scale.

Validity. Validity concerns the extent to which a measure provides an accurate assessment of the construct it is designed to measure. Returning to the bathroom scale example, we will assume that every time I step on the scale it indicates that I weigh 210 pounds. Therefore, it is reliable (i.e., it gives exactly the same answer upon repeated administrations, assuming that the underlying construct has not changed). However, there is still a problem. I do not weigh anywhere near 210 pounds. Although the scale is giving a consistent weight (making it reliable), it is **not** giving an accurate weight. Therefore, it is not a valid measure.

Random Versus Systematic Error. In the bathroom scale example, if the scale was a valid measure of weight and I weighed myself multiple times over a short span of time, the scale readings might vary slightly

FIGURE 10-1. Impact of Random/Systematic Error on Validity and Reliability

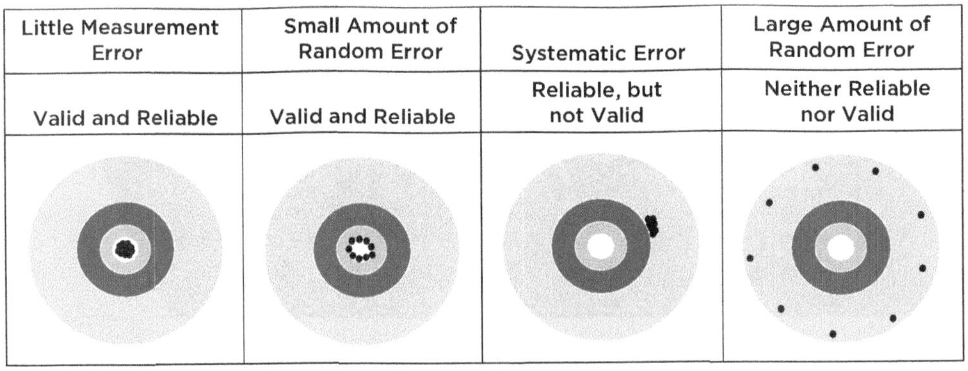

Little Measurement Error	Small Amount of Random Error	Systematic Error	Large Amount of Random Error
Valid and Reliable	Valid and Reliable	Reliable, but not Valid	Neither Reliable nor Valid

(e.g., ± 1–2 pounds) due to **random error**. However, to be valid, some of the readings would have to be slightly above my actual weight, and some would have to be slightly below my actual weight. Thus, if I weighed myself 10 times and calculated the average of the values obtained, the average should be pretty close to my true weight. That is because the random errors above and below my true weight would cancel one another out. Another way of saying this is that if a measure is valid, the sum of the errors will be "0."

In the previous example, if the average of the readings were either much higher or much lower than my actual weight, it would suggest that some type of **systematic error** was affecting the scores. When scores on a measure are affected by systematic error, the **validity** of the measure is called into question. **Systematic errors bias a measure in one direction.** For example, if a self-report measure were used to assess participant weight in a study, weight would probably be underestimated (because people tend to report that they weigh less than they do). This would reflect systematic error. Consequently, the validity of the measure might be less than desired.

Random error primarily affects the reliability of a measure. However, to be valid, a measure must be reasonably reliable. Moreover, just because a measure is reliable does not mean that it is valid. The panels in Figure 10-1 illustrate the impact of random/systematic error on reliability and validity. In the figure, the concept of interest lies in the bull's eye of the targets. Random error is reflected by the spread of the "shots" around the bull's eye. Systematic error is shown in the second panel from the right where most of the errors are in one direction.

Responsiveness. In studies that assess change over time or that compare the amount of change experienced by participants in different groups in addition to being valid and reliable, measures of the primary outcome variables need to be responsive to change. That is, if an experimental medication has the intended effect, investigators need to have measures that are capable of detecting the effect. For example, if the primary outcome of interest in a study was functional ability following a stroke, asking participants how easily they can walk up a flight of stairs would not capture smaller improvements in functional ability (e.g., being able to get out of bed unassisted). Thus, this question may not be sufficiently responsive to change to be used in this study. Nonetheless, it might be sufficiently responsive to use in other studies (e.g., a study of college football players recovering from arthroscopic surgery for knee injury).

Assessing Reliability

Several techniques can be used to assess reliability. The most appropriate technique to use in a particular situation depends on the characteristics of the measure being evaluated as well as the context in which the measure is being used. I describe three of the most commonly used techniques: internal consistency, test–retest, and interrater reliability.

Internal Consistency Reliability

Many measures of subjective phenomena (e.g., experience of depressive symptoms) are assessed via multi-item scales. The notion underlying these scales is not unlike my example of stepping on and off the bathroom scale multiple times. Each item in the scale is designed to measure the same underlying construct (e.g., depression). For example, a measure designed to assess depressive symptoms might include questions asking respondents how often they feel sad, worthless, or like no one likes them. Although each item in the scale will be affected by random error (e.g., on a 10-point scale, a respondent may not be sure whether he is a 4 or a 5, so he picks one of these numbers fairly randomly), when responses to the items are averaged, these errors should cancel out. Thus, by calculating the average of a person's responses across all of the items, the scale score will provide a pretty accurate representation of the extent to which the person experiences depressive symptoms. This assumes, of course, that no systematic biases are operating.

The internal consistency of multi-item scales is usually assessed by Cronbach's alpha. Alpha has a theoretical range from 0 to 1.0. Higher values reflect greater reliability. Alpha can be calculated using the following formula, $\alpha_{Standardized} = \frac{K\bar{r}}{1+(K-1)\bar{r}}$, where K is the number of items in the scale and $\bar{r}$ is the average inter-item correlation. Thus, alpha will be higher when there are more items in the scale and when the items in the scale are more highly correlated. Generally, alpha should be at least 0.70 for a measure to be considered adequately reliable.

Test–Retest Reliability

Test–retest reliability is simply assessed by the correlation of a measure taken at one point in time with the same measure taken at another point in time. When investigators report test–retest reliability, they should provide the time interval between assessments (e.g., 1 week, 1 month). Unfortunately, test–retest reliability can be difficult to interpret because the variable being assessed (e.g., weight, pain severity) may actually change between the two assessments. Consequently, test–retest reliability may underestimate the true reliability of the measure. In contrast, if the time interval is too short, people may simply remember the value that they provided previously and report the same value again (to avoid appearing inconsistent or untruthful). In this case, the reliability of the measure would be overestimated. Because test–retest reliability is evaluated by a correlation, it has a possible range from −1.0 to +1.0. Higher positive values reflect greater reliability. In general, values greater than +0.7 would be considered as evidence of adequate reliability. However, lower values may be acceptable depending on the length of the time interval between assessments and the nature of the variable being assessed.

Interrater Reliability

Interrater reliability is relevant in situations where a variable is assessed by multiple coders. For example, imagine a study in which the primary outcome variable was experience of a vertebral fracture. In this study, multiple radiologists might be used to examine participant x-rays to provide a rating of whether or not a participant had experienced a vertebral fracture (yes/no) or the number of vertebral fractures evident on each participant's x-ray. With this type of design, it is important to verify that different radiologists tend to rate the same x-ray in the same way. The most common statistics used to assess interrater agreement are simple agreement, Cohen's Kappa, and the intraclass correlation coefficient (ICC).

Simple agreement is calculated as the proportion of observations that were coded the same by different coders (i.e., $\frac{\#\ of\ Agreements}{\#\ of\ Observations\ Coded}$).

Cohen's Kappa is similar to simple agreement except that it corrects for the number of agreements that one would expect by chance. Box 10-1 provides an example of the calculations for both simple agreement and Cohen's Kappa. As the example illustrates, simple agreement can suggest interrater reliability is adequate when it is not much higher than one would expect if the raters were just guessing. If you encounter studies that report interrater reliability based only on simple agreement, think about how much

BOX 10-1. Simple Agreement Versus Cohen's Kappa

Imagine that two radiologists are asked to review the same set of 100 x-rays to determine which patients have (and have not) experienced a vertebral fracture. The ratings from their reviews are provided below. Notice that both radiologists coded six patients as having x-ray evidence of a vertebral fracture. However, only two patients were coded as having x-ray evidence of a vertebral fracture **by both radiologists**. This is shown in the shaded box in the top row below. In addition, 90 patients were coded as having **no** x-ray evidence of a vertebral fracture **by both radiologists**. This is shown in the shaded box in the second row below.

	Radiologist #2		
Radiologist #1	**Fracture**	**No Fracture**	**Total**
Fracture	2	4	6
No fracture	4	90	94
Total	6	94	100

Calculating simple agreement:

$$\frac{\text{\# of Agreements}}{\text{\# of Observations Coded}} = \frac{2+90}{100} = \frac{92}{100} = 0.92 * 100\% = 92\%.$$

Calculating Cohen's Kappa:

$$\frac{\text{\# of Agreements} - \text{\# of Agreements Expected by Chance}}{\text{\# of Observations Coded} - \text{\# of Agreements Expected by Chance}}$$

The number of agreements expected by chance is calculated by multiplying the marginal totals and dividing by the grand total (using the multiplication rule for independent events), as shown below.

Number of Agreements Expected by Chance

	Radiologist #2		
Radiologist #1	**Fracture**	**No Fracture**	**Total**
Fracture	0.36		6
No fracture		88.36	94
Total	6	94	100

Plugging these values into the formula for Cohen's Kappa gives us:

$$\frac{92 - 0.36 - 88.36}{100 - 0.36 - 88.36} = \frac{3.28}{11.28} = 0.291 * 100\% = 29.1\%$$

Note how much lower Cohen's Kappa is than simple agreement. This is because when an event is uncommon, a large number of agreements are expected due to chance. Thus, chance-adjusted interrater reliability, as assessed by Cohen's Kappa, will be lower than values obtained on the basis of simple agreement.

the value reported is likely to be influenced by chance agreements. If the authors provide sufficient information, you might even be able to calculate Cohen's Kappa from the information provided. In general, Kappas between 0.60 and 0.74 are considered evidence of good interrater agreement, and Kappas between 0.75 and 1.0 are considered evidence of excellent interrater agreement

The **ICC** is used as a measure of interrater reliability when the variable of interest is measured on a numerical scale. For example, a single person can have multiple vertebral fractures evident on an x-ray. Thus, the outcome variable might be the number of vertebral fractures a person has experienced (0 to ∞), rather than simply whether or not the person has experienced a vertebral fracture (yes/no). Note that ICCs differ from Pearson correlation coefficients discussed in Chapter 7 because Pearson correlation coefficients only capture the direction and magnitude of a linear association between variables. A Pearson correlation coefficient can be 1.0, indicating a perfect correlation between two variables, even when the variables never have the same value. For example, if Y=2X, the Pearson correlation coefficient assessing the relationship between X and Y would be 1.0. Nonetheless, X and Y would always have different values and therefore never "agree." In contrast, ICCs capture both association and agreement, which is required for a measure of interrater reliability. When evaluating the adequacy of interrater reliability in a study where ICCs are reported, one can use the same guidelines as for Kappa.

Assessing Validity

As you read the literature, you will see that investigators often claim to have used "validated" measures. Never take this claim at face value. The validity of measures depends on the context in which they are used. For example, a measure of functional ability may be a valid measure of this construct in older adults but may not be a valid measure of functional ability in adolescents and young adults. To be valid, a measure of functional ability needs to be able to differentiate between people with differing abilities across the entire range of abilities that exist within the target population. In this example, it is likely that the "older adult" measure would include less difficult items (e.g., walking up a flight of stairs) than would be needed to capture the full range of functional ability that exists among adolescents and young adults (e.g., run a marathon). Thus, when investigators talk about measures being "validated," they really should identify the purpose for which the measure is validated. When the measure is used for any other purpose, its validity remains open to question and should be reevaluated.

The major types of validity are face validity, content validity, criterion validity, and construct validity. Face validity and content validity are often confused with one another. **Face validity** is established by having experts in the area of interest review a measure after it has been developed to determine if it looks like it assesses the variable of interest. It provides only very weak evidence of validity. Establishing **content validity** involves much more rigorous procedures. Briefly, content validity is established through the procedures used to develop a measure. This process is easiest to think about in the context of developing a measure to assess knowledge of a particular area. For example, imagine that an investigator wanted to develop a measure to assess knowledge concerning osteoporosis. As a first step, the investigator would need to define the precise knowledge domain(s) of interest. Does he want the measure to assess knowledge of the pathophysiology of osteoporosis, prevention strategies, and treatment approaches? Or are only some of these domains relevant to his interests? Next, he would need to develop a set of questions representative of the universe of questions relevant to the domain(s) of interest. To do this, he might conduct an extensive review of textbooks, the peer-reviewed literature, and guidelines disseminated by professional organizations. He might also consult experts in the field to ensure that important domains are not being overlooked and that the set of questions being developed provide comprehensive coverage of all areas of interest, with no areas inappropriately under- or overemphasized. This is an iterative process that can require multiple rounds of literature searches, question development, review, and revision. Carrying out these types of procedures rigorously provides evidence of content validity. As a reader of the literature, when you are reading papers that claim to have established content validity, be sure to look at the procedures they followed when developing the measure. It is not uncommon for authors to claim to have established content validity when they have done little more than have a few experts look at the measure after it has been developed, with relatively few changes made after the expert review.

Criterion validity is established by correlating a measure with a "gold standard" that is known to be a valid measure of the construct of interest. For example, I might use a well-calibrated scale to assess the validity of self-reported weight. If the two measures are strongly correlated, I would conclude that self-reported weight is a valid measure of actual weight. Unfortunately, the lack of valid "gold standards" for many variables of interest limits the extent to which criterion validity can be used in practice.

Finally, **construct validity** is established by testing hypotheses about how the measure one is attempting to validate should correlate with other measures, none of which are viewed as "gold standards." If the hypotheses are supported, it provides evidence of construct validity. There are two different types of construct validity: convergent and discriminant.

Figure 10-2 shows the conceptual process that underlies the establishment of construct validity. In the figure, I am attempting to validate Measure 1, which is intended to measure Latent Construct 1. Latent constructs are unobserved variables that cannot be measured directly. For example, physical symptoms (e.g., pain, fatigue) and psychological states (e.g., depression, anxiety) experienced by patients are latent variables that cannot be observed directly. Instead, we must infer the presence of these symptoms or states based on how patients respond to questions designed to assess the relevant phenomena. To validate Measure 1, I might hypothesize that Latent Constructs 1 and 2 are correlated. Assuming that I have an established measure of Latent Construct 2 that I am confident is valid and reliable, such as Measure 2 in the figure, I can correlate that measure with Measure 1. If the correlation between the two measures is substantial, it provides evidence of **convergent validity** (i.e., Measure 1 correlates in the way predicted with measures of similar constructs). That helps to erase the question mark shown in the figure, which indicates that I started this process being unsure if Measure 1 was a valid measure of Latent Construct 1.

In the figure, the solid curved lines depict associations hypothesized to be substantial. The dotted curved lines depict associations hypothesized to be small. For example, imagine that Latent Constructs 1 and 2 are depression and anxiety, which we know are highly correlated, and that Latent Construct 3 is

FIGURE 10-2. Establishing Construct Validity

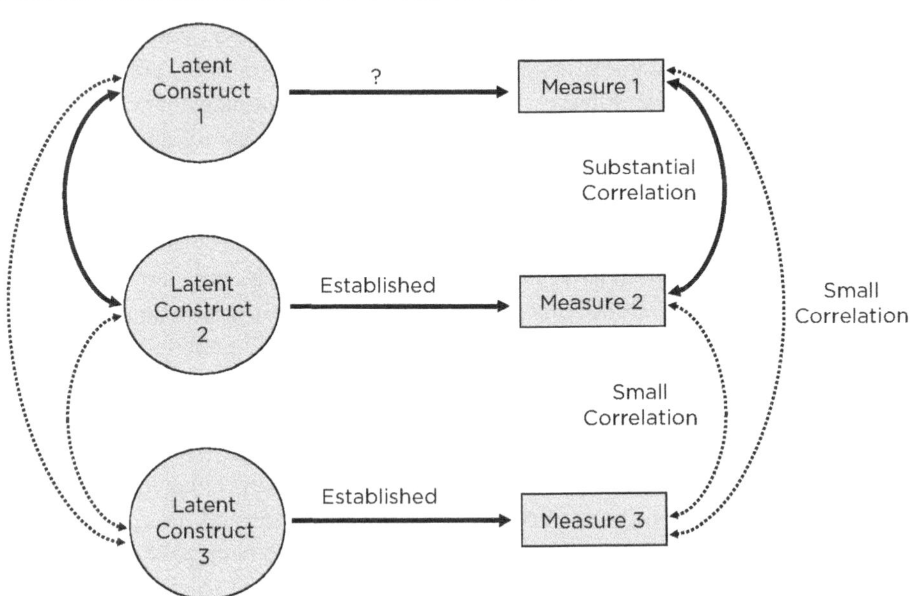

manual dexterity. Thus, the dotted lines in the figure indicate that I am hypothesizing that manual dexterity is uncorrelated with depression and anxiety. Assuming again that I have a measure of Latent Construct 3 that I am confident is valid and reliable, such as Measure 3 in the figure, I can correlate that measure with Measure 1. If the correlation between the two measures is zero or small, it provides evidence of **discriminant validity** (i.e., Measure 1 is uncorrelated or only weakly correlated with measures of distinct constructs).

Assessing Responsiveness

A wide variety of strategies are used to assess the responsiveness of outcome measures in medical research. The specific strategies used vary across clinical areas and are beyond the scope of this book. As you read the literature, some of the statistics that you are likely to see used to assess responsiveness include effect size $\left(\frac{\bar{D}}{SD_{Baseline}}\right)$, standardized response mean $\left(\frac{\bar{D}}{SD_D}\right)$, paired t-test $\left(\frac{\bar{D}}{SD_D/\sqrt{n}}\right)$, relative efficiency $\left(\frac{t_{Measure_1}}{t_{Measure_2}}\right)^2$, and the responsiveness statistic $\left(\frac{\bar{D}(Among\ Improved/Worsened\ Patients)}{SD_D(Among\ Stable\ Patients)}\right)$. In addition, investigators often examine "floor" and "ceiling" effects, both of which make measures less responsive. Ceiling effects occur when values on a measure at baseline are so high that there is little room for them to go higher. For example, in a study evaluating an intervention to improve mobility, if the mobility measure used contained only relatively "easy" items (e.g., ability to get out of bed unassisted), ceiling effects might occur that limit the measure's ability to detect change. To improve the responsiveness of the measure, "harder" items (e.g., ability to walk outside on uneven ground) could be added. Floor effects occur when values on a measure are so low at baseline that there is little room for them to go down. For example, in a study investigating an analgesic, if the pain measure contained only relatively "hard" items (e.g., how many days a week do you have severe pain), floor effects might occur. To improve the responsiveness of the measure, "easier" items (e.g., how many days a week do you have mild or moderate pain) could be added.

Measurement Properties of Diagnostic Tests

In research studies, diagnostic tests may be used to determine if patients meet study eligibility criteria or experience a study end point during the follow-up period. Interpreting the results of diagnostic tests presents special challenges that are important to understand. Table 10-1 presents the generic contingency table usually used to assess the measurement properties of diagnostic tests. The rows indicate whether the results of the test were positive (T+) or negative (T–). The columns indicate whether, in reality, the person

TABLE 10-1. Properties of Diagnostic Tests

	Disease		
Test Result	**Present (D+)**	**Absent (D–)**	**Marginals**
Positive (T+)	True positives	False positives	Total (T+)
Negative (T–)	False negatives	True negatives	Total (T–)
Marginals	Total (D+)	Total (D–)	Total

has the disease (D+) or does **not** have the disease (D–). If the test were perfect, all observations would fall in either the "true positive" or the "true negative" cells. That is, there would be **no** "false negatives" or "false positives." However, for the most part, tests are like people—they are not perfect. Therefore, we have to be able to figure out exactly how good they are and to what extent positive and negative test results can be trusted.

Sensitivity

The sensitivity of a test is the probability that a person who has the disease of interest will test positive for the disease. It is calculated as true positives/total (D+).

To better understand what sensitivity assesses, imagine that you have a group of 100 people all of whom you **know** have Disease X. (Notice the emphasis on the word "**know**" in the previous sentence. I honestly want you to imagine that you **know** these people have Disease X.) Also imagine that you have a new test designed to diagnose Disease X. You give the test to all of the 100 people in your group. You could then calculate the sensitivity of the test by dividing the number of positive test results by 100 (i.e., the number of people tested, remembering that all of the people tested are known to have the disease). The people who test positive correspond to the true positives in the contingency table in Table 10-1. The people who test negative correspond to the false negatives. If 75 of the people in the group tested positive, the sensitivity of the test would be 75%.

If a test is very sensitive, it will yield few false negatives. Therefore, if a patient tests negative, a clinician can be pretty sure that the patient does not have the disease. **Thus, highly sensitive tests help rule out the presence of a disease.**

Specificity

The specificity of a test is the probability that a person who does not have the disease of interest will test negative for the disease. It is calculated as true negatives/total (D–).

To better understand what specificity assesses, imagine that you have a group of 100 people, all of whom you **know do not have** Disease X. (Again, the emphasis is on truly **knowing** this.) Also imagine that you have the new test described previously to diagnose Disease X. You give the test to all of the 100 people in this group. You could then calculate the specificity of the test by dividing the number of negative test results by 100 (i.e., the number of people tested, remembering that all of these people were known to **not have** the disease). The people who test negative correspond to the true negatives in the contingency table in Table 10-1, whereas the people who test positive correspond to the false positives. If 95 of the people in the group tested negative, the specificity of the test would be 95%.

If a test is very specific, it will yield few false positives. Therefore, if a patient tests positive, a clinician can be more confident that the person does have the disease. **Thus, highly specific tests help confirm the diagnosis of a disease.** However, as described below, when a disease is very rare (i.e., very low prevalence), positive results even on a very specific test can be misleading.

Clinical Inferences Based on Test Results

It is relatively easy for researchers to determine the sensitivity and specificity of a diagnostic test. They simply need to assemble two groups of patients—one group that includes only people known to have the disease of interest and one group that includes only people known to **not** have the disease—then test everyone. Unfortunately, sensitivity and specificity do **not** tell clinicians how likely it is that a person who tests positive for a disease actually has the disease or how likely it is that a person who tests negative for a disease actually does **not** have it. This information is provided by the positive predictive value (PPV) and negative predictive value (NPV) of the test, which can also be computed from the contingency table shown in Table 10-1. However, as discussed below, these values vary as a function of the prevalence of the disease in the target population.

PPV

The PPV of a test is the probability that a person who tests positive for a disease does, in fact, have the disease. It is calculated as true positives/total (T+). Notice that whereas the denominators in the calculations of sensitivity and specificity were based on **column totals**, the denominator for PPV is a **row total**.

NPV

The NPV of a test is the probability that a person who tests negative for a disease does, in fact, **not** have the disease. It is calculated as true negatives/total (T–). Notice again that the denominator used to calculate NPV is a **row total**.

Effect of Prevalence on PPV and NPV

PPV and NPV can provide valuable diagnostic information, but the value of these statistics depends on the prevalence of the disease in the target population. Consider the example shown in Box 10-2. The example assumes that the sensitivity and specificity of a diagnostic test for Disease X are 75% and 95%, respectively. Given these values, if the prevalence of Disease X in the population is 40%, the PPV is 90.9%, meaning that a clinician can be over 90% sure that if a patient has a positive test result, the patient actually has Disease X. In contrast, if the prevalence of Disease X in the population is 0.4%, the PPV is

BOX 10-2. Effect of Prevalence on Positive Predictive Value and Negative Predictive Value

Imagine that you have a diagnostic test for Disease X with a sensitivity and specificity of 75% and 95%, respectively. You want to determine the positive and negative predictive values (PPV and NPV, respectively) for the test. You enroll a total of 1,000 people from the target population into a study to evaluate the test. The following examples make different assumptions about the prevalence of Disease X in the target population.

Prevalence of Disease X = 40%

If the prevalence of Disease X in the target population is 40%, you would expect 400 of the people enrolled in the study to have Disease X (D+) and 600 to **not** have Disease X (D–). This is shown in the shaded boxes in the table below. Given that the sensitivity of the diagnostic test is 75%, you would expect 300 of the people with Disease X to test positive (i.e., 400 ∗ 0.75 = 300). Given that the specificity of the test is 95%, you would expect 570 of the people who do **not** have the disease to have negative test results (i.e., 600 ∗ 0.95 = 570).

The remaining two cells can be calculated by subtraction (i.e., false negatives = 400 – 300 = 100; false positives = 600 – 570 = 30).

$$\text{Now it is easy to calculate PPV as true positives}/(\text{T}+) = \frac{300}{330} = 90.9\%$$

$$\text{Similarly, NPV is calculated as true negatives}/\text{T}(-) = \frac{570}{670} = 85.1\%$$

	Disease		
Test Result	**Present (D+)**	**Absent (D–)**	**Marginals**
Positive (T+)	300	30	330
Negative (T–)	100	570	670
Marginals	400	600	1,000

(continued)

BOX 10-2. Effect of Prevalence on Positive Predictive Value and Negative Predictive Value *(Continued)*

Prevalence of Disease X = 4%

If the prevalence of Disease X in the target population is 4%, you would expect 40 of the people enrolled in the study to have Disease X (D+) and 960 to **not** have Disease X (D–). Given that the sensitivity of the diagnostic test is 75%, you would expect 30 of the people with Disease X to test positive (i.e., 40 * 0.75 = 30). Given that the specificity of the test is 95%, you would expect 912 of the people who do not have the disease to have negative test results (i.e., 960 * 0.95 = 912). The remaining cells can be calculated by subtraction.

$$\text{Now, PPV} = \frac{30}{78} = 38.5\% \text{ and NPV is } \frac{912}{922} = 98.9\%.$$

	Disease		
Test Result	**Present (D+)**	**Absent (D–)**	**Marginals**
Positive (T+)	30	48	78
Negative (T–)	10	912	922
Marginals	40	960	1,000

Prevalence of Disease X = 0.4%

If the prevalence of Disease X in the target population is 0.4%, you would expect 4 of the people enrolled in the study to have Disease X (D+) and 996 to **not** have Disease X (D–). Given that the sensitivity of the diagnostic test is 75%, you would expect 3 of the people with Disease X to test positive (i.e., 4 * 0.75 = 3). Given that the specificity of the test is 95%, you would expect 946 of the people who do **not** have the disease to test negative (i.e., 996 * 0.95 = 946). The remaining cells can be calculated by subtraction.

$$\text{Now, PPV} = \frac{3}{53} = 5.7\% \text{ and NPV is } \frac{946}{947} = 99.9\%.$$

	Disease		
Test Result	**Present (D+)**	**Absent (D–)**	**Marginals**
Positive (T+)	3	50	53
Negative (T–)	1	946	947
Marginals	4	996	1,000

5.7%, meaning that very few of the patients who test positive for Disease X actually have the disease. The reason this occurs is that when the prevalence of a disease is low, there are few people in the population who actually have the disease and the false positives identified by testing overwhelm the true positives, resulting in the low PPV.

Figure 10-3 shows the PPV of a diagnostic test assuming that the prevalence of the disease is 0.4%. As you can see in the figure, increasing the sensitivity of the test from 0.75 to 0.99 has very little effect on the PPV. However, increasing specificity from 0.95 to 0.999 has a substantial effect. Thus, as stated previously, **highly specific tests help confirm the diagnosis of a disease** because the high PPV of the test allows clinicians to be reasonably sure that if a patient tests positive for the disease, the patient actually does have the disease. This is especially true when the disease of interest is rare, where false positives can have a major impact on the PPV of the test.

FIGURE 10-3. **Effect of Sensitivity and Specificity on Positive Predictive Value of a Test**

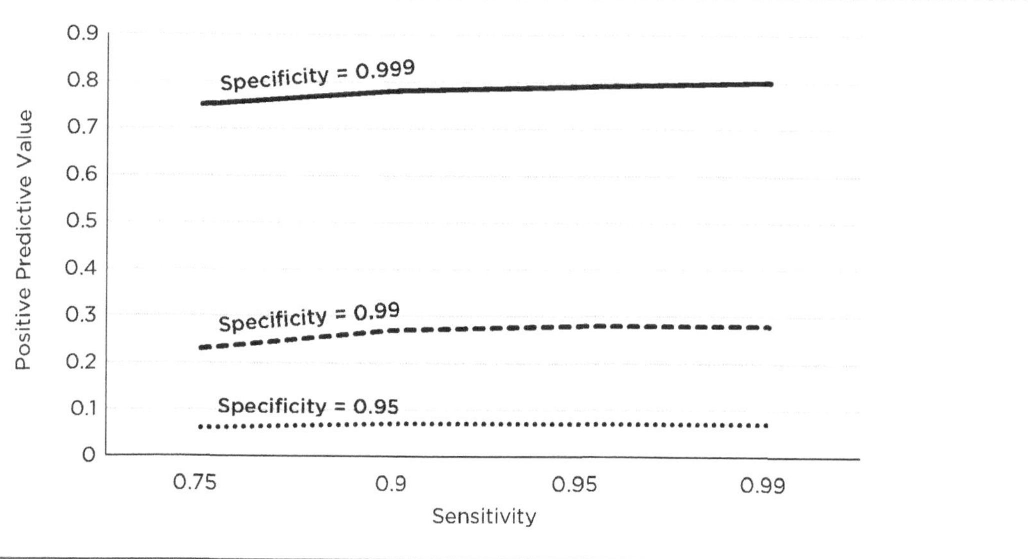

Accuracy

The accuracy of a test is simply the percentage of all test results (both positive and negative) that are correct. As with PPV and NPV, accuracy varies with disease prevalence. Using data from Box 10-2, you can calculate that the accuracy of the test is 87% (i.e., $\frac{(300+570)}{1{,}000}$) when the prevalence of the disease is 40%; 94.2% (i.e., $\frac{(30+912)}{1{,}000}$) when the prevalence of the disease is 4%; and 94.9% (i.e., $\frac{(3+946)}{1{,}000}$) when the prevalence of the disease is 0.4%. As you look at these numbers, think about them for a minute. Remember that the PPV for the test when disease prevalence was 0.4% was only 5.7%. Therefore, although it may sound impressive if you read that a test has 94.9% accuracy, it does not guarantee that one can make strong clinical inferences about the presence of the disease based on the test results.

Likelihood Ratios

Likelihood ratios (LRs) can be used to help decide whether performing a diagnostic test is warranted. There are two types of LRs:

1. LR(+) is the probability of a positive test in someone **with the disease** of interest relative to someone without the disease, calculated as Sensitivity/(1 – Specificity).
2. LR(–) is the probability of a negative test in someone **with the disease** of interest relative to someone without the disease, calculated as (1 – Sensitivity)/Specificity.

LRs can be used to adjust one's estimate of how likely it is that a person has a disease of interest based on the results of testing. In the absence of signs or symptoms that increase clinical suspicion, the prevalence of the disease in the target population is used to calculate the pretest odds of disease. This is the case for screening tests (e.g., mammography) that are performed on a routine basis without reason to think that a particular patient is more at risk than others in the target population (e.g., women over age 50). If a patient has signs or symptoms that increase clinical suspicion, the pretest probability of disease can be adjusted accordingly. By multiplying the LR(+) by the pretest odds of disease, a clinician can determine how likely a patient is to have the disease, assuming that he or she tests positive for the disease. Similarly, by multiplying the LR(–) by the pretest odds of disease, a clinician can determine how likely a patient is to have the disease, assuming that he or she tests negative for the disease. This information can be used to determine if the test is worth doing. Box 10-3 provides an example of using the LR(+) and LR(–) to calculate posttest probabilities.

Often no single test is sufficient to either rule out a disease or confirm a diagnosis. Therefore, multiple tests may be used in combination. There are two general types of testing strategies: parallel or serial. Parallel testing involves performing a series of different tests simultaneously. If any of the tests yields a positive result, the patient is considered a case. (Subsequent tests may be used to confirm this diagnosis.) Parallel testing is performed to increase the sensitivity of testing procedures, decreasing the chances that someone with the disease would be missed due to a false negative. Serial testing (also known as sequential testing) involves performing a single test. If the results of that test are positive, a second test is performed. If the results of the second test are also positive, a third test might be performed. Thus, only one test is performed at a time, and subsequent tests are performed only if the previous one was positive. Serial testing might be used in situations where an inexpensive test is available that is sensitive but not very specific (i.e., yields many false positives). A negative test is used to rule out the disease. A positive test is used to justify the need for a more expensive, more specific test, to confirm the diagnosis.

Effect of Different Cutoff Points on Sensitivity and Specificity

Many diagnostic tests yield scores on a numerical (often continuous) scale. Therefore, it is necessary to determine a value to differentiate positive test results from negative test results. For example, if a test had a possible range from 0 to 100, where higher scores indicated a greater likelihood of the presence of

BOX 10-3. Using Likelihood Ratios to Estimate the Probability of Disease

Imagine that you have a diagnostic test for Disease X with a sensitivity and specificity of 75% and 95%, respectively.

$$LR(+) = \frac{Sensitivity}{1 - Specificity} = \frac{0.75}{0.05} = 15 \qquad LR(-) = \frac{1 - Sensitivity}{Specificity} = \frac{0.25}{0.95} = 0.263$$

Pretest Odds of Disease: Assuming that the prevalence of Disease X is 40% in the target population, the odds of a person in this population having Disease X is: $X = \frac{0.4}{0.6} = 0.667$.

Posttest Odds of Disease: If a person tests positive for Disease X, the odds that he or she has Disease X is:

$$LR(+) * Pretest\ Odds = 15 * 0.667 = 10$$

Posttest Odds of Disease: If a person tests negative for Disease X, the odds that he or she has Disease X is:

$$LR(-) * Pretest\ Odds = 0.263 * 0.667 = 0.175$$

Remember that odds have the form X:1, even though the "1" is often omitted. Thus, the odds calculated previously can be expressed 10:1 and 0.175:1.

You can convert these odds into probabilities by adding the two numbers in each odds back together to form the denominator (i.e., 10 + 1 = 11;0.175 + 1 = 1.175).

Posttest Probability of Disease:

$$\frac{10}{11} = 0.909 * 100\% = 90.9\%$$

Note that this is identical to the positive predictive value calculated previously.

Posttest Probability of Disease:

$$\frac{0.175}{1.175} = 0.149 * 100\% = 14.9\%$$

Note that this is 1 – the negative predictive value (0.851) calculated previously.

Putting it all together, **without the test**, there is a 40% probability that the patient has Disease X (assuming that he or she has no symptoms that increase clinical suspicion). If the patient is tested and tests positive, he or she would have a 91% chance of having the disease. If the patient tests negative, he or she would still have a 15% chance of having the disease.

Should the clinician order the test? You be the judge.

FIGURE 10-4. **Effect of Different Cutoff Points on Sensitivity and Specificity**

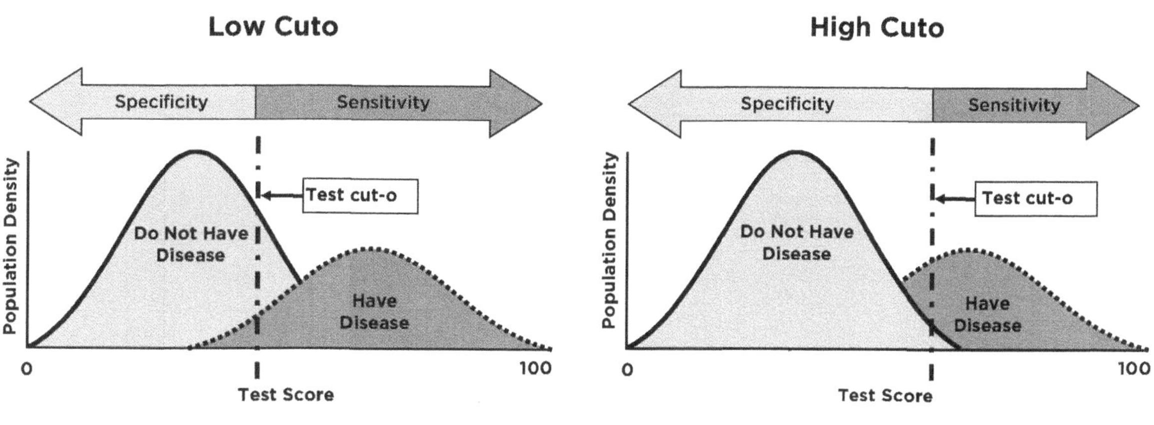

Disease X, a cutoff score of 80 might be used. Scores of 80 or above then would be considered "positive" and scores of 79 or below would be considered "negative."

The value of the cutoff score used to interpret the results of a diagnostic test can have dramatic effects on the sensitivity and specificity of the test. In general, lowering the cutoff score will increase the sensitivity of the test and result in fewer false negatives. However, this will be at the expense of specificity, which will tend to be decreased by lowering the cutoff score. This can be seen visually in the figures shown in Figure 10-4. As the cutoff point for a test is decreased, the test becomes more sensitive but less specific. Conversely, as the cutoff point is increased, the test becomes less sensitive but more specific.

Receiver Operating Characteristic Curves

Receiver operating characteristic (ROC) curves are often used to select the cutoff score for a test that optimizes sensitivity and specificity. As shown in Figure 10-5, the curved blue line drawn across each figure plots the sensitivity of the diagnostic test being evaluated against "1 – the specificity of the test" (i.e., the false positive rate) across a range of possible cutoff scores. The straight line drawn across each figure at a 45° angle represents a hypothetical test with no discriminatory power (i.e., you might as well just guess who does and does not have the disease of interest). The area between the curved line and the straight line is called the "area under the curve." It reflects the extent to which the test helps to discriminate between people with and without the disease of interest. As shown in Figure 10-5, ROC #1 has the greatest discriminatory power.

If there were a cutoff score that could be used to identify people with and without the disease of interest with 100% accuracy, it would be plotted at the upper left-hand side of the curve, designated by the "star" in each chart. At this point, sensitivity and specificity are both 1.0. In reality, a perfect cutoff score never exists. However, in most cases, the optimal cutoff score for a test (i.e., the score that optimizes both sensitivity and specificity) will be near the upper left-hand corner of the curve. For the test shown in ROC #1, the optimal cutoff point is "7," where values on the test had a possible range from 0 to 10. Using this cutoff point, the test would have a sensitivity of 0.91 and a specificity of 0.78.

Choice of the optimal cutoff point also depends on the clinical situation. In some situations, it may be important to have a very sensitive test. In other situations, it may be more important to have a very specific test. For example, imagine that Disease X is curable only if detected early. In this case, you would want a very sensitive test, with very few false negatives. In other cases, high specificity might be more important. For example, if a clinician is going to perform invasive surgery or administer highly toxic medications if a test is positive, it is important that the test be very specific, with very few false positives. Because sensitivity and specificity can be altered by the choice of cutoff scores, it is possible to tailor tests to the needs of these different clinical scenarios.

FIGURE 10-5. Receiver Operating Characteristic Curves

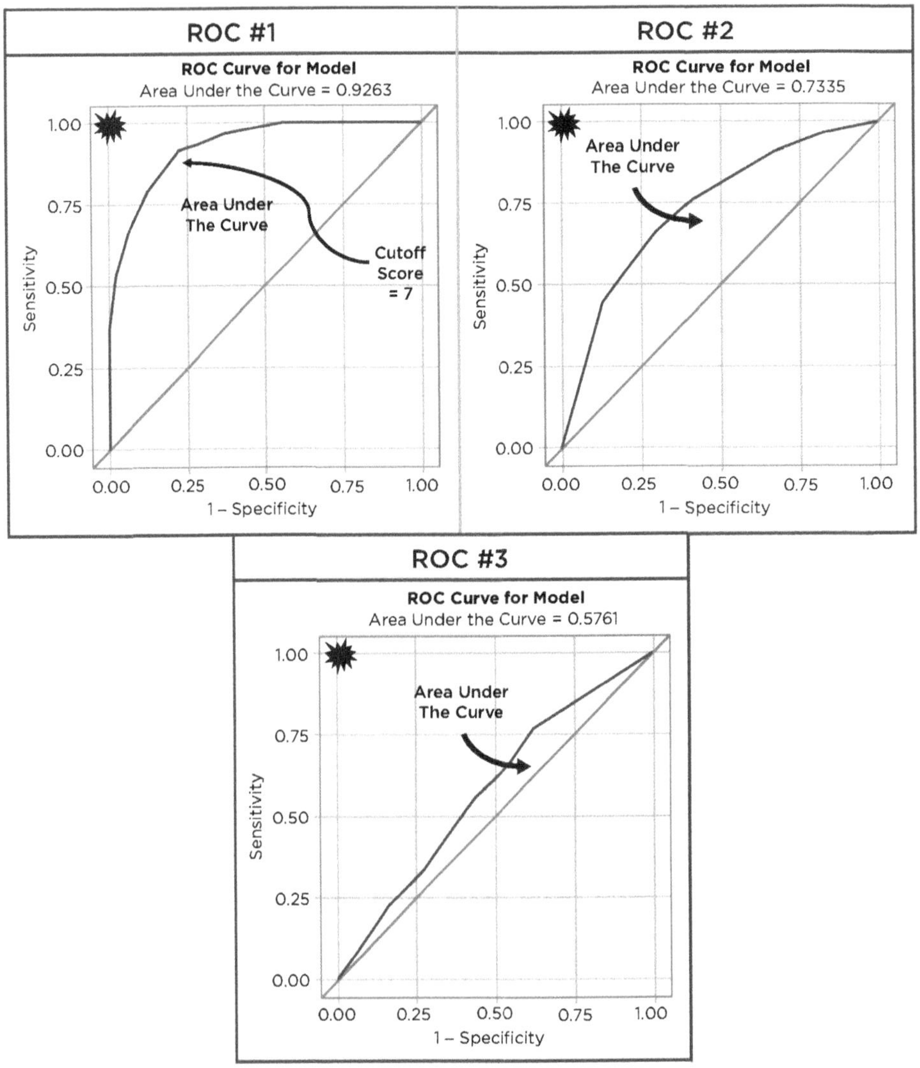

ROC #1

ROC Curve for Model
Area Under the Curve = 0.9263
Area Under The Curve
Cutoff Score = 7
Sensitivity
1.00 0.75 0.50 0.25 0.00
0.00 0.25 0.50 0.75 1.00
1 – Specificity

ROC #2

ROC Curve for Model
Area Under the Curve = 0.7335
Area Under The Curve
Sensitivity
1.00 0.75 0.50 0.25 0.00
0.00 0.25 0.50 0.75 1.00
1 – Specificity

ROC #3

ROC Curve for Model
Area Under the Curve = 0.5761
Area Under The Curve
Sensitivity
1.00 0.75 0.50 0.25 0.00
0.00 0.25 0.50 0.75 1.00
1 – Specificity

ROC, receiver operating characteristic.

Self-Study Questions

1. What is the meaning of the term positive predictive value (PPV)?

   A. Probability of testing positive for the disease if one has the disease
   B. Probability of disease in a patient with a positive test result
   C. Probability of not having the disease when the test result is negative

2. Which of the following is true about the PPV of a test?

   A. It has as its denominator the number of positive test results.
   B. It is sensitive to the underlying prevalence of the disease or condition being tested.
   C. It has as its denominator the number of cases of the disease or condition being tested.
   D. A and B
   E. B and C

3. Is the following statement true or false? Within the context of using multiple diagnostic tests to "confirm" a diagnosis, serial testing usually results in an increase in sensitivity but a decrease in specificity whereas parallel testing has the opposite effect. (True/False)

4. Is the following statement true or false? Changing the cutoff value used for a diagnostic test may change its specificity **and** sensitivity. (True/False)

5. As the prevalence of a disease decreases, the positive predictive validity of a test:

   A. Increases
   B. Decreases
   C. Stays the same

6. Is the following statement true or false? It is always desirable to make a diagnostic test as sensitive as possible. (True/False)

7. If the sensitivity of a new diagnostic test for HIV is 96%, how is this interpreted?

   A. The test will rarely misclassify individuals without HIV infection as being HIV infected.
   B. 96% of individuals with HIV infection will have a positive test for HIV.
   C. 96% of individuals without HIV infection will have a negative test for HIV.

8. Which of the following results has the highest validity?

   A. High random error, low systematic error
   B. Low random error, high systematic error
   C. High overall variability, low systematic error
   D. Low random error, low systematic error

9. Is the following statement true or false? Reliability can be defined as the extent to which a test measures what it is intended to measure. (True/False)

10. Is the following statement true or false? If responses to a measure are influenced by systematic error, but not random error, the measure is reliable but not valid. (True/False)

Use Question Table 10-1 to answer Questions 11 and 12.

QUESTION TABLE 10-1. Results of Tests to Diagnose Cancer

Results of Screening Test	Results of Biopsy: Positive	Results of Biopsy: Negative	Totals
Positive	10	90	100
Negative	1	99	100
Totals	11	189	200

11. Imagine that a test is available to screen for a certain form of cancer. Positive test results are followed-up with a biopsy, which is assumed to provide a definitive diagnosis. Two hundred patients are screened. The results are shown in Question Table 10-1. Based on the information in the table, what is the specificity of the screening test?

    A. 0.10
    B. 0.48
    C. 0.52
    D. 0.99

12. Based on the data in Question Table 10-1, what is the PPV of the screening test?

    A. 0.10
    B. 0.48
    C. 0.52
    D. 0.99

Use Question Table 10-2 to answer Question 13.

QUESTION TABLE 10-2. Validity and Reliability of Blood Glucose Monitoring Devices (Data Fictitious)

Product	Test Results After 10 Repeated Measures (mg/100 mL)	State-of-the-Art Instrument (Gold Standard) (mg/100 mL)
Product A		
Mean (SD)	128 (25)	120
Product B		
Mean (SD)	124 (12)	120

13. A pharmacy is testing two new serum blood glucose monitoring devices to determine which one to recommend to patients. Patients (n = 20) had their blood glucose measured twice, once using Product A and a second time using Product B. Results are shown in Question Table 10-2. Which of the following is true about the validity and reliability of Product B as compared to Product A?

A. Product B is less valid but more reliable.
B. Product B is more valid but less reliable.
C. Product B is less valid and less reliable.
D. Product B is more valid and more reliable.

14. A study is done to determine if a new type of a sphygmomanometer gives the same readings upon repeated administrations. Thirty people are enrolled in the study. Each person has his or her blood pressure measured twice, using the same sphygmomanometer, separated by a 15-minute interval. In this study, is the reliability or the validity of the sphygmomanometer being assessed?

A. Reliability
B. Validity

Use Question Table 10-3 to answer Questions 14–18.

A policy decision was made to screen all men over age 60 for prostate cancer the next time they appeared for an annual physical. A prostrate-specific antigen (PSA) cutoff level of 6.0 was chosen. For men who tested positive, extensive (and expensive) additional testing was done to make a definitive diagnosis. Information found in a review of the records appears in Question Table 10-3.

QUESTION TABLE 10-3. Results of Test to Screen for Prostate Cancer (Data Fictitious)

PSA Value	Prostate Cancer Found	Prostate Cancer Not Found
6.0 +	94	40
<6.0	6	160
Total	100	200

15. What is the sensitivity of the PSA test at this cutoff level?

A. 40%
B. 70%
C. 80%
D. 94%
E. 96%

16. What is the specificity of the PSA test?

A. 40%
B. 70%
C. 80%
D. 94%
E. 96%

17. What is the positive (+) predictive value of the PSA test?

A. 40%
B. 70%
C. 80%
D. 94%
E. 96%

18. If the cutoff level were set at 5.0 instead of 6.0, what would you most likely expect to see happen?

A. Both sensitivity and specificity would increase.
B. Both sensitivity and specificity would decrease.
C. Sensitivity would increase, and specificity would decrease.
D. Sensitivity would decrease, and specificity would increase.

Assessing Equivalence and Noninferiority

11

Throughout this book, we have assumed that investigators are interested in determining if one treatment is **superior** to another. However, sometimes investigators want to demonstrate that two treatments are equally effective or that one treatment is not inferior to another. This situation arises in cases where an effective treatment for a condition already exists. Thus, it would not be ethical to randomize participants in a study to a no-treatment placebo group. In cases where a new treatment has potential advantages over the existing therapy (e.g., less expensive, safer), investigators may wish to demonstrate that the effectiveness of the new treatment is equivalent, or not inferior, to the existing treatment. Unfortunately, the traditional approach to hypothesis testing does not allow investigators to make claims concerning equivalence or noninferiority.

After reading this chapter, you should be able to do the following:

1. Explain why the traditional approach to hypothesis testing cannot be used to support claims of equivalence or noninferiority.
2. Describe the null and alternative hypotheses that are tested in studies designed to support a claim that one treatment is not less effective than another treatment.
3. Describe the null and alternative hypotheses that are tested in studies designed to support claims that two or more treatments are equally effective.
4. Identify major issues that must be considered when interpreting the results of studies claiming to have demonstrated either the equivalence of two or more treatments or the noninferiority of one treatment relative to another.

Traditional Approach: Demonstrating Superiority

Hopefully you remember from Chapter 3 that the traditional approach to hypothesis testing involves stating two different hypotheses. Under the null hypothesis (H_0), the population parameters of interest are assumed to be equal. Under the alternative hypothesis (H_A), the population parameters of interest are assumed to differ. Thus, if H_0 is true and we collect data from two groups, we expect the sample statistics to be the same (e.g., $\bar{x}_1 - \bar{x}_2 = 0$, $\frac{P_1}{P_2} = 1.0$). To test H_0, we can form a 95% confidence interval (CI) around the sample statistic. If the value expected under H_0 is not contained within the 95% CI, we can be 95% confident that the population parameters are **not the same**. Conversely, if the expected value under H_0 is contained within the 95% CI, we cannot rule out the possibility that the population parameters are the same. **Note that in the latter case, we are not 95% confident that the population parameters are the same, only that we cannot rule out the possibility that they are the same.** In fact, if alpha is set at 0.05, we would **not reject** H_0 even if the probability that it is true is as low as 0.051. This is why

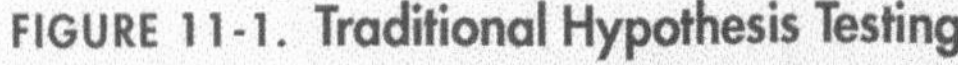

FIGURE 11-1. Traditional Hypothesis Testing

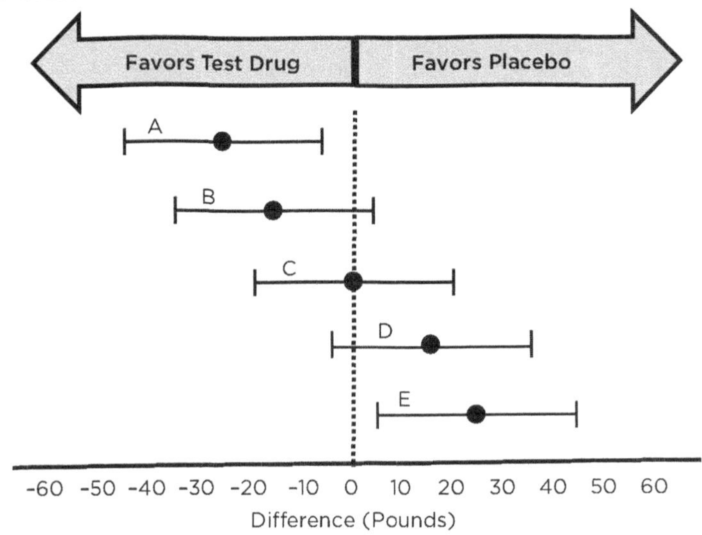

the traditional approach to hypothesis testing cannot be used to demonstrate equivalence or noninferiority with respect to different treatment options.

For example, imagine a study evaluating a weight loss medication. Figure 11-1 shows five different outcomes that could be observed in the study. The difference in mean weight loss between the placebo and experimental drug groups (i.e., $\bar{X}_{WeightLossPlaceboGroup} - \bar{X}_{WeightLossExperimentalDrugGroup}$) is plotted along the x-axis. Thus, positive values indicate that participants in the placebo group lost more weight.

In Scenario A, participants in the experimental drug group lost an average of 30 pounds more than those in the control group. Because 0 is not contained within the 95% CI, we reject the H_0 and can be at least 95% confident that the experimental drug is more effective than placebo.

In Scenario B, participants in the experimental drug group lost an average of about 20 pounds more than those in the placebo group. However, because 0 is contained within the 95% CI, we cannot rule out the possibility that the experimental drug is no more effective than placebo. Therefore, we do not reject H_0.

In Scenario C, participants in the experimental drug group and placebo group lost the same amount of weight. Clearly, we cannot reject H_0.

In Scenario D, participants in the placebo group lost an average of about 15 pounds more than those in the experimental drug group. However, because 0 is contained within the 95% CI, we cannot rule out the possibility that the experimental drug and placebo are equally effective. Therefore, we do not reject H_0.

In Scenario E, participants in the placebo group lost an average of about 25 pounds more than those in the experimental drug group. Because 0 is not contained within the 95% CI, we reject H_0 and can be at least 95% confident that the placebo is more effective than the experimental drug.

Notice that in all of these scenarios, when we fail to reject H_0, we are **not** concluding that the treatments being compared are equally effective or that one treatment is not inferior to the other, but only that there is insufficient evidence to conclude that their effectiveness differs. In order for one to make claims concerning noninferiority and equivalence, H_0 and H_A must be stated differently.

Demonstrating Noninferiority

In studies designed to assess noninferiority, there is usually no placebo group. The control group takes an existing medication that has already demonstrated effectiveness, usually in a placebo-controlled trial. The goal in this type of study is to demonstrate that the new drug being evaluated (i.e., the test drug) is not inferior to an existing medication (i.e., the control drug) by a prespecified amount. This prespecified amount is called the noninferiority margin and is sometimes abbreviated as "M." In a guidance document issued by the Food and Drug Administration (FDA) concerning the design of studies attempting to establish noninferiority, two noninferiority margins are identified (M1 and M2).[1] M1 reflects the difference between the control drug and placebo in previous studies. Thus, it reflects an estimate of the full efficacy of the control drug. M2 is a smaller amount that reflects how much efficacy the investigators are willing to give up in return for other advantages the new drug may offer (e.g., improved safety). In a study designed to demonstrate noninferiority, the null and alternative hypotheses are:

$$H_0: C - T \geq M \text{ and } H_A: C - T < M,$$

where C and T correspond to the sample statistics observed in the study for the control and test drugs, respectively, and M indicates how small the difference between treatments must be in order to reject H_0. Note that framed in this manner, H_0 hypothesizes that the test drug is inferior to the control drug. Thus, rejecting H_0 is equivalent to concluding that the test drug is **not inferior** to the control drug by more than the margin specified.

Returning to the weight loss medication discussed previously, imagine that the investigators had designed the study to assess noninferiority. The test drug was evaluated against a control drug. In a previous placebo-controlled trial, the control drug demonstrated an average weight loss of 30 pounds more than placebo during a 6-month course of therapy. Thus, M1 is 30 pounds. We will assume that the control drug has significant risks. The investigators believe the test drug is much safer (and will do other analyses to demonstrate superior safety). Therefore, they are willing to give up 50% of the effectiveness of the control medication in return for the better safety profile. Thus, they set M2 at 15 pounds. With M2 set, the study hypotheses can be stated as:

$$H_0: C - T \geq 15 \text{ pounds and } H_A: C - T < 15 \text{ pounds.}$$

Figure 11-2 shows five different outcomes that could be observed in the study. In Scenario A, participants in the test drug group lost an average of about 30 pounds more than those in the control drug group. Because M2 is not contained within the 95% CI, we reject H_0 and can be at least 95% confident that the test drug is not inferior to the control drug. In addition, in this scenario, because 0 is not contained within the 95% CI, we can also conclude with 95% confidence that the test drug is superior to the control drug.

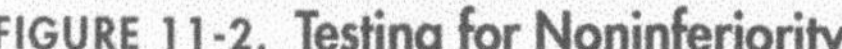

FIGURE 11-2. Testing for Noninferiority

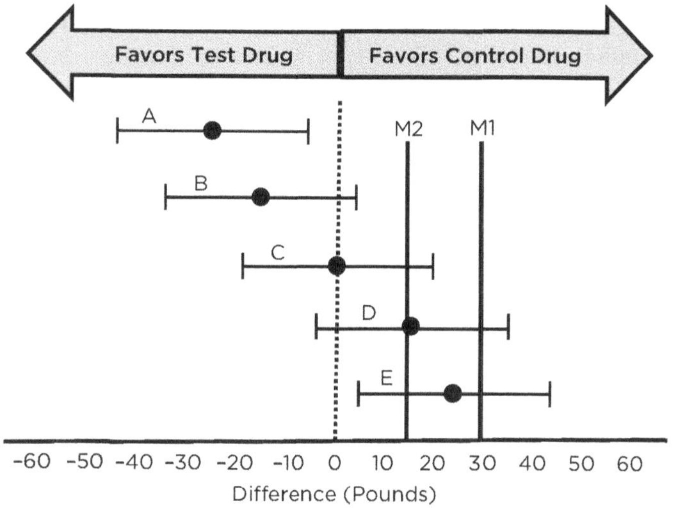

In Scenario B, participants in the test drug group lost an average of about 20 pounds more than those in the control drug group. Again, because M2 is not contained within the 95% CI, we reject H_0 and can be at least 95% confident that the test drug is not inferior to the control drug. However, because 0 is contained within the 95% CI, we cannot claim that the test drug is superior to the control drug.

In Scenario C, participants in the test drug group and control drug group lost the same amount of weight. Nonetheless, because M2 is contained within the 95% CI, we cannot reject H_0. Therefore, we cannot rule out the possibility, with 95% confidence, that the test drug is inferior to the control drug. In other words, we cannot make a claim of noninferiority.

In Scenario D, participants in the control drug group lost an average of about 15 pounds more than those in the test drug group. Because M2 is contained within the 95% CI, we cannot reject H_0. Therefore, we cannot make a claim of noninferiority.

In Scenario E, participants in the control drug group lost an average of about 25 pounds more than those in the test drug group. Because M2 is contained within the 95% CI, we cannot reject H_0. Moreover, because 0 is not contained within the 95% CI, we can conclude with 95% confidence that the control drug is superior to the test drug.

Demonstrating Equivalence

Studies designed to assess equivalence are similar to those designed to assess noninferiority, except that differences in both directions are of interest (i.e., the test drug is neither inferior nor superior to the control drug). Thus, in a study designed to demonstrate equivalence, the null and alternative hypotheses are:

$$H_0: |C - T| \geq |M|, H_A: |C - T| < |M|,$$

where C and T correspond to the sample statistics observed in the study for the control and test drugs, respectively, and M indicates how small the difference between treatments must be in order to reject H_0. Note that, with this set of hypotheses, rejecting H_0 is equivalent to concluding that the test drug and control drug **do not differ** from one another by more than the margin specified.

Returning to the weight loss medication discussed previously, imagine that the investigators had designed the study to assess equivalence. The test drug was evaluated against a control drug. In a previous placebo-controlled trial, the control drug demonstrated an average weight loss of 30 pounds more than placebo during a 6-month course of therapy. Thus, M1 is 30 pounds. As before, we will assume that the control drug has significant risks. Therefore, the investigators are willing to give up 50% of the effectiveness of the control medication in return for the better safety profile. Thus, they set M2 at 15 pounds. With M2 set, the study hypotheses can be stated as:

$$H_0: |C - T| \geq |\pm 15|, H_A: |C - T| < |\pm 15|.$$

Figure 11-3 shows the same five possible study outcomes that we have discussed previously. In Scenario A, participants in the test drug group lost an average of about 30 pounds more than those in the control drug group. Because M2 is contained within the 95% CI, we cannot reject H_0. Thus, we cannot conclude that the two treatments are equivalent. However, because 0 is not contained in the 95% CI, we can conclude with 95% confidence that the test drug is superior to the control drug.

In Scenario B, participants in the test drug group lost an average of about 20 pounds more than those in the control drug group. Again, because M2 is contained within the 95% CI, we cannot reject H_0.

In Scenario C, participants in the test drug group and control drug group lost the same amount of weight. Nonetheless, because M2 is contained within the 95% CI, we cannot reject H_0. A similar conclusion is drawn in Scenario D.

FIGURE 11-3. Testing for Equivalence

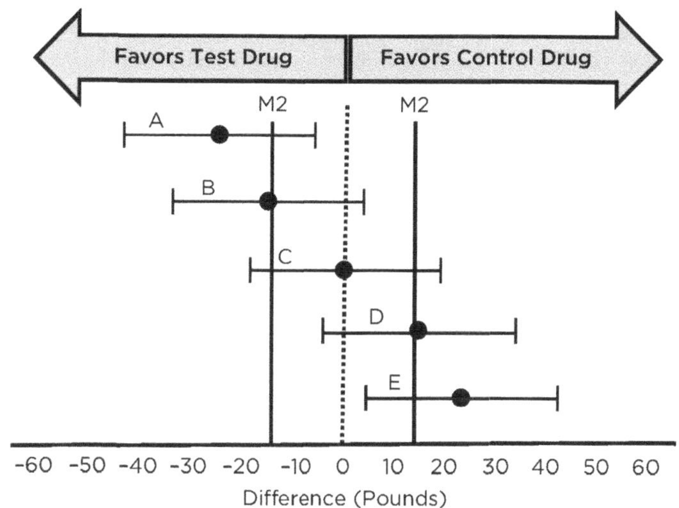

In Scenario E, participants in the control drug group lost an average of about 25 pounds more than those in the test drug group. Because M2 is contained within the 95% CI, we cannot reject H_0. However, because 0 is not contained within the 95% CI, we can conclude with 95% confidence that the control drug is superior to the test drug.

Table 11-1 summarizes the claims that can be made on the basis of the hypothetical study findings described in Scenarios A–E. Note that studies designed to assess noninferiority and equivalence can be used to support superiority claims because in addition to testing whether the 95% CI for the between group difference crosses M2, it is possible to test whether this CI crosses 0. Determining whether the CI crosses M2 is necessary to evaluate noninferiority and equivalence. Determining whether the CI crosses 0 is necessary to evaluate the superiority of one treatment over another.

Important Considerations

When interpreting the results of a study making claims about the equivalence of different treatments or the noninferiority of one treatment relative to another, readers need to consider several issues. First, was the study designed to support claims regarding equivalence or noninferiority? As described previously,

TABLE 11-1. Claims That Can Be Based on Scenarios A—E Using Different Study Designs

	Study Design		
Scenario	**Superiority (Traditional Approach)**	**Noninferiority**	**Equivalence**
A	Test drug superior to placebo	Test drug not inferior to control drug Test drug superior to control drug	Test drug superior to control drug
B	—	Test drug not inferior to control drug	—
C	—	—	—
D	—	—	—
E	Control drug superior to test drug	Control drug superior to test drug	Control drug superior to test drug

—, Findings do not support claims of superiority, noninferiority, or equivalence.

studies designed to demonstrate the superiority of one medication over another cannot be used to support noninferiority or equivalence claims.

Second, do the investigators provide a solid justification for why it is not possible or unethical to conduct a placebo-controlled trial, allowing them to test the null hypothesis that the experimental medication is no more effective than placebo? Ideally, studies would include a placebo arm, even if the investigators are most interested in comparing the effectiveness of two active drugs. The placebo arm provides an opportunity for the investigators to test whether the trial has assay sensitivity, as described in more detail below.

Third, has the control drug demonstrated, in well-controlled clinical trials, that it is more effective than placebo? If not, demonstrating that the experimental (i.e., test) drug is equivalent or not inferior to the control drug does not mean the experimental drug is more effective than placebo. This question concerns assay sensitivity which is "a property of a clinical trial defined as the ability to distinguish an effective treatment from a less effective or ineffective treatment" (p. 7).[2] As outlined in the International Conference on Harmonisation Guideline: "Assay sensitivity is important in any trial but has different implications for trials intended to show differences between treatments (superiority trials) and trials intended to show noninferiority. If a trial intended to demonstrate efficacy by showing superiority of a test treatment to control lacks assay sensitivity, it will fail to show that the test treatment is superior and will fail to lead to a conclusion of efficacy. In contrast, if a trial is intended to demonstrate efficacy by showing a test treatment to be noninferior to an active control, but lacks assay sensitivity, the trial may find an ineffective treatment to be noninferior and could lead to an erroneous conclusion of efficacy" (pp. 7–8).

Fourth, was the choice of M2 well justified? In general, M2 should be the largest difference between the test drug and the control drug that is considered clinically acceptable.[1] The larger M2 is, the easier it is to reject H_0 (i.e., conclude that the test drug is not inferior to the control drug). For example, in Figure 11-4, if M2a were used as the M2 value, H_0 would only be rejected in Scenario A. If M2b were used as the M2 value, H_0 would be rejected in Scenarios A and B. If M2c were used as the M2 value, H_0 would be rejected in Scenarios A, B, and C. Therefore, investigators might try to "stack the deck" in their favor by using an M2 value that is greater than what would be considered clinically acceptable.

Fifth, were the analyses conducted using an intention-to-treat design (i.e., data analyses include all people who enrolled in the study regardless of whether they completed all follow-up procedures or adhered to treatment protocols) or per protocol design (i.e., data analyses are limited to people who completed all follow-up and adhered to treatment protocols)? In studies designed to determine if one treatment is superior to another, intention-to-treat analyses are recommended because they tend to provide the

FIGURE 11-4. Testing for Noninferiority: Importance of M2

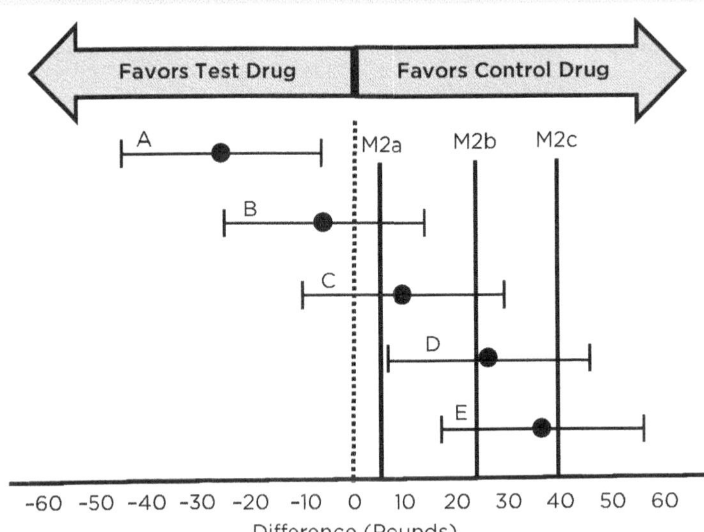

most conservative estimate of between group differences, making it more difficult to reject H_0. However, the reverse is true in studies designed to establish equivalence or noninferiority. For example, if a large proportion of study participants in both groups fails to take the treatment assigned, it would tend to mask any differences between the treatments that might exist, leading to rejection of H_0. Ideally, investigators would report the results of both types of analyses, allowing readers an opportunity to compare the results and assess potential biases when interpreting study findings.[3,4]

Example from the Literature

Hochberg et al[5] used a noninferiority design to compare the efficacy of chondroitin sulfate plus glucosamine hydrochloride (CS+GH) versus celecoxib in patients with knee osteoarthritis who were 40 years of age or older and reported a score of 301 or higher on the pain scale of the Western Ontario and McMaster Universities (WOMAC) osteoarthritis index, indicating severe pain. (This scale has a possible range of 0–500.) A total of 606 patients were enrolled in the study. Patients were randomized using a 1:1 ratio to one of two groups. Patients in the CS+GH group received 400 mg CS and 500 mg GH three times a day. Patients in the celecoxib group received 200 mg celecoxib daily. All patients were treated for 6 months. The primary outcome variable was decrease in the WOMAC pain score from baseline to 6 months.

The investigators set the noninferiority margin (M2) at 40 units on the WOMAC pain scale. However, they provided no justification for the selection of this value. (In this paper, the noninferiority margin is called "delta," which is common in the literature. I have used the term M2 in this chapter to be consistent with the most recent guidance document issued by the FDA.) Thus, the hypotheses tested were:

$$H_0: \bar{X}_{Celebrex} - \bar{X}_{CS+GH} \geq -40 \text{ points and } H_A: \bar{X}_{Celebrex} - \bar{X}_{CS+GH} < -40 \text{ points}$$

In the per protocol analyses, the adjusted mean change on the WOMAC pain scale was −185.7 (95% CI: −200.3 to −171.1) in the CS+GH group compared to −186.8 (95% CI: −201.7 to −171.9) in the celecoxib group. The mean between-group difference was −1.11 (95% CI: −22.0 to 19.8). Because the 95% CI did not include M2, the investigators were able to conclude with 95% confidence that the pain relief provided by glucosamine plus chondroitin is **not inferior** to that provided by celecoxib by more than the margin specified of 40 points on the WOMAC pain scale. The investigators also provided the results of analyses conducted using intention-to-treat principles. These analyses were consistent with those reported previously.

The findings from this study have been questioned due to concerns that the study failed to establish assay sensitivity.[6,7] The investigators responded to these concerns in an editorial to the journal, making for an interesting set of readings for those interested in learning more about some of the challenges involved in designing a rigorous trial to support a noninferiority claim.[8]

Self-Study Questions

1. In a study designed to assess noninferiority, the null hypothesis is:

   A. $H_0: C - T \geq M$
   B. $H_0: C - T = 0$
   C. $H_0: C - T < M$
   D. $H_0: C - T \neq 0$

2. In a study designed to assess superiority, the null hypothesis is:

   A. $H_0: C - T \geq M$
   B. $H_0: C - T = 0$
   C. $H_0: C - T < M$
   D. $H_0: C - T \neq 0$

3. All other things held constant, which of the following noninferiority margins would make it most difficult to reject H_0?

   A. M2 = 1 point on a 100-point scale
   B. M2 = 2 points on a 100-point scale
   C. M2 = 5 points on a 100-point scale
   D. M2 = 20 points on a 100-point scale
   E. This is a trick question; the size of the noninferiority margin has no effect on how difficult it is to reject H_0.

4. If the noninferiority margin in a study was set at 12 units, which of the following 95% confidence intervals would lead to rejection of H_0?

   A. 5 to 11
   B. –11 to –5
   C. –5 to 11
   D. –5 to 14
   E. None of the above

Are the statements in Questions 5–8 true or false?

5. A study that demonstrates that the efficacy of an experimental medication is **not** inferior to a medication that is currently on the market can always be used to infer that the experimental medication is more effective than placebo. (True/False)

6. In a study designed to assess the superiority of one drug over another, if H_0 is **not** rejected, then it is safe to conclude that the two drugs are equally effective. (True/False)

7. In a study designed to assess the noninferiority of one treatment relative to another, it is possible to conclude that one of the treatments is superior to the other. (True/False)

8. In a study designed to assess the noninferiority of one treatment relative to another, it is possible to include a placebo arm in addition to one or more control drug arms. (True/False)

References

1. U.S. Department of Health and Human Services, Food and Drug Administration, Center for Drug Evaluation and Research (CDER), Center for Biologics Evaluation and Research (CBER). Non-inferiority clinical trials to establish effectiveness: guidance for industry. https://www.fda.gov/downloads/Drugs/Guidances/UCM202140.pdf. November 2016. Accessed September 20, 2018.
2. International Conference on Harmonisation. Choice of control group and related issues in clinical trials: E10. https://www.ich.org/fileadmin/Public_Web_Site/ICH_Products/Guidelines/Efficacy/E10/Step4/E10_Guideline.pdf. July 20, 2000. Accessed September 20, 2018.
3. Walker E, Nowacki AM. Understanding equivalence and noninferiority testing. *J Gen Intern Med.* 2011;26(2):192–6.
4. Schumi J, Wittes JT. Through the looking glass: understanding non-inferiority. *Trials.* 2011;12:106.
5. Hochberg MC, Martel-Pelletier J, Monfort J, et al.; MOVES Investigation Group. Combined chondroitin sulfate and glucosamine for painful knee osteoarthritis: a multicenter, randomized, double-blind, non-inferiority trial versus celecoxib. *Ann Rheum Dis.* 2016;75(1):37–44.
6. Meyer R. Does MOVES move the needle? *Ann Rheum Dis.* 2015;74(5):e35.
7. Zeng C, Wei J, Lei GH. Is chondroitin sulfate plus glucosamine superior to placebo in the treatment of knee osteoarthritis? *Ann Rheum Dis.* 2015;74(5):e37.
8. Hochberg M, MOVES Investigation Group. Response to: "Is chondroitin plus glucosamine superior to placebo in the treatment of knee osteoarthritis?" by Zeng et al. *Ann Rheum Dis.* 2015;74(9):e57.

Meta-Analysis

12

Meta-analysis involves a set of statistical procedures used to integrate findings from multiple independent studies, usually with the goal of providing an estimate of treatment effectiveness or safety and examining factors that may lead to variation in treatment effectiveness or safety.[1] Meta-analyses are often conducted in conjunction with a systematic review of the literature. Moreover, the quality of a meta-analysis hinges on the quality of the systematic review upon which the meta-analysis is based. Therefore, in this chapter, I begin by describing the characteristics that differentiate "systematic reviews" from other types of literature reviews. I then discuss the types of statistical procedures involved in conducting a meta-analysis as part of a systematic review.

After reading this chapter, you should be able to do the following:

1. Describe the characteristics of "systematic reviews" that differentiate them from literature reviews that are conducted less systematically.
2. Explain, in general terms, how effect size estimates from multiple studies are combined to compute a pooled effect size estimate.
3. Discuss problems caused by heterogeneity and publication bias.
4. Interpret data presented via forest and funnel plots.

Characteristics of a Systematic Review

The PRISMA (Preferred Reporting Items for Systematic Reviews and Meta-Analyses) statement describes the types of information that should be reported in publications involving systematic reviews and meta-analyses.[2] According to the PRISMA statement, "A systematic review attempts to collate all empirical evidence that fits prespecified eligibility criteria to answer a specific research question. It uses explicit, systematic methods that are selected to minimize bias, thus providing reliable findings from which conclusions can be drawn and decisions made. Meta-analysis is the use of statistical methods to summarise and combine the results of independent studies. Many systematic reviews contain meta-analyses, but not all."

In a systematic review, the objectives of the review are stated very explicitly. The PRISMA statement recommends that authors use the PICOS format to state the objectives of the review.[2] This format specifies (1) the **P**atient population of interest, (2) the **I**ntervention(s) or exposure(s) being examined, (3) the **C**omparators included (e.g., standard care, placebo), (4) the primary **O**utcome(s) of interest, and (5) the **S**tudy designs included. When the PICOS factors are specified, readers are more easily able to assess the generalizability of study findings and their implications for policy or practice.

Systematic reviews involve a comprehensive and methodical search for relevant studies that should be included in the review. In publications, authors should describe their search strategy fully as well as the criteria that studies and study reports needed to meet to be included in the review. Ideally, investigators conducting a systematic review should search for unpublished papers as well as published ones. Unpublished papers tend to be less likely than published papers to report statistically significant findings. This phenomenon is referred to as "publication bias." Therefore, limiting a systematic review to published papers can introduce a bias that inflates estimates of treatment differences.

Systematic reviews use rigorous procedures to screen papers for inclusion in the review. Generally, a systematic search of the literature will yield a large number of papers that **might meet** study inclusion criteria (e.g., in the thousands), whereas only a handful of those papers (e.g., 25 or fewer) **actually meet** study inclusion criteria. This is because the search strategy will usually be fairly broad to avoid missing any papers that should be included. Therefore, the investigators must screen all of the papers identified to determine if they should be included in the review. Ideally, at least two members of the research team, working independently, will screen each paper identified, which minimizes the possibility of excluding a paper accidentally. Many papers can be excluded simply by reviewing their titles and abstracts. For example, many nonempirical papers can be eliminated in this manner. In other cases, the full text of the paper needs to be reviewed to determine whether it meets inclusion or exclusion criteria for the review. The PRISMA statement recommends that authors of systematic reviews report this process of paper selection in a flow chart, such as the one shown in Figure 12-1.[3] This allows readers to easily see the total number of papers identified, the reasons that papers were excluded from the review, and the total number of papers included in the qualitative (i.e., narrative) and quantitative (i.e., meta-analysis) synthesis.

Systematic reviews use rigorous methods to extract data from the papers included in the review. A standardized data collection form should be used by all members of the research team involved in the data extraction process. This data collection form should include information concerning study characteristics (e.g., study design, study setting, sample size, age range of study participants and other relevant participant characteristics, inclusion and exclusion criteria, intervention, comparator, length of follow-up) and study outcomes (e.g., for categorical outcome variables: number improved [not improved] in each treatment group; for numerical outcome variables: mean [standard deviation (SD)] or mean change [SD] in each treatment group). Ideally, at least two members of the research team, working independently, would extract data from each included paper and any discrepancies between the coders would be reviewed and reconciled, minimizing the possibility of error during the data extraction process. In addition, if important data were not included in a study report, the research team should attempt to contact the investigators involved in the original study to obtain the missing data.

Finally, systematic reviews should include an assessment of biases that may have affected the results of the studies included in the review (e.g., lack of randomization to treatment group; failure (or inability) to blind study participants, health care providers, or data collectors). Investigators should also assess the extent to which their review might be biased due to factors such as publication bias. Unless the impact of potential sources of bias are considered when interpreting the results of a review paper, serious inferential errors can be made.

Meta-Analysis

In conjunction with a systematic literature review, meta-analysis may be used to combine information from the studies identified to provide an overall estimate of the effect that the intervention has on the outcome(s) of interest. This is called the "effect size." Outcomes reported in different studies are usually summarized in a forest plot, such as the one shown in Figure 12-2.[3] When the outcome of interest is dichotomous (e.g., died or did not die), risk ratios or odds ratios are usually used to assess the effect size. For outcome variables measured on a numerical scale, effect size can be assessed using either the raw or the

FIGURE 12-1. PRISMA Diagram for Systemic review of the Association Between Polypharmacy and Death

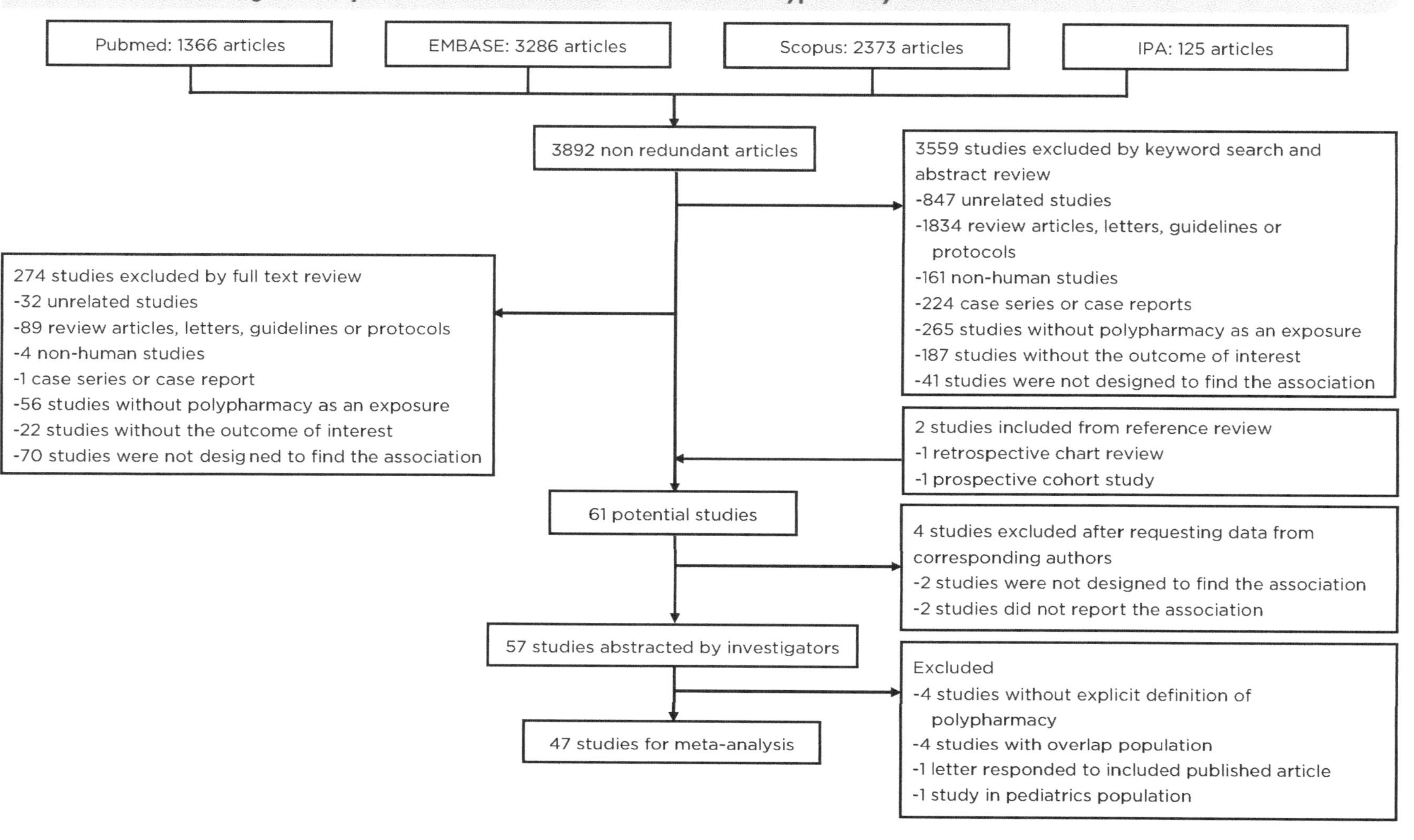

IPA, International Pharmaceutical Abstracts; PRISMA, Preferred Reporting Items for Systemic Reviews and Meta-Analyses.

FIGURE 12-2. Forest Plot of Adjusted Association Between Polypharmacy and Death

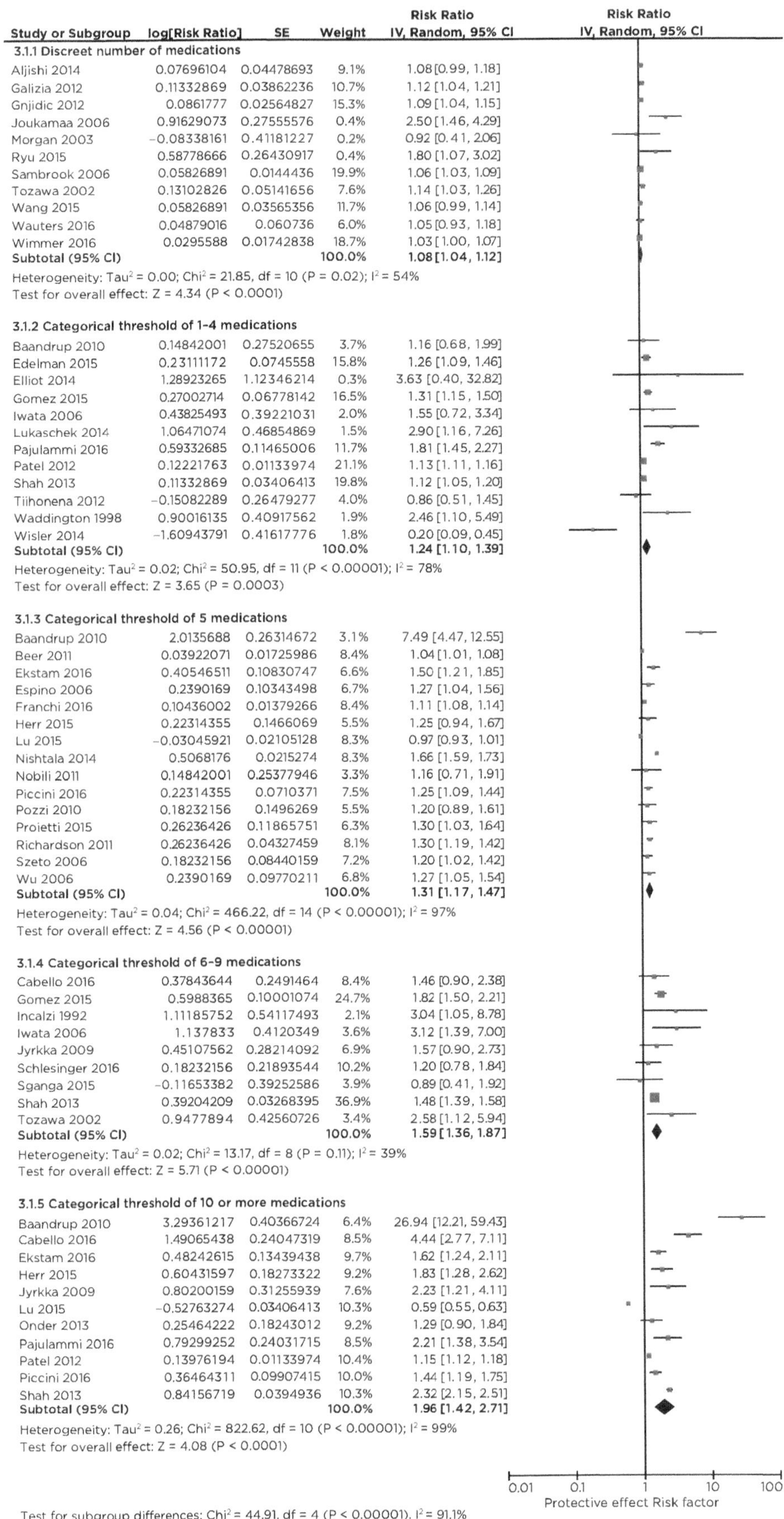

Study or Subgroup	log[Risk Ratio]	SE	Weight	Risk Ratio IV, Random, 95% CI
3.1.1 Discreet number of medications				
Aljishi 2014	0.07696104	0.04478693	9.1%	1.08 [0.99, 1.18]
Galizia 2012	0.11332869	0.03862236	10.7%	1.12 [1.04, 1.21]
Gnjidic 2012	0.0861777	0.02564827	15.3%	1.09 [1.04, 1.15]
Joukamaa 2006	0.91629073	0.27555576	0.4%	2.50 [1.46, 4.29]
Morgan 2003	−0.08338161	0.41181227	0.2%	0.92 [0.41, 2.06]
Ryu 2015	0.58778666	0.26430917	0.4%	1.80 [1.07, 3.02]
Sambrook 2006	0.05826891	0.0144436	19.9%	1.06 [1.03, 1.09]
Tozawa 2002	0.13102826	0.05141656	7.6%	1.14 [1.03, 1.26]
Wang 2015	0.05826891	0.03565356	11.7%	1.06 [0.99, 1.14]
Wauters 2016	0.04879016	0.060736	6.0%	1.05 [0.93, 1.18]
Wimmer 2016	0.0295588	0.01742838	18.7%	1.03 [1.00, 1.07]
Subtotal (95% CI)			**100.0%**	**1.08 [1.04, 1.12]**
Heterogeneity: $Tau^2 = 0.00$; $Chi^2 = 21.85$, df = 10 (P = 0.02); $I^2 = 54\%$				
Test for overall effect: Z = 4.34 (P < 0.0001)				
3.1.2 Categorical threshold of 1–4 medications				
Baandrup 2010	0.14842001	0.27520655	3.7%	1.16 [0.68, 1.99]
Edelman 2015	0.23111172	0.0745558	15.8%	1.26 [1.09, 1.46]
Elliot 2014	1.28923265	1.12346214	0.3%	3.63 [0.40, 32.82]
Gomez 2015	0.27002714	0.06778142	16.5%	1.31 [1.15, 1.50]
Iwata 2006	0.43825493	0.39221031	2.0%	1.55 [0.72, 3.34]
Lukaschek 2014	1.06471074	0.46854869	1.5%	2.90 [1.16, 7.26]
Pajulammi 2016	0.59332685	0.11465006	11.7%	1.81 [1.45, 2.27]
Patel 2012	0.12221763	0.01133974	21.1%	1.13 [1.11, 1.16]
Shah 2013	0.11332869	0.03406413	19.8%	1.12 [1.05, 1.20]
Tiihonena 2012	−0.15082289	0.26479277	4.0%	0.86 [0.51, 1.45]
Waddington 1998	0.90016135	0.40917562	1.9%	2.46 [1.10, 5.49]
Wisler 2014	−1.60943791	0.41617776	1.8%	0.20 [0.09, 0.45]
Subtotal (95% CI)			**100.0%**	**1.24 [1.10, 1.39]**
Heterogeneity: $Tau^2 = 0.02$; $Chi^2 = 50.95$, df = 11 (P < 0.00001); $I^2 = 78\%$				
Test for overall effect: Z = 3.65 (P = 0.0003)				
3.1.3 Categorical threshold of 5 medications				
Baandrup 2010	2.0135688	0.26314672	3.1%	7.49 [4.47, 12.55]
Beer 2011	0.03922071	0.01725986	8.4%	1.04 [1.01, 1.08]
Ekstam 2016	0.40546511	0.10830747	6.6%	1.50 [1.21, 1.85]
Espino 2006	0.2390169	0.10343498	6.7%	1.27 [1.04, 1.56]
Franchi 2016	0.10436002	0.01379266	8.4%	1.11 [1.08, 1.14]
Herr 2015	0.22314355	0.1466069	5.5%	1.25 [0.94, 1.67]
Lu 2015	−0.03045921	0.02105128	8.3%	0.97 [0.93, 1.01]
Nishtala 2014	0.5068176	0.0215274	8.3%	1.66 [1.59, 1.73]
Nobili 2011	0.14842001	0.25377946	3.3%	1.16 [0.71, 1.91]
Piccini 2016	0.22314355	0.0710371	7.5%	1.25 [1.09, 1.44]
Pozzi 2010	0.18232156	0.1496269	5.5%	1.20 [0.89, 1.61]
Proietti 2015	0.26236426	0.11865751	6.3%	1.30 [1.03, 1.64]
Richardson 2011	0.26236426	0.04327459	8.1%	1.30 [1.19, 1.42]
Szeto 2006	0.18232156	0.08440159	7.2%	1.20 [1.02, 1.42]
Wu 2006	0.2390169	0.09770211	6.8%	1.27 [1.05, 1.54]
Subtotal (95% CI)			**100.0%**	**1.31 [1.17, 1.47]**
Heterogeneity: $Tau^2 = 0.04$; $Chi^2 = 466.22$, df = 14 (P < 0.00001); $I^2 = 97\%$				
Test for overall effect: Z = 4.56 (P < 0.00001)				
3.1.4 Categorical threshold of 6–9 medications				
Cabello 2016	0.37843644	0.2491464	8.4%	1.46 [0.90, 2.38]
Gomez 2015	0.5988365	0.10001074	24.7%	1.82 [1.50, 2.21]
Incalzi 1992	1.11185752	0.54117493	2.1%	3.04 [1.05, 8.78]
Iwata 2006	1.137833	0.4120349	3.6%	3.12 [1.39, 7.00]
Jyrkka 2009	0.45107562	0.28214092	6.9%	1.57 [0.90, 2.73]
Schlesinger 2016	0.18232156	0.21893544	10.2%	1.20 [0.78, 1.84]
Sganga 2015	−0.11653382	0.39252586	3.9%	0.89 [0.41, 1.92]
Shah 2013	0.39204209	0.03268395	36.9%	1.48 [1.39, 1.58]
Tozawa 2002	0.9477894	0.42560726	3.4%	2.58 [1.12, 5.94]
Subtotal (95% CI)			**100.0%**	**1.59 [1.36, 1.87]**
Heterogeneity: $Tau^2 = 0.02$; $Chi^2 = 13.17$, df = 8 (P = 0.11); $I^2 = 39\%$				
Test for overall effect: Z = 5.71 (P < 0.00001)				
3.1.5 Categorical threshold of 10 or more medications				
Baandrup 2010	3.29361217	0.40366724	6.4%	26.94 [12.21, 59.43]
Cabello 2016	1.49065438	0.24047319	8.5%	4.44 [2.77, 7.11]
Ekstam 2016	0.48242615	0.13439438	9.7%	1.62 [1.24, 2.11]
Herr 2015	0.60431597	0.18273322	9.2%	1.83 [1.28, 2.62]
Jyrkka 2009	0.80200159	0.31255939	7.6%	2.23 [1.21, 4.11]
Lu 2015	−0.52763274	0.03406413	10.3%	0.59 [0.55, 0.63]
Onder 2013	0.25464222	0.18243012	9.2%	1.29 [0.90, 1.84]
Pajulammi 2016	0.79299252	0.24031715	8.5%	2.21 [1.38, 3.54]
Patel 2012	0.13976194	0.01133974	10.4%	1.15 [1.12, 1.18]
Piccini 2016	0.36464311	0.09907415	10.0%	1.44 [1.19, 1.75]
Shah 2013	0.84156719	0.0394936	10.3%	2.32 [2.15, 2.51]
Subtotal (95% CI)			**100.0%**	**1.96 [1.42, 2.71]**
Heterogeneity: $Tau^2 = 0.26$; $Chi^2 = 822.62$, df = 10 (P < 0.00001); $I^2 = 99\%$				
Test for overall effect: Z = 4.08 (P < 0.0001)				

Test for subgroup differences: $Chi^2 = 44.91$, df = 4 (P < 0.00001). $I^2 = 91.1\%$

IV, inverse variance; CI, confidence interval; SE, standard error; df, degrees of freedom.

standardized mean difference (SMD) between intervention and comparison groups. Differences in raw scores are used when the outcome variable is measured in natural, easily understood units such as mmHg for blood pressure or pounds for weight. The SMD is used when the units of measurement are more abstract and may vary across studies. Conceptually, the SMD is $\frac{\bar{X}_{InterventionGroup} - \bar{X}_{ControlGroup}}{Pooled\ SD}$. By standardizing the raw difference score, one can combine values for studies that used different instruments to measure the outcome of interest. For example, pain can be measured using a wide variety of different instruments. If one instrument assessed pain on a 7-point scale, whereas another instrument assessed it on a 100-point scale, combining difference scores based on the raw values reported would yield meaningless numbers. However, standardizing the raw difference scores converts them to SD units (similar to calculating z-scores). Thus, the higher the standardized difference score is (regardless of the raw scale used), the more SDs it is from 0, which is the expected value for a mean difference under H_0 (i.e., the intervention has no effect on the outcome of interest).

Before the combining of results from different studies, the results from each study are weighted in a way that reflects the precision of the estimates reported. In most cases, the estimate for each study is weighted by the inverse of its variance.[4] This results in large studies (with more precise effect size estimates) being weighted more than small studies where the estimates of effect size are less precise. To assess the precision of the estimates from each study, one can examine the width of the confidence intervals (CIs) shown in the forest plot. The wider the CI, the less precise the estimate of effect size.

The two types of models most commonly used to estimate effect size in meta-analyses are fixed-effects models and random-effects models. Fixed-effects models assume that the effect of the intervention is the same in all of the studies. Thus, any differences observed across studies are assumed to be due to random error, not to differences in sample characteristics, length of follow-up, or other characteristics that differ across studies. In contrast, random-effects models assume that the effectiveness of the intervention may vary across studies. For example, an intervention might have a smaller effect in a study in which participants were sicker at baseline than in a study that used inclusion or exclusion criteria to restrict the study to patients who were healthier at baseline and thought to be more likely to benefit from the intervention.

When conducting a meta-analysis, investigators should evaluate the amount of variability (i.e., heterogeneity) among the effect sizes reported in the studies included in the analysis. When reading a meta-analysis, you can gauge the amount of heterogeneity present by examining the forest plot. The less spread there is in point estimates of the effect size across studies, the less heterogeneity is present. If the amount of heterogeneity present is greater than one would expect due to random variation, a random-effects model should be used to estimate the true effect size. Random-effects models adjust the effect size reported in each study by multiplying it by a factor that reflects the amount of heterogeneity present. Therefore, effect size estimates derived from random-effects models will usually have wider CIs than those derived from fixed-effects models. This makes random-effects models more conservative than fixed-effects models in the sense that wider CIs make it more difficult to rule out the possibility that the intervention has no effect on the outcome(s) of interest.

To determine if the amount of heterogeneity present in a set of studies is greater than one would expect due to random variation, investigators can use Cochran's Q. This statistic follows a chi-square distribution and reflects the magnitude of the difference between (1) the effect sizes reported in the individual studies included in the meta-analysis and (2) the pooled effect size estimate derived when data from the individual studies are combined. If all of the studies included in a meta-analysis reported the same effect size, Cochran's Q would be 0. If Cochran's Q is statistically significant, it indicates that the heterogeneity present among the studies is greater than one would expect due to random variation. However, this statistic has been criticized because it has little power and may fail to detect substantial heterogeneity among effect size estimates.[5]

An alternative statistic to assess the amount of heterogeneity present in a set of studies is I^2. This statistic is designed to reflect the percentage of the total variation in effect size estimates across studies that is greater than one would expect due to random variation.[5] Thus, when I^2 is 0, the variance among effect size estimates is no greater than one would expect due to chance. The formula for I^2 is $\frac{Q - df}{Q} * 100\%$, where Q is Cochran's Q and *df* refers to degrees of freedom. In this context, df is equal to the number of studies included in the analysis minus 1. Although I^2 can have negative values, the statisticians who developed this measure recommended that negative values be reported as 0.[5] Thus, the values of I^2 reported in the literature range from 0 to 100%. The developers provided the following general guidelines for interpreting the value of I^2 reported in meta-analyses: low, 25%; moderate, 50%; and high, 75%.[5] However, they emphasize that these guidelines should not be interpreted rigidly. The amount of heterogeneity that is acceptable may vary, depending on the clinical domain and the specific research questions the investigators are attempting to answer.

Heterogeneity may be caused by both clinical and methodological diversity present among the studies included in a meta-analysis.[2] If a high level of heterogeneity is present, it may not be appropriate to calculate a pooled effect size estimate that combines data from the studies included in the systematic review. That would be akin to mixing apples and oranges. Instead, investigators should attempt to identify the factors that may be causing the heterogeneity. This can be accomplished via subgroup analyses in which the investigators perform separate meta-analyses for subsets of studies that share common characteristics (e.g., stage of disease of study participants, study design, quality of methods employed). Investigators can also conduct sensitivity analyses to determine the extent to which individual studies included in the meta-analysis may have an undue influence on the pooled effect size estimate. When these types of analyses are conducted, investigators should specify which were planned prior to the start of the study.[2] Results of analyses that were not prespecified should be considered exploratory.

Finally, investigators should examine the possibility that they failed to identify all relevant studies (i.e., publication bias). This is often accomplished by examining a funnel plot, such as the one shown in Figure 12-3. In this type of plot, the effect size is plotted on the x-axis and a measure reflecting the

FIGURE 12-3. Funnel Plot of Adjusted Association Between Polypharmacy and Death

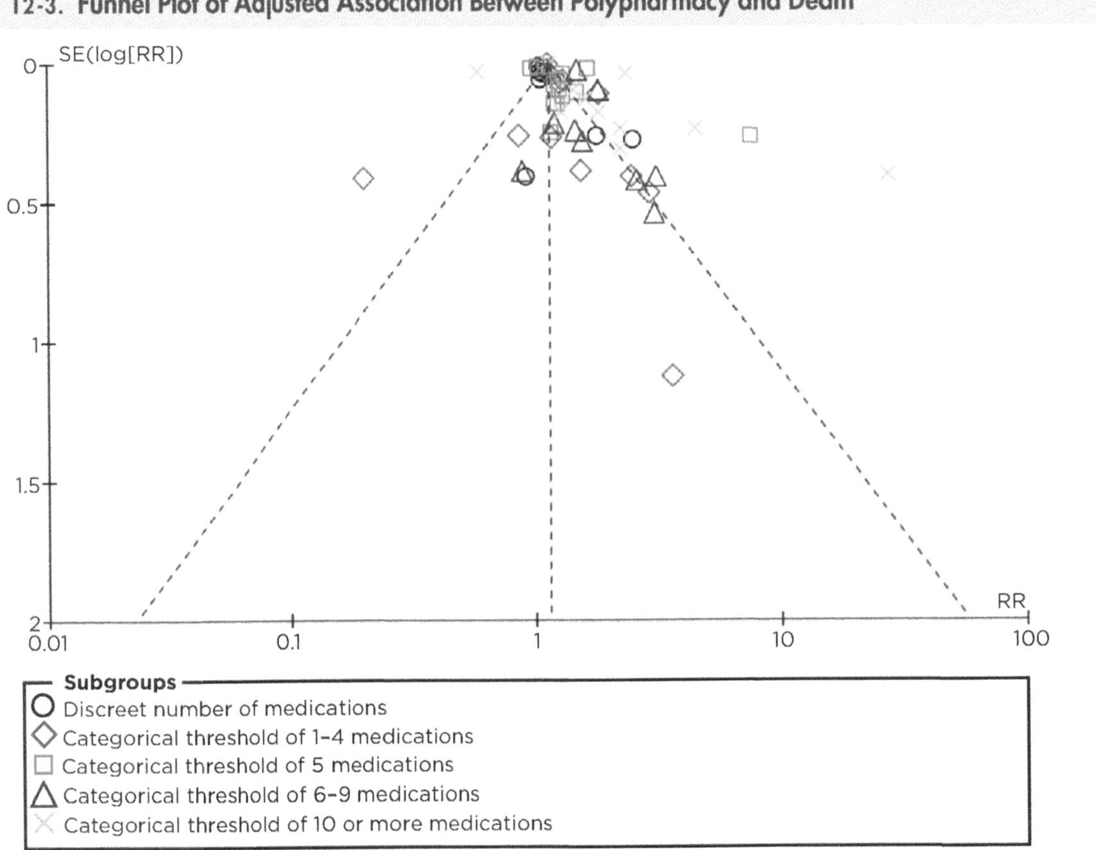

OR, odds ratio; SE, standard error; RR, risk ratio.

precision of the effect size estimate (e.g., standard error [SE] of estimate, sample size upon which estimate is based) is plotted on the y-axis. The studies with the most precise estimates (e.g., smallest SE, largest sample size) appear at the top of the funnel plot. If all studies relevant to the research question have been identified, the distribution of effect size estimates from the individual studies should be symmetrical around the most precise point estimates. Asymmetry in one direction indicates that there are likely studies that were missed by the systematic review. These may be papers where the authors of the original studies never tried to publish their findings, or were unsuccessful in their efforts, because none of their findings were statistically significant.

Example From the Literature

Leelakanok and colleages[3] conducted a systematic review of the literature to examine the association between polypharmacy and mortality. A meta-analysis was conducted in conjunction with the systematic review. The investigators also sought to determine if there is a dose-response relationship between the number of drugs taken and mortality risk. The paper lists specific inclusion and exclusion criteria for the studies included in the review. However, the objectives of the review are not stated in PICOS format. A total of 3,892 papers were identified using electronic databases (see Figure 12-1). Of these, 47 met study inclusion criteria. These included 37 cohort studies (26 prospective and 11 retrospective), 5 case-control studies, 4 clinical trials, and 1 cross-sectional study. Data were extracted from the studies by two members of the research team working independently. Using the Newcastle-Ottawa Scale for quality assessment,[6] 19 of the included studies were classified as medium quality and 28 were classified as high quality.

The investigators created the funnel plot shown in Figure 12-3 to assess the possibility of publication bias. They concluded appropriately, "The funnel plot showed that the SE of log risk ratios was distributed heavily at the top, indicating that smaller studies might have not been published. Study results were distributed around the pooled risk ratio, with more studies being scattered at the positive side (polypharmacy increased the mortality risk), indicating that there may be some publication bias with negative studies not being published" (p. 731). Aside from the issue of publication bias, notice that the authors used causal language in this passage (i.e., "polypharmacy increased the mortality risk"). Because over 90% of the studies included in the review were observational (i.e., cohort, case-control, cross-sectional), only the presence of associations can be examined, and it is not appropriate to make causal inferences. Therefore, it would have been more accurate to state "polypharmacy was associated with an increased risk of mortality."

The investigators used random-effects models to estimate the pooled effect size across studies. A high level of heterogeneity was present among the effect size estimates from the individual studies included in the analysis (I^2 = 91.5%). The investigators attempted to deal with this heterogeneity by stratifying the 47 studies into 5 subsets based on how polypharmacy was defined and conducting a separate meta-analysis within each subset. The findings from these analyses are summarized in the forest plot shown in Figure 12-2. This figure shows the log of the risk ratio estimated in each study with its SE. The weights applied to the individual studies are also shown. You can see that within each set of studies, those with the smallest SEs were weighted most heavily in calculating the pooled effect size estimate. The vertical line on the right of the figure indicates the point on the x-axis where the risk ratio = 1, which is the expected value under H_0 when examining any type of ratio (e.g., risk ratios, odds ratios, hazard ratios). For each study, the square indicates the point estimate for the effect size reported. The size of the square reflects the study sample size (i.e., larger squares indicate larger sample sizes). The horizontal lines drawn from the squares indicate the 95% CI for each point estimate. The longer the lines, the less precise the estimate. For some of the point estimates, no CI is shown. This occurs when the CI is very narrow. Point estimates to the right of the vertical line suggest a positive association between polypharmacy and mortality. Point estimates to the left of the vertical line suggest an inverse association between polypharmacy and mortality. For estimates where the 95% CI includes "1," the relationship between polypharmacy and mortality is not statistically significant. Within each subset of studies, the pooled point estimate is shown by the diamond just below the estimates for the individual studies.

In the forest plot, notice that I^2 is greater than 75% in three of the five meta-analyses shown. Therefore, the pooled effect size estimates should be interpreted with caution. The heterogeneity encountered likely could have been reduced if the investigators had identified study objectives more explicitly using the PICOS format. For example, restricting included studies to those focusing on community-dwelling older adults (aged 65+ years) with no terminal illnesses may have resulted in a more homogeneous set of studies. Similarly, limiting the studies to those that used similar designs (e.g., prospective cohort studies) would have reduced methodological heterogeneity. Nonetheless, of the 47 studies included in the analysis, only four reported an inverse association between polypharmacy and mortality; of these, only two were statistically significant.[7,8] Therefore, the preponderance of the evidence suggests a positive association between polypharmacy and mortality. Keep in mind, however, that this is evidence of an association only. Experimental studies demonstrating that reducing polypharmacy reduces the risk of mortality would strengthen the case for causality.

Self-Study Questions

1. Suppose you are conducting a meta-analysis of studies examining noninvasive strategies to diagnose coronary artery disease. The Forest plot of the included studies shows overlapping confidence intervals (CIs), but the I^2 test is >75%. What approach should you use to calculate an overall pooled estimate for your meta-analysis?

   A. Random-effects model
   B. Fixed-effects model

2. What is a meta-analysis?

   A. A numeric analysis of pooled data from studies of similar design and the same primary hypothesis or outcome measure
   B. The gold standard of study designs
   C. A systematic review of case reports
   D. Both A and C

3. When performing a meta-analysis, one must weight the summary statistics on the basis of the precision of the results. Which studies are given more weight in the pooling?

   A. Less precise studies (wide CIs)
   B. More precise studies (narrow CIs)

4. Which of the following is **not** an important question to ask when critically appraising a systematic review?

   A. Did the authors do a systematic, comprehensive literature search?
   B. Were study eligibility criteria predefined and specified?
   C. Was a meta-analysis conducted? Otherwise, it's not a systematic review.
   D. Did the authors critically appraise (or assess for risk of bias) each study included in the review?
   E. Did at least two reviewers evaluate articles to determine eligibility?

5. Which of the following is **not** an important step in conducting a systematic review?

   A. Developing focused questions
   B. Conducting a comprehensive literature search
   C. Having dual review of abstracts and articles to determine inclusion or exclusion
   D. Assessing heterogeneity
   E. Including only randomized controlled trials because observational studies should never be included

6. Is the following statement true or false? You should have a focused question versus a broad question when conducting a systematic literature review. (True/False)

7. Which of the following combinations of terms describe characteristics of a systematic review?

   A. Broad question, author identification of evidence, methods section, idiosyncratic
   B. Broad question, predefined literature search, methods section, idiosyncratic
   C. Focused question, predefined literature search, methods section, reproducible
   D. Focused question, predefined literature search, no methods section, reproducible

8. Which of the following statements is **false** regarding meta-analysis?

   A. Studies included in a meta-analysis should be derived from a systematic review.
   B. The aim of a meta-analysis is to produce a single estimate of treatment effect.
   C. Meta-analysis usually involves individual patient data from one or more trials.
   D. Populations, interventions, and outcome measures should be similar.

9. Is the following statement true or false? Before you do a systematic review of the literature, you should have a predefined literature search strategy. (True/False)

10. Systematic reviews and meta-analyses have limitations, including threats to validity. Which of the following terms is **not** relevant when thinking about potential threats to the validity of systematic reviews or meta-analyses.

   A. Publication bias
   B. Funnel plots
   C. Heterogeneity
   D. Forest plots

References

1. Haidich AB. Meta-analysis in medical research. *Hippokratia*. 2010;14(Suppl 1): 29–37.
2. Liberati A, Altman DG, Tetzlaff J, et al. The PRISMA statement for reporting systematic reviews and meta-analyses of studies that evaluate healthcare interventions: explanation and elaboration. *BMJ*. 2009;339:b2700.
3. Leelakanok N, Holcombe AL, Lund BC, et al. Association between polypharmacy and death: a systematic review and meta-analysis. *J Am Pharm Assoc*. 2017;57(6):729–38.
4. Egger M, Smith GD, Phillips AN. Meta-analysis: principles and procedures. *BMJ*. 1997;315(7121):1533–7.
5. Higgins JP, Thompson SG, Deeks JJ, Altman DG. Measuring inconsistency in meta-analysis. *BMJ*. 2003;327(7414): 557–60.
6. Wells G, Shea B, O'Connell D, et al. The Newcastle-Ottawa Scale (NOS) for assessing the quality of nonrandomised studies in meta-analyses. www.ohri.ca/programs/clinical_epidemiology/oxford.asp. Accessed January 11, 2018.
7. Wisler JR, Springer AN, Hateley K, et al. Pre-injury neuro-psychiatric medication use, alone or in combination with cardiac medications, may affect outcomes in trauma patients. *J Postgrad Med*. 2014;60(4):366–71.
8. Lu WH, Wen YW, Chen LK, et al. Effect of polypharmacy, potentially inappropriate medications and anticholinergic burden on clinical outcomes: a retrospective cohort study. *CMAJ*. 2015;187(4):E130–7.

Appendices

A Summary of Statistical Tests

Nominal independent variables index membership in a group (e.g., treatment/no treatment; disease/no disease; risk factor/no risk factor).

APPENDIX TABLE A-1. Tests Involving Nominal Independent Variables

	Scale of Measurement of Outcome Variable		
Analytic Situation	**Interval/Ratio**	**Nominal**	**Ordinal**
Tests allowing only one independent variable			
One group, outcome assessed at only one point in time	1-Sample t-test	Binomial test	Sign test
One group, outcome assessed at two points in time	Paired t-test	McNemar test	Wilcoxon signed rank test
Two independent groups, outcome assessed at only one point in time	Independent groups t-test	Chi-square test Fisher's exact test	Wilcoxon rank sum test (AKA Mann–Whitney U)
Three or more independent groups, outcome assessed at only one point in time	1-Way ANOVA	Chi-square test	Kruskal–Wallis ANOVA
Tests allowing multiple independent variables			
Two or more independent groups, outcome assessed at only one point in time	x-Way ANOVA (no interaction term) Factorial ANOVA		
Two or more independent groups, outcome assessed at multiple points in time	Mixed model ANOVA		Friedman 2-way ANOVA by ranks

APPENDIX TABLE A-2. Tests Involving Numerical Independent Variables

Analytic Situation	Scale of Measurement of Outcome Variable		
	Interval/Ratio	**Nominal**	**Ordinal**
Tests allowing only one independent variable			
Only one independent variable, outcome assessed at only one point in time	Pearson correlation Simple linear regression	Chi-square or Fisher's exact test	Spearman correlation
Tests allowing multiple independent variables			
Two or more independent variables, outcome assessed at one or more points in time	Multiple linear regression Polynomial regression ANCOVA GEE	Logistic regression GEE	Logistic regression GEE
Two or more independent variables, outcome assesses time to event		Survival analysis	

ANCOVA, analysis of covariance; GEE, generalized estimating equations

B Answers to Exercises and Self-Study Questions

Chapter 1

TABLE 1-1. Hypothetical Abridged Abstract

Some studies have found that bisphosphonates increase the risk of atypical femur fracture. In this study, we attempted to better quantify the magnitude of this risk. From a large claims database, we identified 100,000 patients who began using an oral bisphosphonate between 2005 and 2010. Bisphosphonate users were matched to 100,000 individuals of similar age and sex but with no history of bisphosphonate use. We compared the risk of atypical femur fracture between these two groups. A total of 214 atypical femur fractures were experienced by study participants between January 1, 2011, and December 31, 2017.

ANSWER: The primary independent variable is use of a bisphosphonate. The primary dependent variable is experience of an atypical femur fracture.

Obesity is a major public health problem. Individuals who are obese are more likely than the nonobese to experience a variety of health problems (e.g., stroke, heart attack, chronic obstructive pulmonary disease) and to die prematurely. This study compared the amount of weight loss experienced by obese individuals who were prescribed either (1) a very low carbohydrate diet, (2) a prescription weight-loss medication, or (3) a placebo. Three hundred obese individuals participated, with 100 of these participants assigned to each arm of the study. Weight of each participant was recorded at the start of the study and at the end of a 6-month treatment period.

ANSWER: The primary independent variable is treatment (very low carbohydrate diet, prescription weight-loss medication, placebo). The primary dependent variable is weight loss.

TABLE 1-2. **Identify the Scale of Measurement (i.e., Nominal, Ordinal, Numerical) for Each of the Following Variables**

Variable	Scale
Age, measured in years	Numerical (continuous)
Age (categorized as: under 18, 18–65, over 65)	Ordinal
Age (categorized as: under 65, 65 or older)	Nominal
Number of broken bones experienced	Numerical (discrete)
Bone mineral density, measured in g/cm^2	Numerical (continuous)
Bone mineral density (normal, osteopenia, osteoporosis)	Ordinal
Sex (male, female)	Nominal
Race (white, African American, Asian, Native American, other)	Nominal
Diagnosed with osteoporosis (yes, no)	Nominal
Taking a bisphosphonate (yes, no)	Nominal

Self-Study Questions

1. Which of the following sets of numbers has the largest SD?

   A. 5, 10, 15, 20, 25
   B. 5, 15, 25, 35, 45
   C. 5, 20, 35, 50, 65
   D. 5, 20, 35, 50, 85

2. Which of the following statistics is most commonly used to describe the central tendency of a normally distributed numerical variable?

   A. Mean
   B. Median
   C. Mode
   D. SD

3. Imagine that you know a person's systolic and DBP. You also know the mean and SD of systolic and DBP in the general population. You use this information to convert the person's blood pressure readings into z-scores. The z-scores obtained are –0.45 for DBP and –0.85 for systolic blood pressure. Based on this information, what would you conclude?

   A. The person appears to have abnormally low blood pressure.
   B. The person appears to have abnormally high blood pressure.
   C. The person's blood pressure appears to be about normal.
   D. These data cannot be correct because z-scores cannot take negative values.

4. The SD of a measure is:

   A. Where the center of the distribution of observations lies
   B. The difference between the median and the mean
   C. The average distance of an observation in a sample from the sample mean
   D. The probability that the measure is normally distributed

5. If data from a sample are normally distributed, approximately 95% of the observations will lie within how many SDs of the mean?

   A. Plus or minus 1
   B. Plus or minus 2
   C. Plus or minus 3
   D. Plus or minus 4

6. If the distribution of a variable is symmetrical, the most appropriate statistics to use to describe the sample are:

   A. Mean and SD
   B. Mean and standard error of the mean
   C. Median and IQR
   D. Median and range
   E. Mode

Chapter 2

Self-Study Questions

1. Imagine that a case-control study is conducted to determine if use of Drug A is associated with an increased risk of sudden cardiac death among people under the age of 40. It is found that "young" adults (i.e., aged 18–39) who died of sudden cardiac death (i.e., the cases) were more likely to have taken Drug A during the 24 hours preceding death compared to control subjects in the same age group who died of noncardiac causes. In this case-control study, which of the following statistics would be most appropriate to use to quantify the increased risk observed?

   A. Relative risk ratio
   B. Odds ratio
   C. Experimental event rate
   D. Control event rate

2. Imagine that a study is conducted examining the risk of falls among older adults taking psychotropic medications compared to older adults not taking such medications. It is found that, among those taking psychotropic medications, the annual incidence of falls is 25.6%, whereas among those not taking psychotropic medications, the annual incidence of falls is 23.2%. Based on these findings, what is the ARI associated with the use of psychotropic medications?

   A. 0.256
   B. 0.232
   C. 0.024
   D. 0.103
   E. 1.103

3. Based on the findings described in Question 2, what is the relative risk (RR) of falls among older adults taking psychotropic medications compared to those not taking psychotropic medications?

   A. 0.256
   B. 0.232
   C. 0.024
   D. 0.103
   E. 1.103

4. Based on the findings described in Question 2, what is the relative risk increase associated with use of psychotropic medications among older adults?

   A. 0.256
   B. 0.232
   C. 0.024
   D. 0.103
   E. 1.103

5. Based on the findings described in Question 2, the number needed to harm is:

   A. 14
   B. 42
   C. 82
   D. 232
   E. 256

6. Is the following statement true or false? If a disease is rapidly fatal, prevalence rates will tend to underestimate the true burden of the disease. (**True**/False)

7. Is the following statement true or false? If a disease is self-limited and usually resolves itself, with or without treatment, within two weeks of onset, prevalence rates will tend to underestimate the true burden of the disease. (**True**/False)

8. Odds ratios provide good estimates of relative risk when:

   A. The disease in question is quite common
   B. The disease in question is quite rare
   C. Odds ratios always provide good estimates of relative risk
   D. Odds ratios never provide good estimates of relative risk

9. A study of a new medication used to prevent myocardial infarctions among those at very high risk reports that the number needed to treat (NNT) is 25. How is this value interpreted?

   A. For every person treated with the new medication, 25 myocardial infarctions will be prevented.
   B. For every 25 people treated with the new medication, 1 myocardial infarction will be prevented.
   C. 25% of people who take the new medication will experience a myocardial infarction.
   D. 25% of people who do not take the new medication will experience a myocardial infarction.
   E. Use of the new medication reduces the risk of myocardial infarction by 25%.

10. Imagine that a Centers for Disease Control and Prevention (CDC) report provided data from two states, Florida and Minnesota, regarding mortality from influenza during the 2017 flu season. Some of the data are presented in Question Table 2-1. For each state, the first column shows the # of patients treated for influenza in each age category, the third column shows the # of deaths among those treated, and the last column shows the age-specific mortality rates among those treated. The crude mortality rates are 8.6 and 5.7 per 1,000 patients treated in Florida and Minnesota, respectively. If the crude rates were adjusted for age, which state would have the highest mortality rate?

   A. Florida
   B. Minnesota
   C. Neither, the adjusted rates would be the same.
   D. The rate cannot be determined from the information provided.

Use Question Table 2-1 to answer Question 10.

QUESTION TABLE 2-1. Fictitious Influenza Mortality for Two States (Original Data)

	Florida				Minnesota			
	Patients Treated		Deaths		Patients Treated		Deaths	
Age	N (in 1000s)	%	#	Rate Per 1,000	N (in 1000s)	%	#	Rate Per 1,000
0–18	6	10	24	4.0	5	25	20	4.0
19–59	6	10	12	2.0	7	35	14	2.0
60–79	48	80	480	10.0	8	40	80	10.0
Total	60	100	516	8.6	20	100	114	5.7

Use Question Table 2-2 to answer Question 11.

QUESTION TABLE 2-2. Fictitious Influenza Mortality for Two States (Revised Data)

	Florida				Minnesota			
	Patients Treated		Deaths		Patients Treated		Deaths	
Age	N (in 1000s)	%	#	Rate Per 1,000	N (in 1000s)	%	#	Rate Per 1,000
0–18	6	10	24	4.0	5	25	20	4.0
19–59	6	10	12	2.0	7	35	21	3.0
60–79	48	80	480	10.0	8	40	120	15.0
Total	60	100	516	8.6	20	100	161	8.1

11. Now, imagine that CDC scientists realized that they made a mistake in the original report. The revised data are shown in in Question Table 2-2. The crude mortality rates are 8.6 and 8.1 per 1,000 patients treated in Florida and Minnesota, respectively. If the crude rates were adjusted for age, which state would have the highest mortality rate?

A. Florida
B. Minnesota
C. Neither, the adjusted rates would be the same.
D. The rate cannot be determined from the information provided.

12. Imagine that a Drug A is suspected to cause Stevens-Johnson Syndrome. A case-control study is conducted. A total of 1,000 patients diagnosed with Stevens-Johnson Syndrome are enrolled in the study. A total of 1,000 control patients without Stevens-Johnson Syndrome are also enrolled. Among the patients with Stevens-Johnson Syndrome, 500 had taken Drug A within the past month. Among the control patients, 400 had taken Drug A within the past month. Based on these findings, what is the relative risk of developing Stevens-Johnson Syndrome among those taking Drug A compared to those not taking Drug A?

A. 1.0
B. 1.2
C. 1.5
D. Cannot determine. Case-control studies do not provide the information needed to calculate the EER and CER, which are needed to calculate RR.

13. Based on the findings described in Question 12, what are the odds of developing Stevens-Johnson Syndrome among patients exposed to Drug A compared to those not exposed?

A. 1.0
B. 1.2
C. 1.5
D. 0.103
E. 1.103

14. Is the following statement true or false? NNT/NNH can be computed from data obtained from a case-control study. (True/**False**)

Chapter 3

Self-Study Questions

1. Imagine that a new drug is available to treat a rare and aggressive form of cancer. A study is conducted. A total of 500 people receive the new medication. A total of 1,500 people receive standard care. All patients are followed for 1 year. Among the people receiving the new medication, 200 die before the end of the follow-up period. Among the people receiving standard care, 200 die before the end of the follow-up period.

A. In this example, is survival independent of the medication taken?
B. What is the conditional probability of surviving if a person receives the new medication?
C. What is the conditional probability of surviving if a person receives standard care?

	Die		Survive		Total
New Medication	200	A	300	B	500 (0.25)
Standard Care	200	C	1,300	D	1,500 (0.75)
Total	400 (0.20)		1,600 (0.8)		2,000

In this example, the joint probability of surviving **and** taking the new medication is 300/2,000 = 0.15.

To determine if survival is independent you have to determine if this joint probability is equal to the product of the marginal probabilities. The product of the marginals (in Cell B) is: 0.8 ∗ 0.25 = 0.20. They are not equal, suggesting that the events are **not** independent. (You should do this for all cells. However, if you find one cell where they are not equal, it means that the events are not independent.)

Conditional probability of surviving if a person receives new medication is: 300/500 = 0.60.

Conditional probability of surviving if a person receives standard care is: 1,300/1,500 = 0.867.

The fact that these conditional probabilities differ also tells you that the two events are **not** independent.

2. Imagine that it is thought that Medication A causes birth defects when women take it during pregnancy. Data from a cohort of 100,000 women are available. Among these women, 10,000 took Medication A during pregnancy and 10 of these women gave birth to babies with one or more birth defects. Among the 90,000 women who did **not** take the medication during pregnancy, 90 gave birth to babies with one or more birth defects.

   A. In this example, are birth defects independent of whether Medication A was taken during pregnancy?
   B. What is the conditional probability of having a baby with a birth defect among women who took Medication A during pregnancy?
   C. What is the conditional probability of having a baby with a birth defect among women who did **not** take Medication A during pregnancy?

	Birth Defect		No Birth Defect		Total
Medication A	10	A	9,990	B	10,000 (0.10)
No Medication A	90	C	89,910	D	90,000 (0.90)
Total	100 (.001)		99,900 (.999)		100,000

In this example, the joint probability of having a baby with a birth defect **and** taking Medication A is 10/100,000 = 0.0001.

To determine if having a baby with a birth defect is independent of having taken Medication A during pregnancy, you have to determine if this joint probability is equal to the product of the marginal probabilities. The product of the marginals (in Cell A) is: 0.001 ∗ 0.1 = 0.0001. They are equal, suggesting that the events are independent. (You should do this for all cells. In this case, you will find that they are all the same—again, meaning that the events are independent.)

Conditional probability of having a baby with a birth defect if Medication A was taken during pregnancy is: 10/10,000 = .001.

Conditional probability of having a baby with a birth defect if Medication A was **not** taken during pregnancy is: 90/90,000 = .001.

The fact that these conditional probabilities are the same also tells you that the two events are independent. So what does it mean that the events are independent? In this case, it means that whether or not a woman has a baby with a birth defect was not affected by whether or not she took Medication A during pregnancy.

3. Imagine that you collected data concerning weight in a sample of 36 people. The mean weight in the sample is 180 pounds with an SD of 20 pounds.

   A. Assuming that the variable is normally distributed, about how many people in the sample weigh between 160 and 200 pounds? **(Answer: 24–25)** About how many weigh between 140 and 220 pounds? **(Answer: 34)**
   B. Using the data provided, calculate the standard error (SE) of the mean for weight. **(Answer: 3.33)**
   C. Calculate a 95% confidence interval (CI) for the mean. **(Answer: 173.3–186.7)**
   D. What would you tell someone who asked, "What is the average weight in the population from which this sample was drawn?" **(Answer: I am 95% confident that the mean weight in the population from which the sample was drawn is between 173.3 and 186.7 pounds.)**

E. Calculate a 99% CI for the mean. Why is the 99% CI wider than the 95% CI? **(Answer: 171.3–188.7. It is wider than the 95% CI because the critical value is larger. More generally, whenever you make an estimate of anything, if you want to be more confident that your answer includes the correct answer, you must include a wider range in your estimate.)**

F. Now, what would you tell someone who asked, "What is the average weight in the population from which this sample was drawn?" **(Answer: I am 99% confident that the mean weight in the population from which the sample was drawn is between 171.3 and 188.7 pounds.)**

G. Imagine that data had been available for 400 people, but that mean weight was still 180 pounds. and the SD was still 20 pounds. Do you think the CIs for weight would become wider or narrower? Why? Compute the 95% CI using these data to check your answer. **(Answer: 95% CI: 178–182. Thus, as sample size increases the CIs becomes narrower, assuming everything else is held constant.)**

H. Imagine that you want to determine whether the mean weight in the population from which this sample was drawn was 175 pounds. Further, you only want to conclude that the mean weight is different than 175 pounds if you are at least 95% certain that it is different.
   i. Based on the data from the sample where N = 36, what would you conclude? **(Answer: You cannot rule out the possibility with 95% confidence that population mean is 175.)**
   ii. Based on the data from the sample where N = 400, what would you conclude? **(Answer: Reject null. Population mean is unlikely to be 175.)**

I. In the sample of 400 people, imagine that the mean weight was still 180 pounds but that the SD was 40 pounds. Compute the 95% and 99% CIs for weight using these data. **(Answer: 95%: 176–184; 99%: 174.8–185.2)**
   i. Based on the 95% CI, would your conclusion be the same as in part h (ii)? **(Answer: Yes, you would still reject null.)**
   ii. What if you only wanted to conclude that the mean weight is different than 175 pounds, if you were at least 99% certain that it is different. What would you conclude? **(Answer: You cannot rule out the possibility with 99% confidence that population mean is 175.)**
   iii. If the SD had been 20 pounds, would your conclusion have been different? **(Answer: 99% CI: 177.4–182.6. Reject null. Population mean is unlikely to be 175.)**

J. Assume that the mean in the population from which the sample was drawn was **not** 175. Based on all of the above, what set of conditions (i.e., sample size, SD, type of CI) provided the greatest power to rule out the possibility that the true population mean could be 175? **(Answer: Power increases as sample size increases. Power decreases as the SD of observations increases. You have less power when you set alpha at 0.01 rather than 0.05)**

4. Imagine that you collected data concerning weight in a sample of 36 people. The mean weight in the sample is 180 pounds with an SD of 20 pounds. Now, imagine that you want to test the hypothesis that the mean in the population from which this sample was drawn is different from 175 pounds.

   A. What is the null hypothesis? **(Answer: Population mean is 175.)**
   B. What is the alternative hypothesis? **(Answer: Population mean is NOT 175.)**
   C. Compute a z-score to determine whether you should reject the null hypothesis. **(Answer: 1.5)**
   D. What do you conclude? **(Answer: You cannot rule out the possibility with 95% confidence that population mean is 175.)**
   E. If the sample size had been 400, would that have changed your conclusion? **(Answer: The z-score would be 5.0. You would reject null hypothesis. Population mean is unlikely to be 175.)**

5. Is the following statement true or false? Population parameters can be calculated from the data collected in a study. **(Answer: False)**

6. The SE of a variable:

   A. Indexes the amount of variance among observations in a sample
   B. Indexes the amount of variance that would be observed in the means of different random samples (of a fixed sample size) that are drawn from the same population
   C. Decreases as sample size decreases
   D. A and B
   E. A and C

7. Probabilities can:

A. Range from −1 to +1
B. Be 0
C. Range from 0 to +1
D. Take any value

8. If the probability that an event will happen is 0.8, the probability that it will **not** happen is:

A. −0.2
B. 0.2
C. 0.5
D. 0.7
E. 1.0

9. Which of the following statements is true with respect to the binomial distribution?

A. It is appropriate to use when analyzing proportions
B. It can only be used with dichotomous variables
C. The value calculated by the binomial formula is a probability
D. It can be used to analyze problems even if the sample size is quite small
E. All of the above

10. Imagine that 40% of patients who begin therapy with lipid-lowering drugs discontinue therapy (without the knowledge of their physician) within 1 year of therapy initiation. A pilot study is conducted to determine if a pharmacist-directed lipid management program can improve medication adherence. Ten patients are enrolled into the pilot study. At the end of a 1-year follow-up period, all 10 patients are still taking their medication as prescribed by their physician. What is the probability that all 10 patients would still be complying with their lipid medications if the disease management program had no effect on compliance?

A. 0.05
B. 0.01
C. 0.006
D. 0.0001

11. Imagine that 20% of patients who begin therapy with lipid-lowering drugs discontinue therapy (without the knowledge of their physician) within 1 year of therapy initiation. A pilot study is conducted to determine if a pharmacist-directed lipid management program can improve medication adherence. Ten patients are enrolled into the pilot study. At the end of a 1-year follow-up period, all 10 patients are still taking their medication as prescribed by their physician. What is the probability that all 10 patients would still be complying with their lipid medications if the disease management program had no effect on compliance?

A. 0.01
B. 0.05
C. 0.11
D. 0.20
E. 0.0001

12. The SE of the mean of a variable is affected by:

A. The SD of the variable
B. The number of people in the sample from which the mean was calculated
C. A and B

13. The SE of the mean is:

A. The average distance of individual observations in a sample from the sample mean
B. Given a specific sample size, the average distance of all possible sample means from the true population mean
C. The probability of incorrectly rejecting the null hypothesis
D. The probability of incorrectly accepting the null hypothesis
E. The probability of incorrectly rejecting the alternative hypothesis

14. Two events are independent if:

A. They cannot occur at the same time
B. The probability of one event does not alter the probability of the other event
C. The probability of each event is 0.5
D. The probabilities of all possible outcomes are equal
E. None of the above

15. You are reading a study that involves 1,000 patients with diabetes. In total, 250 of these patients receive a new experimental medication thought be superior to existing therapy in achieving long-term glycemic control. The remaining 750 patients receive an existing medication. All patients are evaluated bi-monthly. Among the patients receiving the experimental medication, 150 are consistently rated as being within guidelines for glycemic control. Among patients receiving the existing medication, 300 are consistently rated as being within guidelines for glycemic control. Based on the multiplication rule for independent events, does glycemic control appear to be independent of the type of medication the person is taking?

- **A.** Yes, glycemic control appears independent of the type of medication taken.
- **B. No, glycemic control does NOT appear independent of the type of medication taken.**

16. You are reading an article in a journal. The article reports that patients receiving an experimental medication were more likely to report gastrointestinal distress compared to patients receiving a placebo ($P = .08$). If alpha was set at $P < 0.05$, what would you conclude from this information?

- **A.** The difference between patients taking the experimental medication versus placebo was statistically significant.
- **B. The difference between patients taking the experimental medication versus placebo was NOT statistically significant.**

17. In a sample of 2,000 people, 100 people were taking Drug A. Of these people, 10 died. In this sample, what is the **joint probability** of taking Drug A and dying?

- **A. 0.005**
- **B.** 0.05
- **C.** 0.10
- **D.** 0.20
- **E.** 0.30

18. In a recent paper, investigators report that participants in a study who were given a new drug for weight control lost an average of 3 pounds over a 1-month period. The 95% CI for this mean estimate was 0.8 to 5.2 pounds. Based on this information only, what would you conclude?

- **A. The reported results are statistically significant.**
- **B.** The reported results are **not** statistically significant.
- **C.** A conclusion cannot be reached because no *P* value is given.
- **D.** A conclusion cannot be reached because no information about power is provided.
- **E.** C and D

19. If all other things are held constant, when sample size increases, the SE of estimates based on data from the sample will:

- **A. Decrease**
- **B.** Stay the same
- **C.** Increase

20. Suppose that there is a study showing that the mean bone density of women is 1.00 ± 0.15 g/cm^2, and the mean bone density of men is 1.07 ± 0.09 g/cm^2. The 95% confidence level for the difference between these means is 0.02 to 0.14 g/cm^2. How is this information interpreted?

- **A.** The true difference in the mean bone density of men and women is 0.07 g/cm^2.
- **B.** Because the 95% CI does not include "1," the difference is statistically significant.
- **C. There is 95% chance that the true difference in the mean bone density of men and women is between 0.02 and 0.14 g/cm^2. (Note, however, that when the difference in means is expressed in this manner, one must look at the sample means to determine which mean is higher and which is lower.)**
- **D.** A *P* value is needed to determine whether the difference is statistically significant.

21. If an investigator sets alpha at 0.05, we know that:

   A. The chance that the investigator will make a Type I error is 5%
   B. The chance the investigator will make a Type II error is 5%
   C. Power is 0.95
   D. Power is 0.05

22. Imagine that you are reading a paper that reports the mean bone mineral density in a sample and the 95% CI for the point estimate of the mean. What percentage of the time would you expect the true population mean bone density to be captured within the 95% CI?

   A. 5% of the time
   B. 95% of the time
   C. 99% of the time
   D. 100% of the time

23. Is the following statement true or false? A 95% confidence interval will always be narrower than a 99% CI. **(Answer: True)**

24. When one performs a hypothesis test, the null hypothesis is that:

   A. The means in the samples being compared are the same
   B. The means in the populations from which the samples were drawn are the same
   C. The means in the samples being compared are different
   D. The means in the populations from which the samples were drawn are different

25. When an investigator writes in a paper that one treatment is more effective than another *(P* <0.05), this indicates that:

   A. He is absolutely certain that the treatment is more effective than the other
   B. The chance that the treatments are equally effective is less than 5%
   C. He cannot completely rule out the possibility that the treatments are equally effective
   D. A and B
   E. B and C

26. If a team of scientists conclude that there is no evidence that either of two treatments is superior to the other, what type of error might they be making?

   A. Alpha (Type I) error
   B. Beta (Type II) error
   C. They could be making either alpha or beta error
   D. This is a trick question; scientists don't make mistakes . . . especially when they are working in a team.

27. Imagine that a study is conducted among 3,000 people with flu-like symptoms. In total, 1,000 people receive penicillin. The remainder receive placebo. Among the people who receive penicillin, 800 report feeling better within 2 days of the initiation of therapy. Among the people who receive placebo, 1,000 report feeling better within 2 days of therapy initiation. Based on this information, what is the conditional probability of feeling better within 2 days of the initiation of therapy given that the patient received penicillin?

   A. 0.40
   B. 0.50
   C. 0.80
   D. 1.0
   E. The probability cannot be determined from the information provided.

28. Based on the information in the previous question, does recovery (i.e., feeling better within 2 days of the initiation of therapy) appear to be independent of treatment?

   A. Yes, recovery appears to be independent of treatment.
   B. No, recovery appears to depend on the type of treatment received. People who take penicillin appear to recover more quickly.

Chapter 4

Self-Study Questions

1. In ANOVA, as the difference in observed means increases, what happens to the between groups sums of squares (SS)?

   A. The between groups SS increases.
   B. The between groups SS stays the same.
   C. The between groups SS decreases.

2. Is the following statement true or false? Addition of predictor variables to an ANOVA has no effect on the F-test associated with predictor variables that have been added previously. (True/**False**)

3. Is the following statement true or false? A variable involved in an interaction is sometimes called an effect modifier. (**True**/False)

4. As predictor variables are added to an ANOVA, which of the following tend to decrease?

   A. Error SS
   B. Between groups SS
   C. Total SS
   D. Error SS *and* total SS

5. In a journal article, the authors perform an ANOVA and report that F(2,298)=0.84, ns. (The abbreviation "ns" means Not Significant.) The next step in the analysis is to:

   A. Perform a Tukey's honestly significant difference test
   B. Perform a Student-Newman-Keuls test
   C. Perform a Bonferroni correction
   D. Stop; no further analyses should be performed since the overall F test was not significant

6. Imagine that you are given the data from a trial that randomly assigned 400 participants to one of four treatments for hypertension. The outcome that was being studied in this trial was blood pressure, measured in mmHg. Given just this information, what type of statistical analysis would be most appropriate to assess treatment effect?

   A. A 1-sample t-test
   B. A 1-way ANOVA
   C. A paired t-test
   D. Factorial ANOVA

7. In an ANOVA, the between groups SS reflects:

   A. The portion of variance in the independent variable that is explained by the dependent variable
   B. The portion of variance in the dependent variable that is explained by the independent variable
   C. The portion of variance in the independent variable that is NOT explained by the dependent variable
   D. The portion of variance in the dependent variable that is NOT explained by the independent variable

8. Assume that a team of investigators is studying the impact of lifestyle modifications on weight loss. They assign 300 subjects to one of the following three options: exercise only, low-carbohydrate diet only, and low-fat diet only. During the course of the study each participant is assigned to one of the treatment arms for one month and then their weights are assessed. After this month, they are switched to one of the other two treatment arms for an additional month and have their weight assessed again. Finally, they enter the third treatment arm and have their weight assessed at the end of that month. At the end of the trial, each of the 300 participants has tested each of the lifestyle modifications for one month. To analyze these data, the investigators would probably use:

   A. 1-Way ANOVA
   B. Factorial ANOVA
   C. Repeated measures ANOVA
   D. Kruskal-Wallis ANOVA

9. If all other things are held constant, as alpha error increases:

   A. Power decreases
   B. The chance of missing a true effect increases
   C. The chance of incorrectly rejecting the null hypothesis increases
   D. Beta error decreases
   E. Both C and D

10. Which of the following would usually be considered an acceptable level of power in a study?

A. 0.05
B. 0.60
C. 0.80
D. 0.90
E. Both C and D

11. All other things held constant, as sample size increases:

A. Alpha error usually decreases
B. Power usually decreases
C. Power usually increases
D. The magnitude of the true difference usually increases

12. Imagine that a study is conducted examining the effect of a new medication on bone density. Individuals in the study are randomly assigned to receive either the new medication or placebo. Individuals then are followed for 1 year, and bone density is assessed at the end of the year. In the results of the paper reporting study findings, the authors write that the bone density of people taking the new medication was greater than those taking placebo and that the mean difference was 0.04 g/cm^2 (95% CI: –0.02 to 0.10 g/cm^2). Based just on these findings, what would you conclude?

A. The difference between people taking placebo versus the new medication was statistically significant.
B. The difference between people taking placebo versus the new medication was NOT statistically significant.
C. The difference between people taking placebo versus the new medication was clinically meaningful.
D. There is insufficient information presented to draw any conclusions.

13. Another study assessed the effect of the same medication discussed in the last question. This time a before-after study design was used. All 100 people in the study took the new medication. Bone density was assessed at two points in time: before the initiation of therapy and again 6 months later. The mean difference in bone density between these two time periods was 0.15 g/cm^2 (SD = 0.2 g/cm^2). What is the 95% CI for the difference score?

A. 0.13 to 0.17 g/cm^2
B. –0.05 to 0.35 g/cm^2
C. 0.11 to 0.19 g/cm^2
D. –0.25 to 0.55 g/cm^2
E. The 95% CI cannot be determined from the information provided.

14. Which of the following statistical tests would be most appropriate to use to analyze the data in the study described in Question 13?

A. 1-Sample t-test
B. Paired t-test
C. Independent groups t-test
d. ANOVA

15. Imagine that the same set of data is analyzed using both CIs and an appropriate t-test. How will the conclusions drawn using these different approaches compare?

A. They will ALWAYS lead to the same conclusion with respect to whether the null hypothesis should be accepted or rejected.
B. They will USUALLY (but NOT always) lead to the same conclusion with respect to whether the null hypothesis should be accepted or rejected.
C. As a general rule, they will lead to different conclusions with respect to whether the null hypothesis should be accepted or rejected.

16. Is the following statement true or false? A difference observed in a study can be statistically significant without being clinically meaningful. (**True**/False)

17. T-tests assume that the dependent variable is measured on what type of scale?

- **A.** Nominal
- **B.** Dichotomous
- **C.** Ordinal
- **D. Numerical**
- **E.** Either C or D

18. When one looks at a figure presenting results of a factorial ANOVA, interactions are usually detected by:

- **A.** The point at which different lines intersect the y-axis
- **B.** The point at which different lines intersect the x-axis
- **C. A lack of parallelism among the lines corresponding to the different groups**
- **D.** Either A or B

19. Imagine that you are reading a paper. It states that the sample size was determined so that the study would have 80% power to detect a change in blood pressure of 10 mmHg. Which of the following is a correct interpretation of this statement?

- **A.** If the drug alters blood pressure by less than 10 mmHg, the investigators have an 80% chance of correctly identifying this effect.
- **B.** If the drug alters blood pressure by 10 mmHg or more, the investigators have an 80% chance of correctly identifying this effect.
- **C.** If the drug alters blood pressure by 10 mmHg or more, the investigators have a 20% chance of failing to detect this effect.
- **D. Both B and C**
- **E.** Both A and C

20. Imagine that you are reading a paper. It states that the study had 50% power to detect a change in blood pressure of 10 mmHg. Which of the following is a correct interpretation of this statement?

- **A.** If the drug alters blood pressure by less than 10 mmHg, the investigators had a 50% chance of correctly identifying this effect.
- **B.** If the drug alters blood pressure by 10 mmHg or more, the investigators had a 50% chance of correctly identifying this effect.
- **C.** If a change in blood pressure of 10 mmHg is clinically meaningful, the study was NOT sufficiently powered.
- **D. Both B and C**

21. When performing a t-test, the null hypothesis is rejected when:

- **A.** The t-statistic is greater than the critical value
- **B.** The investigators conclude that the medication under investigation is effective
- **C.** The difference between the means being compared is unlikely to be "0"
- **D. All of the above**

22. A study states: "Postintervention cases had shorter hospital stays compared with preintervention cases (median 6 vs 7 days, respectively, $P = 0.026$)." If alpha was set at 0.05, would the investigators conclude that this difference was statistically significant?

- **A. YES, they would conclude that the difference is statistically significant.**
- **B.** NO, they would NOT conclude that the difference is statistically significant.
- **C.** Statistical significance cannot be determined from the information provided.

23. If alpha is set at 0.05 in a study, how likely is it that the investigators will conclude that a medication is effective when it is not?

- **A. They have a 5% chance of concluding that it is effective if it is not.**
- **B.** They have a 95% chance of concluding that it is effective if it is not.
- **C.** They have an 80% chance of concluding that it is effective if it is not.
- **D.** This is a trick question; they would never conclude that it is effective if it is not.
- **E.** The likelihood cannot be determined from the information provided.

24. Clinicians often prefer CIs over hypothesis testing because:

- **A.** CIs are more likely to lead to the correct conclusion
- **B.** CIs are easier to compute
- **C. CIs provide more useful information**
- **D.** A and B
- **E.** All of the above

25. Imagine that you are reading a journal article. It states that t = 4.25, $P < 0.04$. On the basis of this test, the authors conclude that there is a statistically significant difference between the treatments being evaluated. The value "$P < 0.04$" means that:

A. The investigators were willing to accept a 5% chance of incorrectly rejecting the null hypothesis
B. The probability is less than 4% that a difference as large as the one observed would have occurred if, in reality, the treatments did not differ (i.e., in reality, the null hypothesis is true)
C. The study is adequately powered to identify the smallest clinically meaningful difference
D. The difference between the treatments is clinically meaningful

26. Performing multiple t-tests is a problem because:

A. It increases error variance
B. It inflates alpha error
C. It takes more time
D. It leads to computational errors
E. This is a trick question; performing multiple t-tests is not a problem

27. In the formulas for t-tests, the denominator term indexes:

A. The observed difference in means
B. Alpha error
C. Beta error
D. Sampling error
E. Power

28. What is the probability of making at least one alpha error if you perform five separate independent groups t-tests with alpha set at 0.01 for each test?

A. 1%
B. 5%
C. 10%
d. 15%
E. 20%

29. Which of the following is NOT an assumption of ANOVA?

A. The variance in the all groups is approximately equal
B. The dependent variable is assessed on a numerical scale
C. All predictor variables have no more than two groups
D. Observations are independent of one another

30. Which of the following is NOT an assumption of t-tests?

A. The outcome variable is measured on an ordinal scale.
B. The outcome variable is normally distributed, or the sample size is large enough to assume that the sampling distribution is normally distributed.
C. There cannot be more than two groups.

Chapter 5

Self-Study Questions

1. Imagine that you are reading a paper. Fifty people with arthritis are given a medication. Patients rate their pain on a 5-point scale before the initiation of therapy and again 2 months later. There is no control group. Pain is rated on a 4-point scale (i.e., 1 = no pain, 2 = mild pain, 3 = moderate pain, 4 = severe pain). Assume that this pain scale had ordinal (but not interval) properties. What is the most appropriate statistical test to use to analyze these data?

A. 1-Sample t-test
B. Paired t-test
C. 1-Way ANOVA
D. Wilcoxon signed rank test

2. Is the following statement true or false? Parametric procedures are appropriate to use in small samples when the dependent variable is not normally distributed. (True/**False**)

3. Imagine that you are an investigator who is testing a new relaxation technique on older adults (>65 years). Your technique has already been tested on people in other age groups, and you know that the average score on a 10-point scale is 7 points. On this scale, 1 = feel totally relaxed and 10 = feel totally wired. You want to determine if older adults rate your relaxation techniques differently than people in other age groups. You give the rating scale to 15 older adults. What type of test would you use to analyze these data?

A. 1-Sample t-test
B. Sign test
C. Wilcoxon rank sum test

4. What is the null hypothesis for the relaxation study described in Question 3?

   A. There is no difference in ratings between older adults and other age groups.
   B. There is a difference in ratings between older adults and other age groups.
   C. Older adults score higher than other age groups.
   D. Older adults score lower than other age groups.

5. Imagine that an investigator wants to compare the effectiveness of Tylenol and Ecotrin. Sixty patients with chronic pain are recruited into the study. Half receive Tylenol, and half receive Ecotrin. Following 2 weeks of therapy, subjects rate their pain on a 5-point scale where 1 = no pain, 2 = mild pain, 3 = moderate pain, 4 = severe pain, and 5 = excruciating pain. Assume that this pain scale had ordinal (but not interval) properties. Which of the following is the most appropriate test to use in comparing the effectiveness of the two medications?

   A. Binomial test
   B. 1-Way ANOVA
   C. Independent groups t-test
   D. Wilcoxon rank sum test

6. Imagine that a cross-over study is conducted evaluating the effect of a new analgesic on chronic pain. People are randomly assigned to receive either the medication or a placebo for 7 days. At the end of the 7-day period, all individuals undergo a 14-day washout period. At the end of the washout period, individuals who took the medication during the first period receive the placebo for a second 7-day period, and individuals who took the placebo during the first period receive the medication for the second 7-day period. Pain is assessed on a 5-point scale where 1 = no pain, 2 = just a little pain, 3 = a moderate amount of pain, 4 = a lot of pain, and 5 = excruciating pain. Which of the following statistics would be most appropriate to use to analyze the data from this study?

   A. Binomial test
   B. Independent groups t-test
   C. Wilcoxon signed rank test
   D. 1-Sample t-test

7. If the dependent variables in a study are measured on ordinal scales, they should be analyzed using what type of statistical procedures?

   A. Parametric procedures
   B. Nonparametric procedures (If you are reading a paper that used parametric procedures to analyze an ordinal dependent variable, the investigators have assumed that the distance between adjacent points on the scale is the same. As a reader of the literature, consider whether this assumption is warranted.)
   C. Either type (It really does not matter.)

Chapter 6

Self-Study Questions

1. Imagine that you are reading a paper. Fifty people with hypertension are given an experimental medication. The investigators want to know whether the medication is effective in controlling blood pressure. Blood pressure is measured before the initiation of therapy and again 2 months later. Assume that, at both time points, blood pressure is dichotomized as either 1 = within normal range or 2 = NOT within normal range. Given that blood pressure was dichotomized, what is the most appropriate statistical test to use to analyze these data?

   A. 1-Sample t-test
   B. Paired t-test
   C. McNemar test
   D. Kappa statistic

2. Imagine that there is a disease that has a 1-year survival rate of 20% with current treatment. In a trial of a new medication, 10 patients took Medication A, and 70% of these patients survived over a year. What statistical test should be used to determine whether the new treatment is more effective than the current one?

   A. 1-Sample t-test
   B. Chi-square test
   C. Binomial test
   D. Z approximation

3. Imagine that you are reading a study in which the investigators examined the effect of an experimental medication on survival following an acute myocardial infarction. Two thousand individuals participated in the study: 1,000 in the experimental group and 1,000 in a placebo control group. Nine hundred people in the experimental group survived compared to 700 people in the control group. Which of the following tests would be most appropriate to use to analyze the results of this study?

   A. Binomial test
   B. Chi-square test
   C. Wilcoxon rank sum test
   D. Wilcoxon signed rank test
   E. Fisher's exact test

4. Is the following statement true or false? The McNemar test is used as an alternative to a chi-square test when you have a small sample size. (True/**False**)

5. Is the following statement true or false? Probabilities calculated by nonparametric procedures used to analyze nominal data require that raw data be converted to ranks. (True/**False**)

6. Is the following statement true or false? Imagine that a study is conducted to evaluate the effect of a new weight loss medication. A total of 100 people take part in the study. Prior to the initiation of therapy, each participant is classified as either (1) overweight or (2) not overweight. Each participant then is followed for 6 months. At the end of the follow-up period, each participant is again classified as either (1) Overweight or (2) Not overweight. What type of statistical test would be used to determine if the proportion of participants who were overweight changed over the course of the study?

   A. Fisher's exact test
   B. Paired t-test
   C. McNemar's test
   D. Chi-square test

7. Imagine that there is a study that assesses the effect of a new weight loss medication. In the study, 50 patients take a placebo, and 50 patients take the new medication. If the outcome is measured as whether patients lose weight or not (weight loss: yes/no), what kind of statistical test would be most appropriate for the investigator to use?

   A. Independent group t-test
   B. Chi-square test
   C. Paired t-test
   D. Wilcoxon signed rank test

8. Based on the study described in Question 7, if the outcome had been measured as the number of pounds that a patient lost, which of the following statistical tests would be most appropriate to use?

   A. Independent group t-test
   B. Chi-square test
   C. Paired t-test
   D. Wilcoxon signed rank test

9. What type of statistical test is an alternative to a chi-square test when the sample size requirements for a chi-square test are not met?

   A. Binomial test
   B. Fisher's exact test
   C. Wilcoxon rank sum test
   D. Wilcoxon signed rank test

Chapter 7

Self-Study Questions

1. In a multiple regression analysis, R^2 is:

   A. The proportion of variance in the dependent variable explained by the independent variables
   B. The proportion of variance in the dependent variable NOT explained by the independent variable(s)
   C. The proportion of variance in the independent variable explained by the dependent variable
   D. Greater if error variance is greater

2. A paper states that the correlation between two variables is 0.34 with a standard error of 0.08. This correlation is based on a sample size of 500. If alpha were set at 0.05, would this correlation be considered statistically significant?

   A. Yes, it would be considered statistically significant.
   B. No, it would not be considered statistically significant.
   C. Statistical significance cannot be determined from the information provided.

3. In linear regression analysis, calculation of error variance is based on:

   A. The difference between individual observations and predicted values on the regression line
   B. The difference between individual observations and the overall mean
   C. The difference between predicted values and the overall mean
   D. None of the above

4. In linear regression analysis, the regression line is drawn in a way that:

   A. Maximizes the slope of the regression line
   B. Minimizes the slope of the regression line
   C. Minimizes error variance
   D. Maximizes error variance

5. In linear regression analysis, the regression coefficient:

   A. Indexes the magnitude of the effect of the independent variable on the dependent variable
   B. Indexes the slope of the regression line
   C. Increases as the regression sums of squares increases
   D. Both A and B
   E. A, B, and C

6. Is the following statement true or false? The possibility of confounding can be controlled through the use of multivariate statistical methods AFTER data for a study have been collected. (**True**/False)

Use Question Table 7-1 to answer Questions 7–9.

QUESTION TABLE 7-1. Regression Analysis Predicting Diastolic Blood Pressure (mmHg)

Predictor Variable	Regression Coefficient (SE)	95% CI
Intercept	30.82 (12.45)	5.92, 55.72
Female	3.31 (1.12)	1.07, 5.55
Body mass index (BMI)	0.34 (0.07)	0.2, 0.48
Smoker	5.78 (2.95)	–0.12, 11.68

Data in this table are fictitious. Regression coefficients are unstandardized. The reference groups for sex and smoking status are male and nonsmoker, respectively.

7. Question Table 7-1 shows the results of a linear regression analysis predicting diastolic blood pressure. How do you interpret the regression coefficient for "Female"?

   A. Controlling for BMI and smoking status, the average blood pressure of females is 3.31 points higher than males.
   B. Controlling for BMI and smoking status, the average blood pressure of males is 3.31 points higher than females.
   C. Controlling for BMI and smoking status, the relationship between sex and blood pressure is not statistically significant.
   D. A and C
   E. B and C

8. How do you interpret the regression coefficient for BMI in Question Table 7-1?

   A. On average, controlling for sex and smoking status, for every 1-unit increase in blood pressure, BMI goes up 0.34 units.
   B. On average, controlling for sex and smoking status, for every 1-unit increase in BMI, blood pressure goes up 0.34 units
   C. On average, controlling for sex and smoking status, for every 1-unit increase in blood pressure, BMI goes down 0.34 units.
   D. On average, controlling for sex and smoking status, for every 1-unit increase in BMI, blood pressure goes down 0.34 units.

9. Based on the data reported in Question Table 7-1, is the relationship between "Smoker" and blood pressure statistically significant?

   A. Yes, it is statistically significant,
   B. No, it is not statistically significant.

Use Question Table 7-2 to answer Questions 10–12.

Imagine that you are a pharmacist working in an ambulatory care clinic. A 62-year-old white female with newly diagnosed hypertension and diabetes asks you about treatment options for her elevated blood pressure. After counseling her about antihypertensive therapy, she asks whether she should take a new drug called Notapril. The woman heard about the drug while listening to a cardiologist on a morning news show. During the show, the cardiologist described results from a recent clinical trial that was published in the current issue of the *New England Journal of Medicine*. You tell the woman that you will find out more about Notapril and discuss it with her before she leaves the clinic. While the patient is having her blood drawn, you go online and retrieve the article. It contains Question Table 7-2.

QUESTION TABLE 7-2. Effect of Notapril on Systolic Blood Pressure (mmHg)

Predictor Variable	Regression Coefficient	*p*
Intercept	47.44	0.01
Male	3.25	0.02
Smoking status		
1 pack/day	2.57	0.03
>2 pack/day	4.22	0.01
Age (yr)	0.56	0.04
Presence of diabetes	15.32	0.03
Weight (lb)	0.97	0.01
Notapril	−9.53	0.02

Regression coefficients are unstandardized. Reference groups are females, nonsmokers, and patients who took a placebo.

10. Based on Question Table 7-2, how is the coefficient for sex interpreted?

    A. Controlling for the other variables in the model, the average blood pressure of men is 3.25 points higher than women.
    B. Controlling for the other variables in the model, the average blood pressure of women is 3.26 points higher than men.
    C. Controlling for the other variables in the model, the difference in blood pressure between men and women is not statistically significant if alpha is set at 0.05.

11. Based on Question Table 7-2, how is the coefficient for diabetes interpreted?

    A. After adjusting for other factors, diabetics require 15.32 mg more Notapril to obtain the same effect as nondiabetics.
    B. After adjusting for other factors, the blood pressure of diabetics is 15.32 mmHg higher than nondiabetics.
    C. After adjusting for other factors, the blood pressure of diabetics is 15.32 mmHg lower than nondiabetics.
    D. After adjusting for other factors, diabetics require 15.32 mg less Notapril to obtain the same effect as nondiabetics.
    E. After adjusting for other factors, the relationship between diabetes and systolic blood pressure is not statistically significant if alpha is set at 0.05.

12. The woman in the scenario in Question Table 7-2 is concerned that, because she has diabetes, Notapril may have less effect on her blood pressure than it has on the blood pressure of people without diabetes. Is there any information contained in Question Table 7-2 that would support her concern?

    A. Yes, there is information in Question Table 7-2 that supports her concern.
    B. NO, there is no information in Question Table 7-2 that supports her concern.

Chapter 8

Self-Study Questions

1. Which of the following statements are true with respect to logistic regression?

   A. The goal is to predict the probability that individuals in the sample will experience the outcome of interest.
   B. In a well-fitting model, most predicted probabilities will be close to either 1 or 0.
   C. In a well-fitting model, the difference between expected and observed probabilities will be small.
   D. All of the above

Use Question Table 8-1 to answer Questions 2–5.

QUESTION TABLE 8-1. Logistic Regression Predicting Development of Lung Cancer (Data Fictitious)

Variable	Regression Coefficient	OR	95% CI
Age (yr)	0.1521	1.16	1.06–1.89
Female	–0.3001	0.74	0.64–0.96
White	0.5489	1.73	0.92–3.11
Smoker	1.578	4.85	3.82–6.74

Reference groups: male, nonwhite, nonsmoker.

2. What is the outcome variable in this study?

   A. Racial classification
   B. Average age
   C. Development of lung cancer
   D. A and B
   E. None of the above

3. In what way is race associated with lung cancer risk?

   A. The odds of lung cancer are 1.73 times higher among individuals who are nonwhite compared to those who are white.
   B. The odds of lung cancer are 1.73 times higher among individuals who are white compared to those who are nonwhite.
   C. The relationship between race and the development of lung cancer is not statistically significant.

4. How is the odds ratio for age interpreted?

   A. The risk of developing lung cancer increases 16% for each 1-year increase in age.
   B. The risk of developing lung cancer decreases 16% for each 1-year increase in age.
   C. People over the age of 65 are 16% more likely to develop lung cancer than younger people.
   D. The relationship between age and development of lung cancer is not statistically significant.

5. Is the following statement true or false? After controlling for age, sex, and race, the relationship between smoking and development of lung cancer is not statistically significant. (True/**False**)

Use Question Table 8-2 to answer Questions 6–10.

Reference: Qato DM, Wilder J, Zenk S, Davis A, Makelarski J, Lindau ST. Pharmacy accessibility and cost-related underuse of prescription medications in low-income Black and Hispanic urban communities. *J Am Pharm Assoc.* 2017;57:162–9.

QUESTION TABLE 8-2. Logistic Regression Examining Individual and Pharmacy Characteristics of Cost-Related Medication Underuse

Table 3

Individual and pharmacy characteristics associated with cost-related underuse among prescription medication users on Chicago's South Side (n = 169)

Characteristic	Estimated prevalence, % (95% CI)	Unadjusted OR (95% CI)	Adjusted OR (95% CI)
Pharmacies			
Primary pharmacy type			
Retail independent (n = 12)	15.5 (3.5-47.8)	Reference	Reference
Retail chain (n = 109)	11.2 (6.4-18.7)	0.69 (0.12-3.8)	1.3 (0.19-8.5)
CHC or clinic (n = 23)	9.2 (3.2-23.5)	0.55 (0.08-3.9)	0.42 (0.04-4.1)
Distance traveled to primary pharmacy		0.21 (0.16-0.27)*	1.1 (0.94-1.2)
<1 mile (n = 95)	8.7 (4.9-15.2)	Reference	Reference
≥1 mile (n = 58)	14.3 (6.4-28.9)	1.7 (0.59-5.2)	2.1 (0.62-6.9)
Individuals			
Household income			
25k/y (n = 66)	14.4 (7.9-27.2)	Reference	Reference
≥25k/y (n = 77)	9.1 (4.5-17.5)	0.55 (0.20-1.5)	0.90 (0.26-3.1)
Insurance status			
Uninsured (n = 31)	18.9 (7.4-40.4)	Reference	Reference
Private insurance (n = 64)	5.0 (1.7-13.6)	0.22 (0.05-1.0)	0.13 (0.02-0.68)*
Medicare (n = 50)	13.4 (6.3-26.3)	0.67 (0.17-2.6)	0.46 (0.10-2.2)
Medicaid (n = 18)	10.4 (3.0-30.2)	0.50 (0.09-2.7)	0.29 (0.05-1.8)
Other Insurance (n = 4)	0 (0-0)	—	—

CI, confidence interval; CHC, community health clinic; OR, odds ratio.
Logistic regression was used to examine individual and pharmacy characteristics associated with cost-related underuse. Adjusted model includes pharmacy and individual characteristics plus age and number of prescription medications.
*Statistically significant difference at $P < 0.05$.

6. What is the prevalence of cost-related medication underuse among people who used retail independent pharmacies, retail chain pharmacies, and community health clinics (CHCs)?

   A. 18.9%, 5.0%, 13.4%, respectively
   B. 15.5%, 11.2%, 9.2%, respectively
   C. 14.4%, 9.1%, 18.9%, respectively
   D. Prevalence cannot be determined from the information provided.

7. Is the difference in the prevalence of cost-related medication underuse among people who used CHCs versus those who used retail independent pharmacies statistically significant?

   A. Yes, it is statistically significant in both the adjusted and unadjusted models.
   B. No, it is not statistically significant in either model.
   C. It is statistically significant in the adjusted model but not the unadjusted one.
   D. It is statistically significant in the unadjusted model but not the adjusted one.

8. In the adjusted model, which of the following is true?

   A. Individuals with private insurance were significantly less likely than those with no insurance to experience cost-related medication underuse.
   B. Individuals with Medicare were significantly less likely than those with no insurance to experience cost-related medication underuse.
   C. Individuals with Medicaid were significantly less likely than those with no insurance to experience cost-related medication underuse.
   D. All of the above

9. In the unadjusted model, which of the following is true?

   A. Individuals with private insurance were significantly less likely than those with no insurance to experience cost-related medication underuse.
   B. Individuals with Medicare were significantly less likely than those with no insurance to experience cost-related medication underuse.
   C. Individuals with Medicaid were significantly less likely than those with no insurance to experience cost-related medication underuse.
   D. None of the above

10. How is the adjusted OR for private insurance interpreted?

A. The odds of cost-related medication under-use is 13% lower among those with private insurance compared to those with no insurance.
B. The odds of cost-related medication underuse is 87% lower among those with private insurance compared to those with no insurance.
C. The odds of cost-related medication underuse is 13% lower among those with private insurance compared to those with Medicaid.
D. The odds of cost-related medication underuse is 87% lower among those with private insurance compared to those with Medicaid.

Chapter 9

Self-Study Questions

1. Results of a study involving survival analysis are often depicted diagrammatically using which of the following?

A. Kapla–Meier Curve
B. Scatterplot
C. Box plot
D. Histogram

2. The outcome of interest in a study examining a new cancer medication is 5-year survival. Patients who are alive 5 years after diagnosis are coded as "1." Patients who die prior to this time are coded as "0." Of the following choices, which type of analysis would be most appropriate to use in analyzing these data?

A. Logistic regression
B. Linear regression
C. Analysis of variance
D. Survival analysis

3. The outcome of interest in a study examining a new cancer medication is 5-year survival. The primary outcome variable is time to death, measured in days from study enrollment. Of the following choices, which type of analysis would be most appropriate to use in analyzing these data?

A. Logistic regression
B. Linear regression
C. Analysis of variance
D. Survival analysis

4. When survival analysis is used to analyze between group differences, which of the following tests can be used to assess the statistical significance of differences observed?

A. McNemar test
B. Independent groups t-test
C. Logrank test
D. F-test
E. None of the above

5. Which of the following is NOT an assumption of survival analysis?

A. A dichotomous outcome is being analyzed
B. Loss to follow-up is not associated with the outcome.
C. At least 5% of study participants experience the outcome.
D. There are no secular trends that affect the probability of the outcome.
E. This is a trick question; all of the above are assumptions of survival analysis.

6. Is the following statement true or false? It is possible to control for confounding factors when survival analysis is used. (**True**/False)

Chapter 10

Self-Study Questions

1. What is the meaning of the term positive predictive value (PPV)?
   A. Probability of testing positive for the disease if one has the disease
   B. Probability of disease in a patient with a positive test result
   C. Probability of not having the disease when the test result is negative

2. Which of the following is true about the PPV of a test?
   A. It has as its denominator the number of positive test results.
   B. It is sensitive to the underlying prevalence of the disease or condition being tested.
   C. It has as its denominator the number of cases of the disease or condition being tested.
   D. A and B
   E. B and C

3. Is the following statement true or false? Within the context of using multiple diagnostic tests to "confirm" a diagnosis, serial testing usually results in an increase in sensitivity but a decrease in specificity whereas parallel testing has the opposite effect. (True/**False**)

4. Is the following statement true or false? Changing the cutoff value used for a diagnostic test may change its specificity AND sensitivity. (**True**/False)

5. As the prevalence of a disease decreases, the positive predictive validity of a test:
   A. Increases
   B. Decreases
   C. Stays the same

6. Is the following statement true or false? It is always desirable to make a diagnostic test as sensitive as possible. (True/**False**)

7. If the sensitivity of a new diagnostic test for HIV is 96%, how is this interpreted?
   A. The test will rarely misclassify individuals without HIV infection as being HIV infected.
   B. 96% of individuals with HIV infection will have a positive test for HIV.
   C. 96% of individuals without HIV infection will have a negative test for HIV.

8. Which of the following results have the highest validity?
   A. High random error, low systematic error
   B. Low random error, high systematic error
   C. High overall variability, low systematic error
   D. Low random error, low systematic error

9. Is the following statement true or false? Reliability can be defined as the extent to which a test measures what it is intended to measure. (True/**False**)

10. Is the following statement true or false? If responses to a measure are influenced by systematic error, but not random error, the measure is reliable but not valid. (**True**/False)

Use Question Table 10-1 to answer Questions 11 and 12

QUESTION TABLE 10-1. Results of Tests to Diagnose Cancer

Results of Screening Test	Results of Biopsy: Positive	Results of Biopsy: Negative	Totals
Positive	10	90	100
Negative	1	99	100
Totals	11	189	200

11. Imagine that a test is available to screen for a certain form of cancer. Positive test results are followed up with a biopsy, which is assumed to provide a definitive diagnosis. Two hundred patients are screened. The results are shown in Question Table 10-1. Based on the information in the table, what is the specificity of the screening test?
   A. 0.10
   B. 0.48
   C. 0.52
   D. 0.99

12. Based on the data in the Question Table 10-1, what is the PPV of the screening test?

A. 0.10
B. 0.48
C. 0.52
D. 0.99

Use Question Table 10-2 to answer Question 13.

QUESTION TABLE 10-2. Validity and Reliability of Blood Glucose Monitoring Devices (Data Fictitious)

Product	Test Results After 10 Repeated Measures (mg/100 mL)	State-of-the-Art Instrument (Gold Standard) (mg/100 mL)
Product A		
Mean (SD)	128 (25)	120
Product B		
Mean (SD)	124 (12)	120

13. A pharmacy is testing two new serum blood glucose monitoring devices to determine which one to recommend to patients. Patients (N = 20) had their blood glucose measured twice, once using Product A and a second time using Product B. Results are shown in Question Table 10-2. Which of the following is true about the validity and reliability of Product B as compared to Product A?

A. Product B is less valid but more reliable.
B. Product B is more valid by less reliable.
C. Product B is less valid and less reliable.
D. Product B is more valid and more reliable.

14. A study is done to determine if a new type of a sphygmomanometer gives the same readings upon repeated administrations. Thirty people are enrolled in the study. Each person has his or her blood pressure measured twice, using the same sphygmomanometer, separated by a 15-minute interval. In this study, is the reliability or the validity of the sphygmomanometer being assessed?

A. Reliability
B. Validity

Use Question Table 10-3 to answer Questions 15–18.

A policy decision was made to screen all men over age 60 for prostate cancer the next time they appeared for an annual physical. A prostate-specific antigen (PSA) cutoff level of 6.0 was chosen. For men who tested positive, extensive (and expensive) additional testing was done to make a definitive diagnosis. Information found in a review of the records appears in Question Table 10-3.

QUESTION TABLE 10-3. Results of Test to Screen for Prostate Cancer (Data Fictitious)

PSA Value	Prostate Cancer Found	Prostate Cancer Not Found
6.0 +	94	40
<6.0	6	160
Total	100	200

15. What is the sensitivity of the PSA test at this cutoff level?

A. 40%
B. 70%
C. 80%
D. 94%
E. 96%

16. What is the specificity of the PSA test?

A. 40%
B. 70%
C. 80%
D. 94%
E. 96%

17. What is the positive (+) predictive value of the PSA test?

A. 40%
B. 70%
C. 80%
D. 94%
E. 96%

18. If the cutoff level were set at 5.0 instead of 6.0, what would you most likely expect to see happen?

A. Both sensitivity and specificity would increase.
B. Both sensitivity and specificity would decrease.
C. Sensitivity would increase, and specificity would decrease.
D. Sensitivity would decrease, and specificity would increase.

Chapter 11

Self-Study Questions

1. In a study designed to assess noninferiority, the null hypothesis is:

A. H_0: $C - T \geq M$
B. H_0: $C - T = 0$
C. H_0: $C - T < M$
D. H_0: $C - T \neq 0$

2. In a study designed to assess superiority, the null hypothesis is:

A. H_0: $C - T \geq M$
B. H_0: $C - T = 0$
C. H_0: $C - T < M$
D. H_0: $C - T \neq 0$

3. All other things held constant, which of the following noninferiority margins would make it most difficult to reject H_0?

A. M2 = 1 point on a 100-point scale
B. M2 = 2 points on a 100-point scale
C. M2 = 5 points on a 100-point scale
D. M2 = 20 points on a 100-point scale
E. This is a trick question; the size of the noninferiority margin has no effect on how difficult it is to reject H_0.

4. If the noninferiority margin in a study was set at 12 units, which of the following 95% confidence intervals would lead to rejection of H_0?

A. 5 to 11
B. –11 to –5
C. –5 to 11
D. –5 to 14
E. None of the above

Are the statements in Questions 5–8 true or false?

5. A study that demonstrates that the efficacy of an experimental medication is NOT inferior to a medication that is currently on the market can always be used to infer that the experimental medication is more effective than placebo. (True/**False**)

6. In a study designed to assess the superiority of one drug over another, if H_0 is NOT rejected, then it is safe to conclude that the two drugs are equally effective. (True/**False**)

7. In a study designed to assess the noninferiority of one treatment relative to another, it is possible to conclude that one of the treatments is superior to the other. (**True**/False)

8. In a study designed to assess the noninferiority of one treatment relative to another, it is possible to include a placebo arm in addition to one or more control drug arms. (**True**/False)

Chapter 12

Self-Study Questions

1. Suppose you are conducting a meta-analysis of studies examining noninvasive strategies to diagnose coronary artery disease. The Forest plot of the included studies shows overlapping confidence intervals (CIs), but the I^2 test is >75%. What approach should you use to calculate an overall pooled estimate for your meta-analysis?

A. Random-effects model
B. Fixed-effects model

2. What is a meta-analysis?

A. A numeric analysis of pooled data from studies of similar design and the same primary hypothesis or outcome measure
B. The gold standard of study designs
C. A systematic review of case reports
D. Both A and C

3. When performing a meta-analysis, one must weight the summary statistics on the basis of the precision of the results. Which studies are given more weight in the pooling?

A. Less precise studies (wide CIs)
B. More precise studies (narrow CIs)

4. Which of the following is NOT an important question to ask when critically appraising a systematic review?

   A. Did the authors do a systematic, comprehensive literature search
   B. Were study eligibility criteria predefined and specified?
   C. Was a meta-analysis conducted? Otherwise, it's not a systematic review.
   D. Did the authors critically appraise (or assess for risk of bias) each study included in the review?
   E. Did at least two reviewers evaluate articles to determine eligibility?

5. Which of the following is NOT an important step in conducting a systematic review?

   A. Developing focused questions
   B. Conducting a comprehensive literature search
   C. Having dual review of abstracts and articles to determine inclusion or exclusion
   D. Assessing heterogeneity
   E. Including only randomized controlled trials because observational studies should never be included

6. Is the following statement true or false? You should have a focused question versus a broad question when conducting a systematic literature review. (**True**/False)

7. Which of the following combinations of terms describe characteristics of a systematic review?

   A. Broad question, author identification of evidence, methods section, idiosyncratic
   B. Broad question, predefined literature search, methods section, idiosyncratic
   C. Focused question, predefined literature search, methods section, reproducible
   D. Focused question, predefined literature search, no methods section, reproducible

8. Which of the following statements is FALSE regarding meta-analysis?

   A. Studies included in a meta-analysis should be derived from a systematic review.
   B. The aim of a meta-analysis is to produce a single estimate of treatment effect.
   C. Meta-analysis usually involves individual patient data from one or more trials.
   D. Populations, interventions, and outcome measures should be similar.

9. Is the following statement true or false? Before you do a systematic review of the literature, you should have a predefined literature search strategy. (**True**/False)

10. Systematic reviews and meta-analyses have limitations, including threats to validity. Which of the following terms is NOT relevant when thinking about potential threats to the validity of systematic reviews or meta-analyses.

   A. Publication bias
   B. Funnel plots
   C. Heterogeneity
   D. Forest plots

Index

Page numbers followed by *b*, *f*, or *t* indicate material in boxes, figures, or tables, respectively.

T

U

V

W

Z